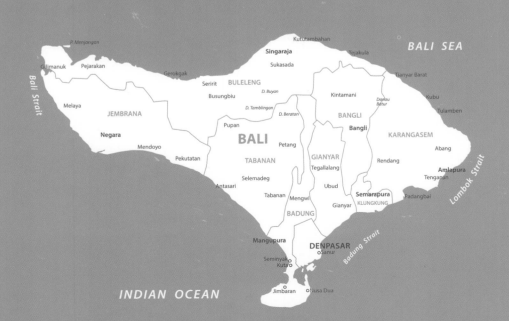

HEALING HERBS
OF PARADISE

Published by:

Al Sears, MD

11905 Southern Blvd.

Royal Palm Beach, FL 33411

www.AlSearsMD.com

ISBN 978-0-9968102-1-0

The author would like to extend special thanks to I Made Westi and Ni Wayan Lelir for their invaluable contributions and contagious enthusiasm in the creation of this book.

Warning-Disclaimer: Dr. Al Sears wrote this book to provide information in regard to the subject matter covered. Every effort has been made to make this book as complete and accurate as possible. The purpose of this book is to educate. The author and publisher shall have neither liability nor responsibility to any person or entity with respect to any loss, damage or injury caused or alleged to be caused directly or indirectly by the information contained in this book. The information presented herein is in no way intended as a substitute for medical counseling or medical attention.

CONTENTS

INTRODUCTION

BY AL SEARS, MD

My plane swept in low, over open ocean. Through the jet's tiny window, I could just catch a glimpse of what lay ahead. It was green as far as I could see. A deeper, richer green than I'd ever seen before. The jungles of Asia.

After 30 hours in the air, I was about to fulfill a dream I'd had since I was a child. I was about to stand on the island of Bali.

My dream began with my father's stories from World War II. I was fascinated by his tales of the island beaches... impenetrable jungles... and the warm, generous people who lived there.

The island that enchanted him most was Bali. An island with a unique culture and a beauty he never felt he could quite describe. This was too much for my young imagination. I had to visit Bali someday.

And now, here I was. About to realize my dream.

I've been to jungles before... in India, Jamaica, and the Amazon. But none of them compare with Bali. The island boasts shades of green I've never seen anywhere else on the planet.

Bali has a rich and unique herbal tradition. In fact, "Balian" is the local word for their healers.

My journey would take me deep into the interior. To the foot of Bali's volcano, far away from the beaches of my father's stories.

And it was there, in the city of Ubud, that I met a married couple dedicated to preserving Bali's herbal traditions.

I Made Westi is the son of traditional rice farmers. Spry and energetic, Westi is in his early 40s. But when it comes to herbs, he has the enthusiasm of a teenager.

Westi is an unusual farmer. And not just because he grows herbs instead of rice. He's also been to college. And he sees that modern farming methods are destroying the island he loves.

Westi's wife is *Ni Wayan Lelir.* A petite woman with dark hair and sparkling eyes, her energy matches her husband's. And so does her knowledge of herbs.

Lelir's parents were traditional herbal healers. In fact, she can trace the herbal tradition in her family back for at least five generations. And she's following in the family footsteps, studying traditional Indian medicine — called Ayurveda — at a nearby university.

Westi has converted the family's rice fields into a huge herb garden. He leads "herbal walks" through the fields and rice paddies near their home. Lelir runs a shop where she prepares and sells herbal medicines and cosmetics. Between them, they may know more about cultivating, preparing and using Bali's traditional herbs than anyone else on Earth.

Bali is one of Earth's unique places. An ancient culture that has drawn from its neighbors, yet retains a flavor all its own. Bali has its own language, its own customs... and its own healing system.

But that system is rapidly disappearing. Western medicine is pushing Bali's rich herbal tradition into the background. Young Balinese are becoming modern... and leaving the old ways behind.

Westi and Lelir are working tirelessly to preserve Bali's rich herbal traditions.

This book is an extension of their life's work. It's filled with herbal wisdom little known in the West. They've recorded traditions, personal stories and recipes.

You'll Discover More than Herbs. You'll Discover Bali's healing Secrets.

When Westi and I first talked about publishing a book, he envisioned a "materia medica" — a what, where and how of Bali's herbs. But as our discussions went on, it became clear this book would become much more than that.

You'll travel with us to some of Bali's most beautiful and unusual places. Places like the Sacred Monkey Forest Sanctuary, an ancient forest temple complex that's now home to hundreds of monkeys.

And every chapter will introduce you to one of Bali's many useful plants. Some will be familiar — with unfamiliar uses. Others will be strange and new. Many have remarkable properties that Western science is only now discovering... centuries after Bali's healers understood their use.

Many chapters include recipes for herbal teas and other healing preparations. I can speak from personal experience that some of them are remarkably effective.

I also share some of my experiences, personal research and recommendations with you.

But Is It Practical?

The answer is "yes." Some of these plants are readily available in supermarkets. You can buy pineapple and ginger, for instance, almost anywhere.

Others are available in many Asian markets. They may take a little more effort to find, but the effort will be worth it.

You can read this book from cover to cover, just as you would a novel. Believe me, this isn't your high school botany text.

You can also use the book as a reference by reading each chapter individually. You don't need to read any particular chapter before any other. Each one stands on its own.

However you decide to read this book, please do read it. You'll find answers for many common — and some not so common — health problems. You'll find simple instructions for preparing delicious and healthful teas and drinks.

And you'll encounter a rich herbal tradition almost unknown in the Western world.

To Your Good Health,

Al Sears, MD, CNS

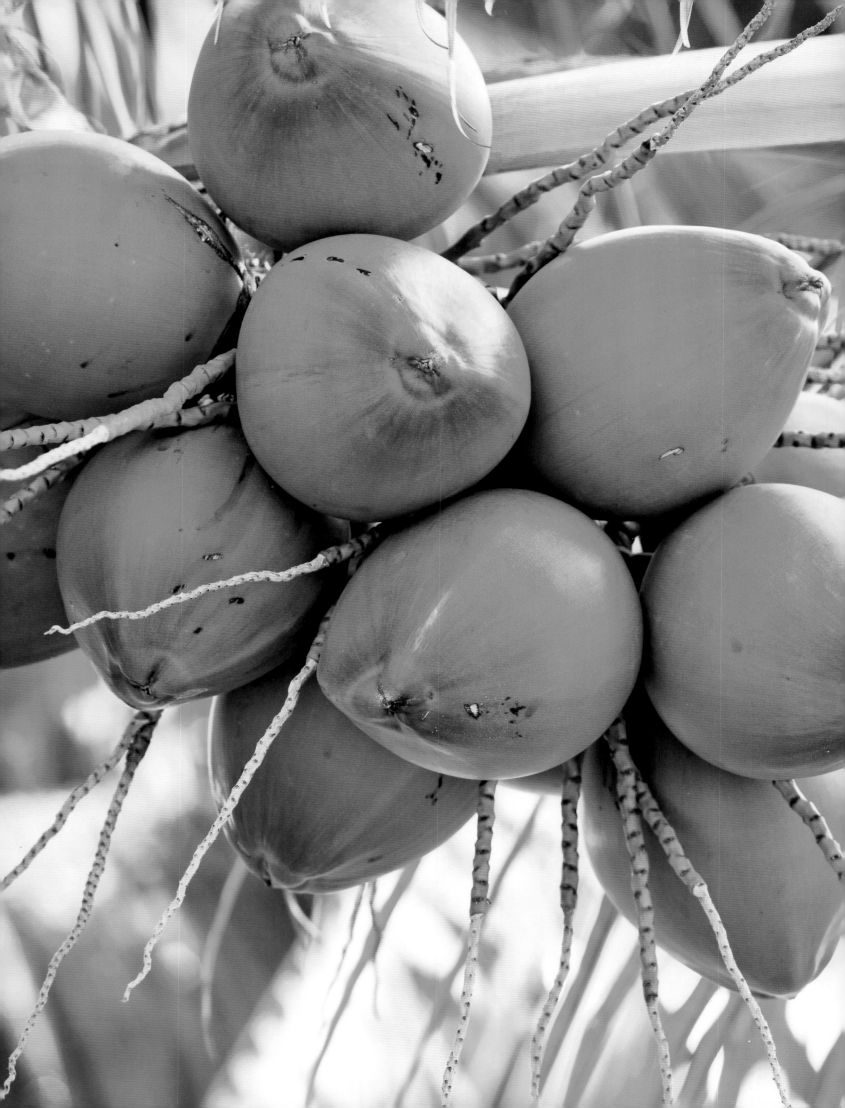

FAT–FILLED MIRACLE FOOD

The sweat was pouring off us in the heavy midday heat of Bali.

After hiking in the low mountains around the garden and rice paddies passed down from his father, we were a little tired from the hundred-degree heat... and from walking all afternoon. And we were about as thirsty as you can get.

Just at the moment, that we stopped to look out over the plateau. A girl who worked on one of the nearby plantations came walking by with a bundle of coconuts.

"May I have two of those?" Westi asked her.

She gave us two of the coconuts.

Westi set them on the ground, and produced what looked like a narrow meat cleaver.

"We call this a Bali knife. Very useful."

Turns out, Westi is the master of understatement. I discovered he uses it for *everything.*

He handed it to me.

"That's incredibly beautiful."

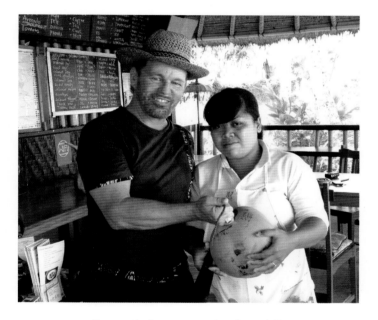

Coconuts have zero starch and the brain-healthy nutrient, choline.

I'd never seen anything like it. I gave it back to him... and then my new friend did something I had never seen before.

He sat down on the ground and grabbed a coconut. With incredible speed and ease he shaved off a little piece and set it aside. Then he chopped a V-shaped hole with his heavy knife, chopped a slit next to it, picked up the shaved piece, bent it a little, and made a spout.

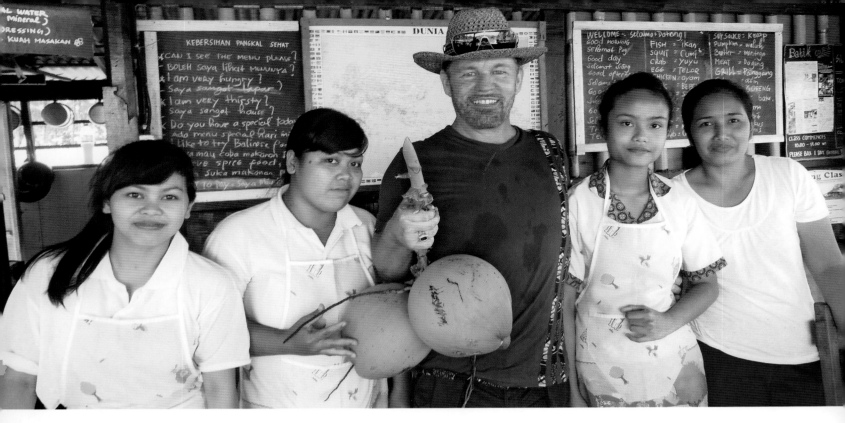

Buying coconuts at a small, roadside shop on the edge of the forest.

An Instant Refresher

In a few seconds we were drinking cool, refreshing coconut water right from the source.

Everywhere I've traveled they had a different way of opening coconuts, and Westi's method was the best I'd ever seen.

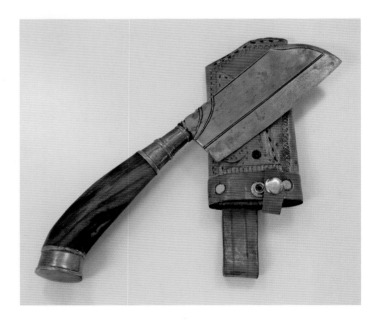

The "half knife-half hatchet" given to me by my friend Westi for cutting open coconuts the "Bali" way.

I really appreciated the cool drink at the time in the heavy heat and altitude...

On the day I was to leave, Westi made a little presentation of giving me my own Bali knife as a present.

It's like a half-knife, half-hatchet. The Balinese use them as all-purpose tools.

He grabbed a coconut off a nearby tree so I could film him using my new knife to demonstrate how to make a drinking cup out of a coconut.

Here I was, struggling for years to cut open coconuts at my house in Florida... and now I've got a Bali knife.

I've managed not to cut myself too badly using it in my yard, too.

It's great, because I used to spill the water all over the place when I chopped open coconuts. But I'm getting the hang of my Bali knife. Now I can drink coconut water straight from the source — with almost no spillage.

We have coconut palms here in South Florida. Seeing them always gives me the feeling of lazy afternoons at the beach and warm tropical breezes.

Luckily, I have coconut trees in my yard. I love to eat them... but until I got my Bali knife, it always involved a great deal of care and difficulty to get them open.

Now I don't have to worry about it anymore, thanks to Westi.

Of course, I still have to get the coconuts down from the tree, which isn't easy. Climbing a straight, smooth coconut palm is a trick. You can tie your feet together with a rope and shimmy up, and I've done that. But it's no picnic!

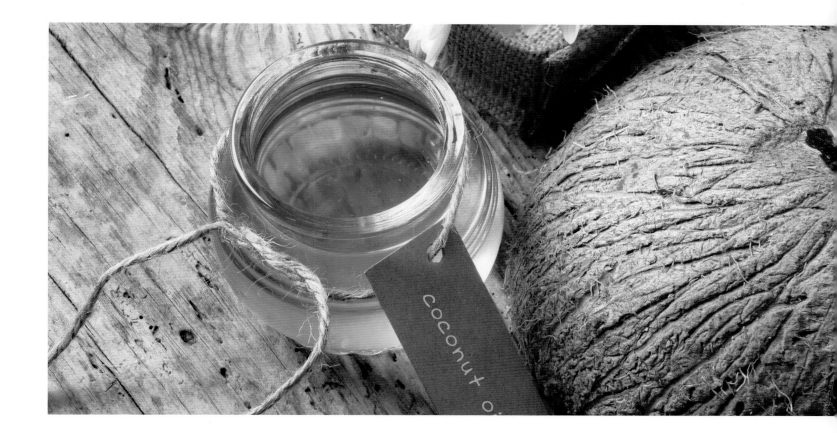

Coconuts Provide "All the Necessities of Life"

In Jamaica, they seem to be able to literally run up the palm trees. It's a lot harder than it looks, and I still haven't quite mastered the art. I tried it when I was in Jamaica, because we would gather coconuts constantly. They use coconuts for almost everything. . In fact, I think of them as a staple food now.

When I traveled to India, the home of Ayurvedic medicine (the world's oldest health care system), I learned their name for the coconut palm tree. They call it *kalpa vriksha,* which means, "the tree which provides all the necessities of life." It's a fitting name — the tree of life.

Coconuts are an excellent way to get protein and natural fiber. They also have zero starch, as well as the brain-healthy nutrient, choline.

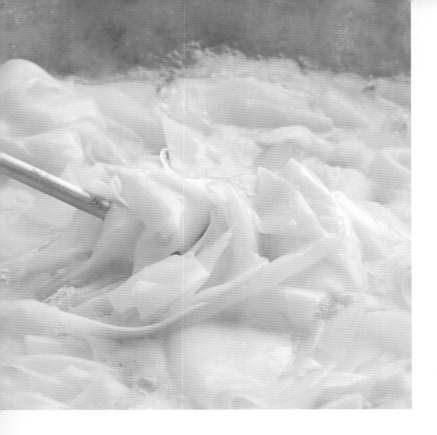

Rasta, my friend in Jamaica, showed me how to scrape the coconut out of the shell and mash it up like the locals. We used a grater, like you would use for cheese.

Then I put the shredded coconut in a big pot of water — a lot of water, like maybe ten times as much as the coconut — and boiled it.

It looked to me like a kind of coconut stew and bubbled like a cauldron. It eventually looked like lava bubbling slowly. When it stopped bubbling, all the water was gone. There was only coconut oil. We put the coconut oil into jars to cool at room temperature until it was solid. And to make it a liquid again, we just put the jar outside in the heat.

I like nuts cooked in coconut oil. Peanuts are really good. Almonds are very popular in Jamaica, too. Almond trees are all over the place. They take the almonds, dry them in the oven and then char them a little in coconut oil.

Coconut Oil "De-Ages" and Beautifies Your Skin

When I went to Jamaica, I learned that they press the flesh of the coconut to make oil to use on their skin. It doesn't take too much coconut flesh. You can put it on a flat surface and just roll a round coffee cup over it and get some oil.

Lelir, Westi's wife, makes a lip balm out of coconut oil. She uses Balinese bitter orange leaves and infuses them with the coconut oil. And she makes moisturizing oil they call "Sweet Dream." It is coconut oil-based and takes an entire month to brew.

Jamaicans use coconut oil both internally and externally. They use it in makeup as a base, and as a skin and hair conditioner. Warm coconut oil can cure dry and damaged hair.

They also flavor foods with it, and use it as cooking oil. It's always around the house; it's in every kitchen — and probably every bathroom.

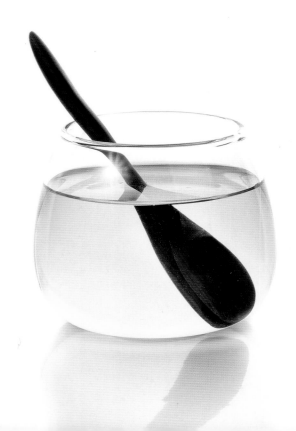

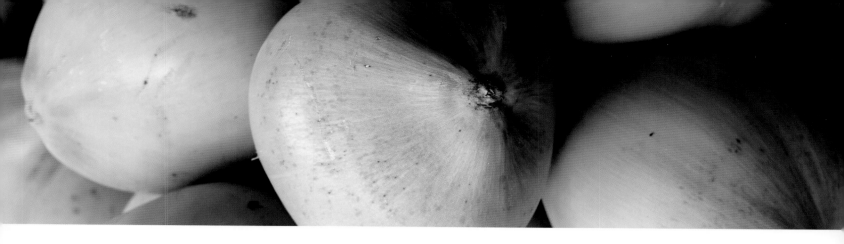

Two Prized Fats Fight Inflammation

Coconut oil is also useful when you cook with it because it, slows down the digestion of food, which helps you feel fuller after you eat.

It also stabilizes blood-sugar levels, which can help people with diabetes and those who are trying to lose weight. It has also been found to help in thyroid disease and in women with symptoms associated with menopause and PMS.

Coconuts also have unique kinds of fats that you'll find in less than a half-dozen foods anywhere in the world. They're called *medium chain fatty acids* (or medium-chain triglycerides — MCTs).

These fats — capric acid and lauric acid — are very rare. They are *only* found in human breast milk, the milk of cows and goats, and coconut and palm kernel oil (which is not the same as palm oil). And these fats have great benefits for your brain, and are also among the heart-healthiest fats you can get from any food. MCTs reinforce your skin and strengthen your immunity to fight infection from bacteria and viruses.

MCTs also fight depression and inflammation, two major brain-robbing conditions. Scientists are studying these fats, because they also have the potential to fight Alzheimer's disease. Animal studies have shown that these fats can protect neurons from injury and cell death.

Nursing babies get about 1 gram of lauric acid per kilogram of body weight each day. You can get about two grams of lauric acid from one tablespoon of dried coconut. Quality coconut milk will contain about three and a half grams for every two ounces. Coconut oil has almost seven grams per tablespoon.

When you consume MCTs, your body converts them into monoglycerides and medium-chain fatty acids.[1] These fats are very different from the fats in vegetable oils. When you eat lauric acid, it boosts your immune system to help the body fight infections and diseases.[2] Lauric acid is known to be antiviral, antifungal and antibacterial.

Cosmetic companies are starting to lust after coconuts, because the oil is such an effective moisturizer and skin softener.

Let me explain:

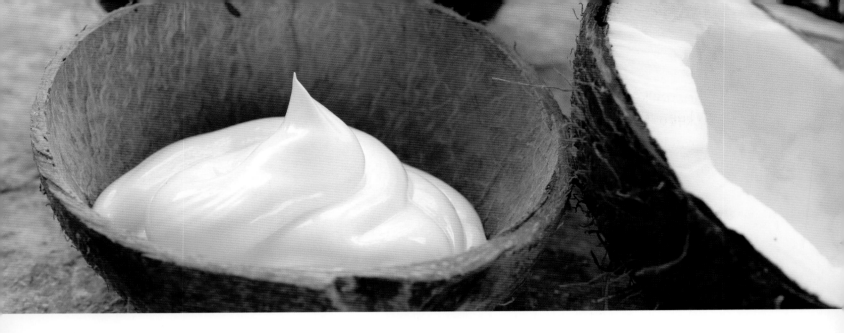

Nature's Most Effective Moisturizer

The outer layer of your skin is partly made of fat. And keeping this layer water-tight and healthy not only keeps your skin firm and smooth, but it's your best defense against all the environmental toxins and pollutants produced by the modern world.

This skin barrier is called your "acid mantle." It's made up of skin cells and fats called *sebum* that protect you from environmental dangers like toxins, viruses, bacteria and other attackers.

This barrier also works as an antioxidant. It protects skin from water loss, and it maintains the correct hardness of the water-holding protein, *keratin,* in your skin.

MCTs in coconut oil reinforce your protective skin barrier and increase the proteins that hold onto water.

What MCTs also do is help maintain your skin's *pH* balance. In order to stay water-tight and healthy, your skin needs to be slightly acidic (which is why the barrier is called an "acid" mantle). These MCTs have an alkalizing effect in your body as well.

"COCONUT OIL FIGHTS INFECTIONS BY SUPPORTING YOUR IMMUNE SYSTEM"

The problem with many so-called "mild" soaps and commercial products is that they damage your skin barrier by stripping away too much of your fatty sebum. What's worse is that they reverse your skin's natural *pH* so it's no longer mildly acidic.

These products then leave your skin open to infection, unable to retain moisture. That means you're more prone to developing rashes and breakouts.

Also, most cosmetics loosen your keratin fibers, creating gaps in the protective covering, so they can artificially hydrate your skin.

This looks good for a little while. But when the artificial hydration wears off, it makes your skin even more prone to water loss, damage, infections and pollutants.

The MCTs in coconut oil react naturally with your skin, unlike many commercial products, to keep it hydrated and firm. They increase your acid mantle and keep your skin protein intact. One study showed that MCTs significantly increase skin hydration, compared with drugs and other mixtures.[3]

MCT fatty acids also gently dissolve dead skin cells, leaving behind a fresher, more even complexion. This will prevent wrinkles from forming and will help to soften wrinkles that are already present.

Coconut oil can penetrate underneath your protective layer, too, going deep down to heal underlying skin damage. By massaging coconut oil into your skin, you can improve the connective tissue deep below the surface. Coconut oil has been proven in clinical studies to mimic the skin's natural repair mechanisms.[4]

Coconut oil also protects against overexposure to the sun, which is why it's used in suntan lotion.

Coconut oil works well as a delivery system, because MCTs like lauric acid are easily absorbed by your skin cells. Commercial skin-care products use synthetic versions of these acids, but the man-made versions aren't even close to being as effective.

In your body, lauric acid transforms into a substance called *Monolaurin,* which can strengthen your immunity and fight infections from bacteria and viruses.

Lauric acid has antiviral, antifungal, antibacterial and antiprotozoal properties that help bulletproof your immune system.

Unlike longer-chain fatty acids, the medium-chain fatty acids in coconut oil are tiny enough to enter your cells' mitochondria directly.

This means that your cells use the fat from coconut oil for energy instantly, instead of storing it for later use.

Another study found that coconut oil can help reduce the symptoms of type 2 diabetes

Using Coconut Oil For Skin Care:

- Makes your skin soft and smooth to the touch
- Gives your skin an overall healthy glow
- Helps your complexion keep its natural moisture
- Firms your skin
- Prevents breakdown of natural collagens
- Promotes healthy new skin cells
- Prevents liver spots
- Prevents wrinkles

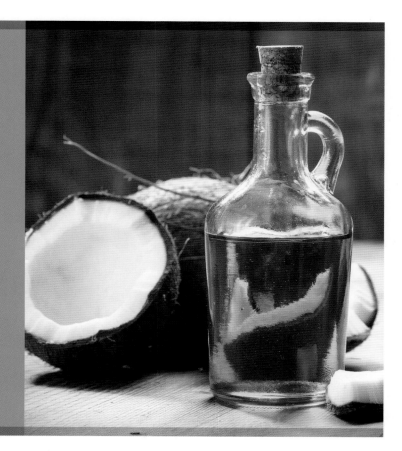

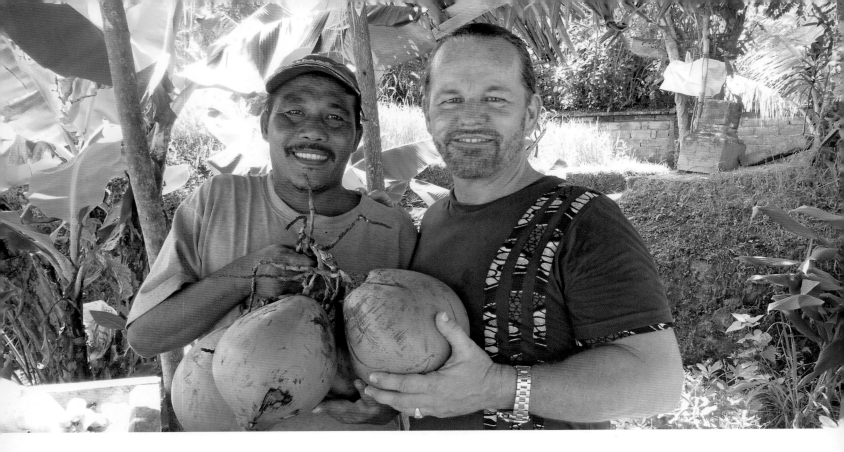

Getting ready to carve up some freshly cut coconuts.

and that people who incorporate medium-chain fatty acids, such as those found in coconut oil, into their diets can lose body fat.[5]

It controls your hunger by leaving you feeling satisfied longer.[14] More about that in a moment.

Coconut oil also helps improve your HDL to LDL ratio ("good" vs. "bad" cholesterol), and reduces the amount of fat your body stores.[6]

In fact, in Sri Lanka, about 50% of calories from the typical diet come from coconut oil. Heart disease there, as in Bali, is virtually non-existent.

Researchers, perplexed by this, decided to see what happened when they took a group of young Sri Lankan men and had them substitute corn and soybean oil for coconut oil.

The results weren't pretty.

Their HDL level plunged 42% — which put them far below what's considered healthy. Their LDL/HDL ratio increased 30%.[7] That's a recipe for heart disaster.

These results simply confirm what countless studies are finding. Coconut oil is good for your heart and helps increase your good HDL cholesterol.

For example, a study published in the *Journal of Nutrition* studied 25 women. They were given three different diets. A diet high in coconut oil, a low-fat diet with small amounts of coconut oil, and a diet high in polyunsaturated fats. Each diet lasted three weeks.

As you might guess, the highest increase in HDL was seen in the women who ate the high fat, coconut oil diet.[8]

Coconuts Replace Vital Minerals

One thing coconuts *don't* have is a lot of vitamins.

Many so-called skin care and health experts keep telling you that coconuts are healthy because they are "high" in this or that vitamin, but it's just not true.

A cup of raw coconut only has 0.2 mg of vitamin E, 2 mg of vitamin C, no vitamin A, almost zero B vitamins, and 0.2 mcg of vitamin K.[9]

What coconuts do have are lots of minerals. A cup of coconut has a good amount of iron, zinc, copper, selenium and potassium.

Besides making drinking vessels, the Balinese do something else I'd never seen before... Once we drank all the coconut water, Westi swiftly and deftly chopped the coconut in two with my new Bali knife and made a spoon out of the shaving we had used as a spout. Then he expertly used the sharp edge to scoop out the delicious coconut jelly about as fast as I've ever seen it done.

You might be asking yourself, why go to all that trouble? As it turns out, the water and jelly of young coconuts are rich in magnesium.

We don't get much magnesium any more. The mineral content of vegetables today has dropped by more than 80% in some cases. Commercial farming technology and powerful fertilizers practically *sterilize* the soil — leaving it with almost no mineral content.

Magnesium content in vegetables has dropped between 25-80% since before 1950.[10] Sadly, we're not getting it from other foods either.

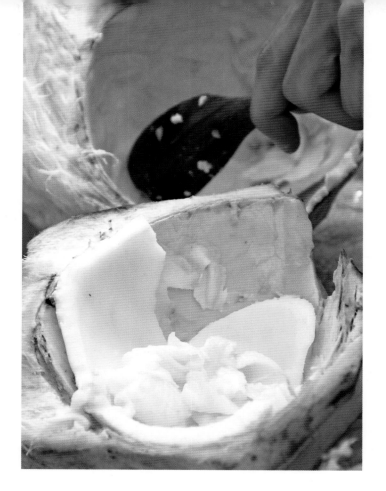

Coconut jelly is delicious and rich in magnesium.

- Refined grains remove 80-97% of magnesium.
- Refined oils remove *all* magnesium.
- Refined sugar removes *all* magnesium.

I've pored over years' worth of clinical studies, health records and surveys and what I've found mirrors what I see with my own patients. A majority of people get nowhere near enough magnesium.[11]

This is bad news, because magnesium is one of your body's master minerals. You need it to make antioxidants, and it helps fight anxiety and fatigue. It also tones blood vessels, enhancing circulation in the tiny vessels in your eyes and ears, giving you sharper hearing and vision.

You need magnesium for healthy blood sugar and bone building. Magnesium is especially important for your heart.

Did you know that magnesium is unique in that it helps maintain a healthy electrical balance required for normal heart rhythm?[12]

Your heart works because of electricity... a tiny bioelectric current that keeps it beating steadily. Without magnesium, the electrical impulses would stop.

Recent research shows that people who get the least amount of magnesium have a 50% higher risk of heart problems.[13]

Magnesium used to be in your drinking water. But water with a high mineral content — "hard" water — fell out of favor because most people don't like the taste.

And, as you get older, not only do you lose magnesium from the place where you store most of it — your bones — but magnesium stored in bones isn't completely bioavailable as you age.[14]

However, you can change all that by drinking coconut water. And it has other health benefits as well.

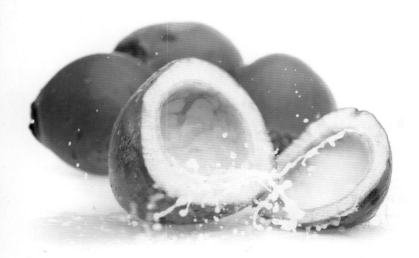

Coconut Water is Packed with Energizing Nutrients

Young, green coconuts produce the coconut water Westi and I drank in Bali... but it's not just for drinking. It's also naturally sterile. In tropical countries where coconut trees grow wild, they use a combination of coconut water and coconut oil to heal skin injuries.

Take a drink and you'll be re-vitalized almost immediately. Within five minutes, you'll feel a burst of energy, have clarity of mind and a sense of well-being.

One of the reasons for this is that coconut water can boost thyroid function. Having your thyroid work efficiently is essential for boosting your metabolism and energy production.

Coconut water is also loaded with potassium, which is an electrolyte. That makes it a pretty good substitute for those sugary "sports drinks." I recommend it after a workout with my PACE exercise program.

A study was done on eight participants who exercised for a certain duration of time. Then, after the workout, they were each given different beverages. Coconut water was found to rehydrate and also be better absorbed by the body rather than water and carbohydrate-electrolyte beverages.[15]

The coconut has many other traditional uses, too, as Lelir, who is a fifth-generation herbalist, told me...

Nature's Cure All

Whenever a woman comes into our shop carrying an infant, I'm reminded of my childhood...

I come from a very large family. I'm the 5th of 11 children. Our house was crowded... but very happy. In Bali, having many brothers and sisters means you have many friends.

My brothers, sisters and I were all born at home. No doctor or nurse ever came to help my mother. Not even a midwife. Instead, my father gave her herbs.

Our home was small — a few rooms huddled under a thick thatched roof. Because no room had more than one window, it always felt a little dark, but this kept us cool.

When mother was ready to deliver the baby, our father would chase everyone out of their bedroom, except one or two of the older girls. They would stay to assist father.

The rest of us would sit on our beds or in the kitchen and wait. We'd strain to be first to hear our new little brother or sister cry.

We usually didn't have to wait long. Father's herbs worked so well, most of us were born pretty quickly.

When my mother was pregnant, she would drink young coconut juice twice a day. Every morning and every afternoon, my father would give her some juice from young green coconuts to drink.

When she was ready to give birth, my mother would also take 3 tablespoons of cold-pressed coconut oil. The oil helps make birth easier.

In the U.S., coconut juice is called "coconut water." Coconut water comes only from young coconuts. Mature coconuts produce coconut milk, which is very different. Coconut water is packed with vitamins and minerals, so it's very healthy for both the mother and baby.

Coconut has many other uses. It's the most important tree in Bali. They grow all over the island. Westi knows more than 10 varieties. But green coconut is the most useful of all.

Sometimes tourists get what we call "Bali belly." This comes from eating unfamiliar foods... or from microbes in the water. Stomach trouble is a big problem anywhere in the world where there are lots of tourists.

But in Bali, we have a cure. Green coconut water is very good for Bali belly. When you feel it coming on, start drinking green coconut water regularly. Your stomach will feel better quickly.

Coconut water is good for almost any kind of upset stomach. Pregnant women in Bali say it cures even the worst morning sickness.

Coconut oil is good for your skin, too. It's very gentle, so we use it to keep our babies' skin soft and smooth. It clears up rashes, too.

To get rid of cold sores, we burn coconut leaves. Then we apply the cooled ashes to the sore. This works within a few days.

We have so many uses for coconuts. The wood is good for building. We make charcoal from coconut shells... and rope and baskets from the husks. And, of course, coconut plays a big part in our cooking.

We even make palm wine – called "tuak" – from coconut palms. Tuak is a very mild wine. It's only about 5% alcohol... about as strong as American beer. But it's inexpensive, natural and easy to make. So it's very popular for celebrations.

We also make coconut sugar to sweeten our food. To make the sugar, you cut slits in the buds of coconut flowers before they open and collect the sap. (This is different from palm sugar, which you make from sap collected from the stems of sugar palms.)

You boil the coconut bud sap until it's thick and crystallizes, and you have 100% natural sugar. Coconut sugar is naturally brown. My mother always used it to bake her cakes, because the sugar gave her cakes a lovely brown color.

Coconut sugar is much healthier than the table sugar used in the West. Coconut sugar is all natural, and not processed like table sugar. It's more like maple sugar.

In the West, most people avoid eating a lot of coconut. That's because the oil is full of saturated fat. Most people think all saturated fat is bad and will clog your arteries.

But we Balinese have always eaten lots of coconut without any heart problems.

— Lelir

My Own Research and Discoveries

The saturated fats in coconut, or MCTs, are different from saturated animal fats. MCTs don't cause fatty build-up in your blood. Studies show they help get rid of fats in the blood, which is why the Balinese rarely suffer from heart disease.

Coconuts can even help you lose weight.[16]

Swapping out other fats in your diet for MCTs could not only help you get lean, it could boost your health in other ways, too.

I found some interesting research on MCTs done by doctors in China, just a couple of years ago.

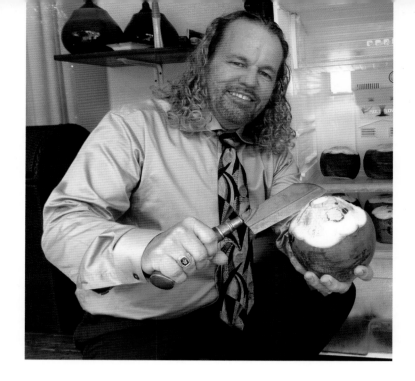

At home, I now use my Bali knife to cut the coconuts from the trees in my back yard. Once I get the coconuts down, I shave them a bit until I see the white coconut meat at the top. Then I refrigerate them, so I can have a drink whenever I want.

They looked at 112 women with high levels of triglycerides in their blood. They kept half of the women on the diets they'd been eating. But they switched some of the fat in the second group's diet for MCTs. After just eight weeks, the MCT group had lost weight — and inches of fat from their bodies.[17]

They weren't dieting. They weren't exercising more. The only change was replacing one kind of fat with another. They were slimmer and sexier without making any effort.

MCTs Seem to Act Like an "Anti-Fat Fat."

How does it work? MCTs — like those in coconut oil — tell your body to burn fat for fuel, instead of storing it.

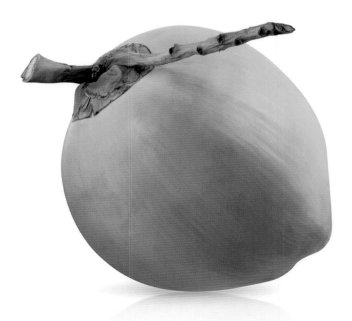

In another study, Canadian researchers looked at a group of overweight men. And sure enough, eating more MCTs put their metabolism into high gear... and started them burning more fat. In just four weeks, they lost an average of about 2.5 pounds.[18]

As I mentioned earlier, this group didn't diet nor exercise. The only change was swapping out unhealthy fats for MCTs.

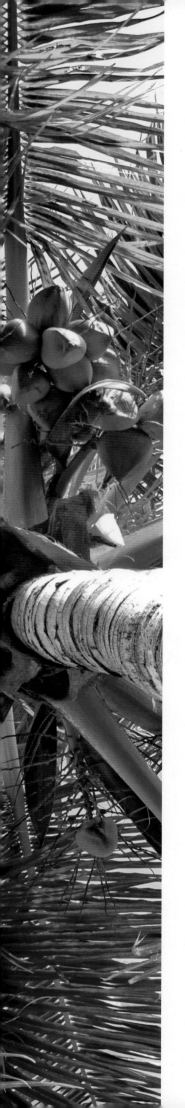

I also discovered something else when reading through the study... the thinner the men were, the better MCTs worked. It's sort of like a snowball effect. So your results could just keep getting better and better.

Research also supports using green coconut water for an upset stomach and diarrhea. Sometimes, it's hard to drink much water when your stomach is upset. But you need lots of water to rehydrate when you have diarrhea. That's one thing that's great about coconut water. It's just as good as plain water for rehydration... but it's gentler on your stomach, so you can drink more.

Coconut water is also cleaner than most other water. So it's often safer to drink than the local water when you're traveling. In fact, coconut water is so pure, I've sometimes seen it used as an emergency IV fluid in surgery.

If you don't have coconut trees in your yard like I do, you can still get coconut water. Many health food stores sell fresh coconuts now. The raw, fresh water will always be the best tasting coconut water you can get.

The next best thing is pre-packaged, "virgin" or no sugar added coconut water. There are quite a few companies selling it now, so it's easy to get at your local grocery store or health foods store.

The three most popular brands are Vita Coco, Zico and O.N.E. They all use Brazilian coconuts, which have a different but equally refreshing taste compared to Southeast Asian coconuts like the ones I tried on Bali.

All three brands have flavored versions of their coconut water, so be sure to find a brand labeled 100% pure coconut water with nothing added. You can find them in most grocery stores.

Some others brands that are worth looking a little harder for are:

• Harmless Harvest – It's made with 100% raw, organic coconut water.

• Taste Nirvana – All their coconuts come from one place: Samui Island in Thailand.

• Nature Factor – The first to be certified organic.

• Blue Monkey – They make sure their coconuts come from local Southeast Asian groves that use sustainable farming practices.

• Naked Pure Coconut Water – Also made from Brazilian green coconuts.

• C2O Pure Coconut Water – Made from inland coconuts grown in fresh water conditions, which taste a bit different from either Brazilian or Thai coconuts.

Avoid beverages that are "coconut juice" or "coconut drink," because they usually have added sugar and flavors.

Here is What I Recommend

When you're looking for coconut oil, try to find unrefined oil such as virgin coconut oil. Most oils are refined, bleached and deodorized (RDB) and are processed with chemicals. Three to four tablespoons a day of coconut oil will provide enough lauric acid to build the immune system.

It's not hard to put coconut oil to work for you, either. You see, it's solid at room temperature... about the consistency of soft margarine. So it's easy to work with.

For most recipes, you can simply add an equal amount of coconut oil in place of butter, margarine or shortening. You can also use coconut oil in place of butter when you sauté.

The taste is a little different, so you may want to experiment a bit. I think coconut oil's mild flavor is delicious, though, and love to use it in my recipes.

Coconut

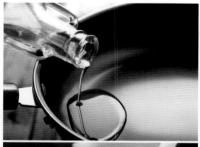

Fry with it. Coconut oil has a high smoke point. That means that it won't degrade at high temperatures – leaving all the fatty acids intact. It's especially great for pan searing. If you do cook with it, consider getting it with no flavor. This is known as "expeller-pressed" coconut oil.

Take it to go. If you've got a very busy schedule, you can eat a snack with coconut oil already in it.

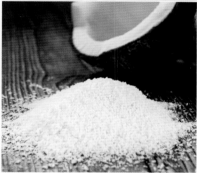

Another great favorite of mine is to grab a banana. Dip it in plain yogurt. Then roll it in finely chopped coconut. Afterward, I store it in the freezer and eat it whenever I want a quick snack.

Make a smoothie. Scoop a healthy serving of coconut oil (it'll probably be solid, but that's okay) into the blender. Mix in your favorite fresh fruits. Maybe even add some protein powder. Add organic milk and a little ice. Blend it all and enjoy a tasty, heart-healthy smoothie.

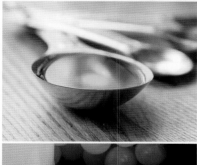

Bake with it. If you are going to bake, just substitute expeller-coconut oil for vegetable oil. Not only will everything taste better, but most of the fat you'll be eating will get burned off right away.

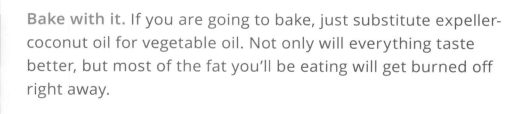

Eating raw coconut is a great way to get protein, natural fiber and healthy fats.

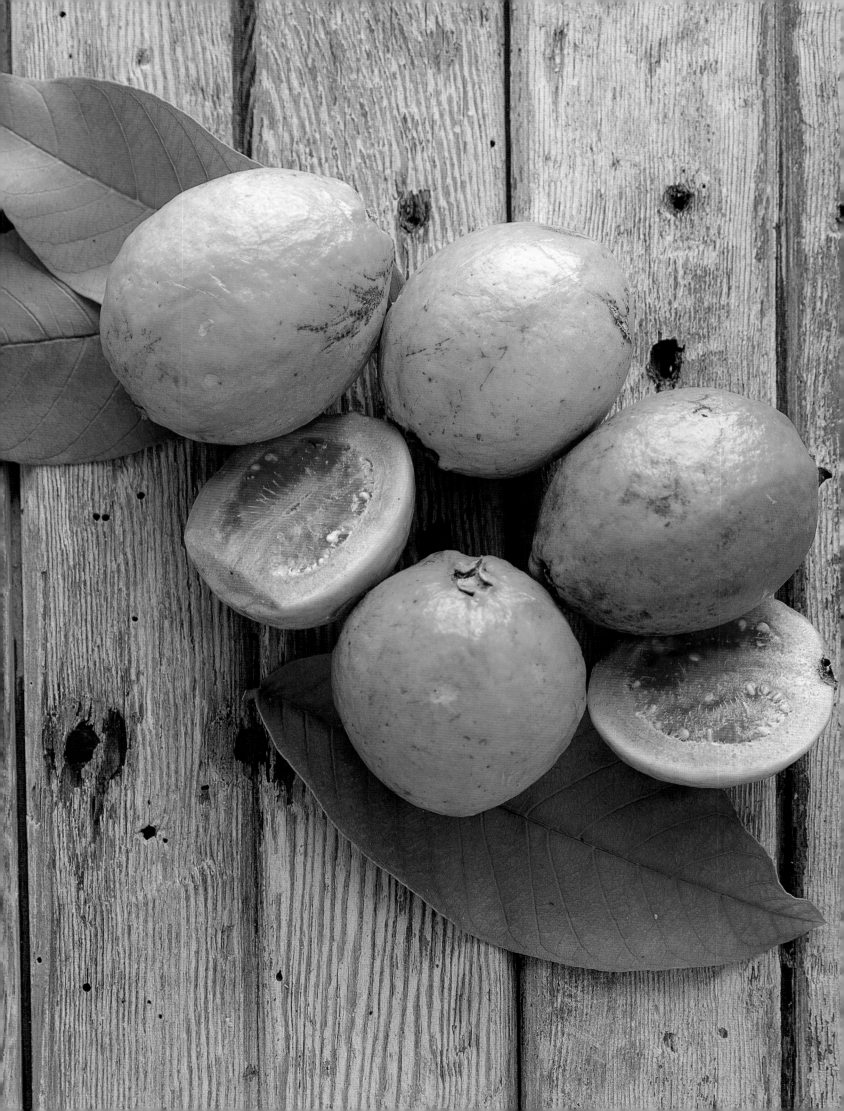

BRAIN–BOOSTING BALI FRUIT ALSO BEATS CANCER

The first time I went to Bali, I tried every new food I could, but I never got an upset stomach or any type of indigestion.

Normally, I don't experience much of that anyway, wherever in the world I travel. I like to challenge my body, because I know it will help my immune system become stronger.

Lelir had me eat guava every day for breakfast and I never thought twice about what I ate for my entire visit. Lelir's family has been using guava to relieve upset stomachs and to cure diarrhea for as long as they've been herbal healers.

Jamaicans use guava in much the same way. They usually eat it as a fresh desert fruit. But they also use guava to make jam and jelly, and as a sweet base for syrup or wine.

Guava leaves are also used in "bush baths" to relieve rashes and treat skin diseases.

Guavas are rich in dietary fiber, vitamins A and C, folic acid, potassium, copper and manganese. Those alone are enough of a benefit, because they power up your immune system.

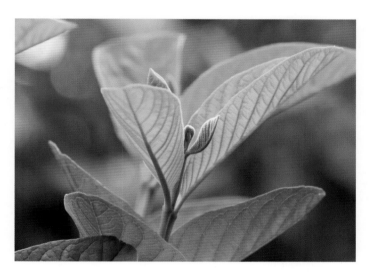

Guava leaves can be used fresh or dried in the sun, and simmered in water to make a tea.

A Potent Cancer Cell Killer

The leaves also have another surprise... they have anticancer properties...

Guava extracts have been shown to suppress tumor growth, and in animal studies can suppress leukemia. Guava is especially good for men, because it can interrupt the pathways by which prostate cells become cancerous, and it can induce apoptosis, or cell death, in prostate cells that have already become cancerous.[1]

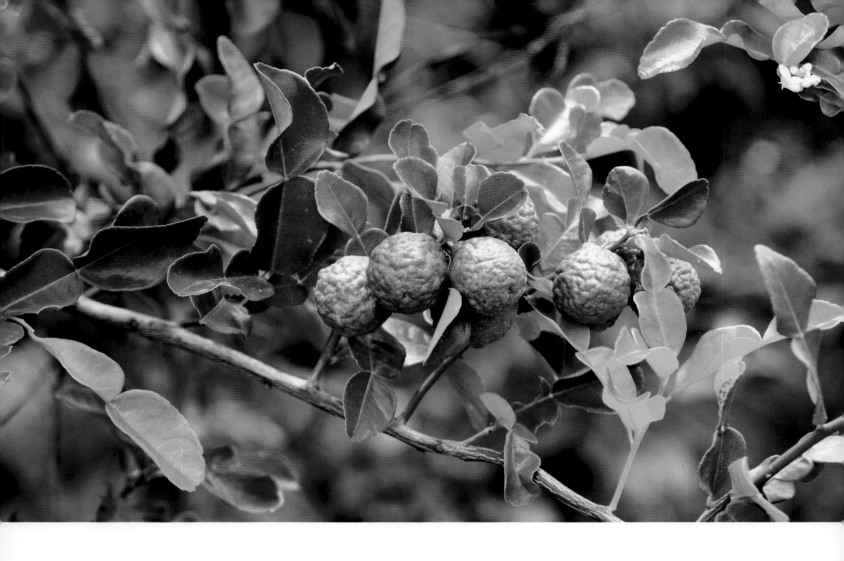

Scientists are studying 60 compounds from guava for their possible anticancer effects. Part of guava's anticancer power comes from its leaves, which are a rich source of a little-known flavonoid called *morin*.

Research shows that morin can block the growth of tumor cells,[2] and kill off colon[3] and breast[4] cancer cells.

Guava leaves can also boost your brain health. Morin can shield your neurons and those important brain cells called *oligodendrocytes*.

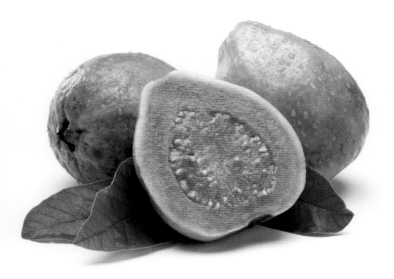

A study in the journal, *Glia*, found that free-radical damage from inflammation was much higher in glial cells not protected with morin.[5]

The reason this is so important is that glial cells not only support other brain cells, but they also detoxify and carry waste away from your brain while you sleep. This helps prevent the buildup of altered proteins, like the amyloid protein we see in people with Alzheimer's disease.

Wipe Out Bacteria, Fungus and Viruses

Guava leaf also has antibacterial, antiviral, and antifungal effects.[6] It even works against the H1N1 "bird flu" virus strain.[7]

When guava leaves were tested for their free radical scavenging and antioxidant activity, they proved to be surprisingly potent.[8]

The leaves also improve your intestinal health. Guava fruit has what we call "prebiotic activity." Prebiotics are non-digestible ingredients that power up the good bacteria in your gut. When these bacteria are strengthened, it improves your digestion, and you can absorb essential minerals better, improving your immune system.

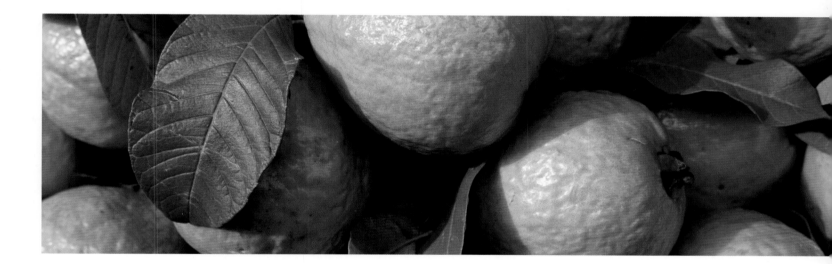

Diabetes Destroyer

Even better in today's world, guava may help fight blood sugar problems and diabetes.

Components found in the leaves, stems and the fruit can help block digestion of carbohydrates. This means producing less insulin, and having better blood sugar control.[9, 10, 11, 12]

In one study, 15 pre-diabetic men took a guava extract at every meal for 12 weeks. They all experienced reduced blood sugar, and a noticeable decrease in fats and triglyceride levels in the blood, which shows that their bodies were processing the carbohydrates more efficiently.

A second study done over a period of eight weeks looked at people who were diabetics and on diabetes medications. After supplementing with guava extract, they had reduced insulin production and lower blood sugar levels as well.

Another benefit of guava comes from the essential oils. They are anti-inflammatory.[13,14] Guava can strengthen your heart and kidneys, which is extremely important if you have diabetes.[15, 16]

So there's a lot more to guava than just the fruit. Plus, as Lelir explained to me, guava has a highly beneficial traditional use that might have you visiting the produce section of the grocery store instead of the drug store...

Quick Relief for an Embarrassing Problem

In the last few years, Ubud has become a popular spot for more adventurous visitors. They're looking for the "real" Bali. So they head away from the tourist beaches and into the interior.

Some of these intrepid visitors wind up in our shop. It's always fun to chat with them. They're interested in discovering the real Bali, and Westi and I are happy to tell them about our corner of the island.

But some of our visitors arrive at our shop a little uncomfortable. Unfamiliar food and water can loosen your bowels. And that's distressing when you're in a new place and don't know where the nearest restroom is.

I remember a curious young American couple dropped into our shop a couple of years ago. They were very nice, but the wife seemed on edge.

After we had talked about herbs for a few minutes, she asked if there was a restroom nearby. She'd had mild diarrhea for a couple of days.

Once we helped them with their problem, we showed them how to relieve her problem without using drugs.

Here in Bali, we've used the leaves of a plant we call Jambu Batu or Jambu Biji to relieve diarrhea for hundreds of years. It is guava – and it grows throughout the Pacific islands.

For our new young friend, I washed about an ounce of young guava leaves. Then I mashed them with a mortar and pestle.

Next, I added a cup of clean water to the mash and then squeezed the water out of the leaves. Finally, I added just a little honey and salt and gave it to her to drink.

This is the same recipe we used for our son when he was little. Any time he got diarrhea, we'd mix up a cup for him and have him sip it. It always cleared up his diarrhea quickly.

Guava is also very nutritious, and delicious. Guava trees grow wild in sunny spots all over the island. But if you want to try it, you won't have to find a tree. Any market in Bali will have guava available in season.

But be sure you don't eat too much. Guava fruit is famous for causing constipation.

But that's also good news. Because you probably can't find young guava leaves where you live. Instead, when you feel a bout of diarrhea coming on, eat some guava fruit. Eating a little guava every day when you have a stomach bug will help you avoid the discomfort of diarrhea.

— *Lelir*

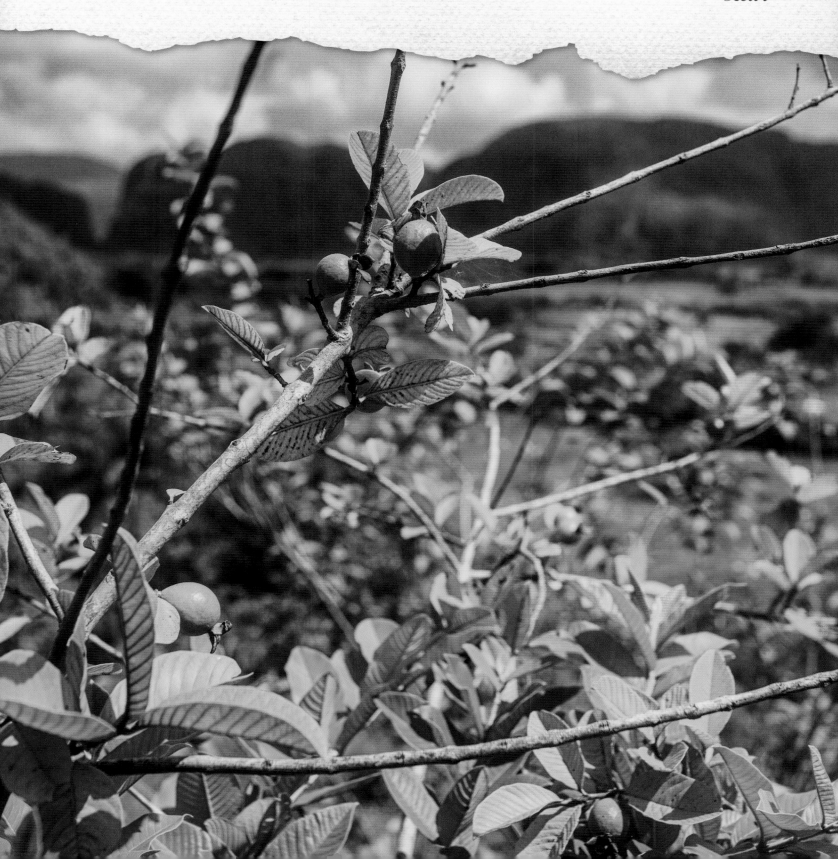

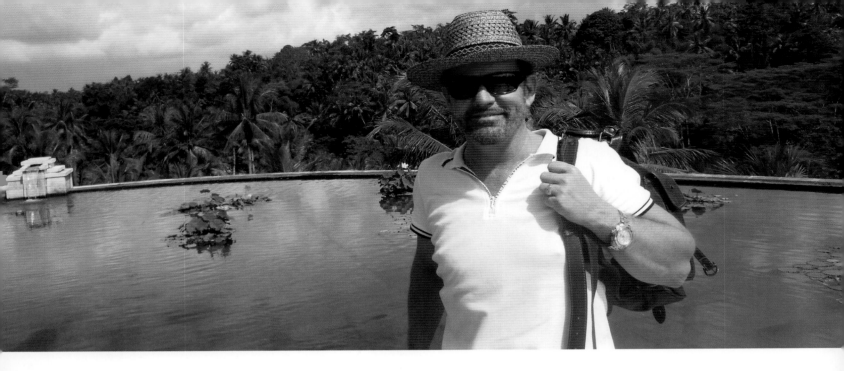

Going for a hike in the palm forests outside Ubud, Bali in May 2013.

My Own Research and Discoveries

Science backs up guava's use in traditional medicine.

Not long ago, researchers in China tested guava leaf. They confirmed that the leaf contains compounds that have a strong antidiarrhea effect.[17] A number of studies prove guava's effectiveness against diarrhea.[18, 19, 20]

And guava leaves are strong enough that they not only relieve stomach problems, but they can also cure ulcers. In fact, the leaf and its extracts are so powerful that they can block giardia, the parasite that can give you a virulent form of diarrhea.[21,22]

Guava fruit is in season from September through December. When it's in season, you don't have to look too hard to find it.

It usually smells nice and sweet when it's ripe, and should be slightly soft when you press on the rind. And when a guava fruit is ripe, you can eat it just like an apple. Eat the seeds, too! They're crunchy and have a lot of nutrients in them.

You may want to freeze your guava if you want to have it during the summer, because ripe guava only lasts about two days in the refrigerator.

"GUAVA LEAVES ARE STRONG ENOUGH THAT THEY NOT ONLY RELIEVE STOMACH PROBLEMS, BUT THEY CAN ALSO CURE ULCERS."

You may have to search a bit for the leaves. You can often find sellers on places like Amazon.com or Localharvest.org. Occasionally, you'll see the fresh leaves at a health food store, but you're more likely to find the dried leaves. And that's okay because they make more potent teas and decoctions anyway. Fresh leaves contain more water, so you need to almost double the amount to dried leaf infusions.

TO MAKE A DECOCTION OF GUAVA LEAVES,
WHICH CAN HELP CURE BAD BREATH, GINGIVITIS, MOUTH AND
STOMACH ULCERS, AND RELIEVE INDIGESTION AND DIARRHEA,
HERE'S WHAT LELIR RECOMMENDS:

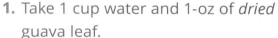

Guava

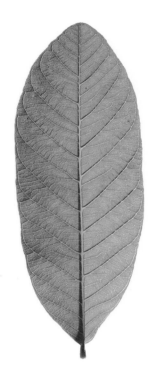

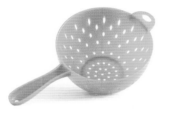

2. Cut or crush the herb or root and add it to the water in the pot.

Turn on the heat to medium. Simmer your decoction with the lid off until the volume of water is reduced by one-quarter (so, three-quarters remains).

1. Take 1 cup water and 1-oz of *dried* guava leaf.

Place the water into a pot made from non-reactive metal (such as stainless steel or enamel; do not use aluminum).

3. Cool and strain. Store in the fridge for no more than 72 hours.

Take in divided doses, according to use. Swish three times a day.

To make a tea, take 1 teaspoon of the decoction above and add it to 8 oz. of water. Add honey or stevia for a bit of sweetness.

If you use fresh guava leaves, you may need to add 2-4 teaspoons of the decoction to an 8 oz. glass of water.

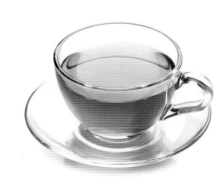

Also, if you want some guava leaf tea, remember that the time of year that leaves are harvested plays a role in their free-radical scavenging activity, or how high their antioxidant strength is.

Leaves harvested between May and August, a bit before the fruit is usually harvested, have higher levels of antioxidant power.[23]

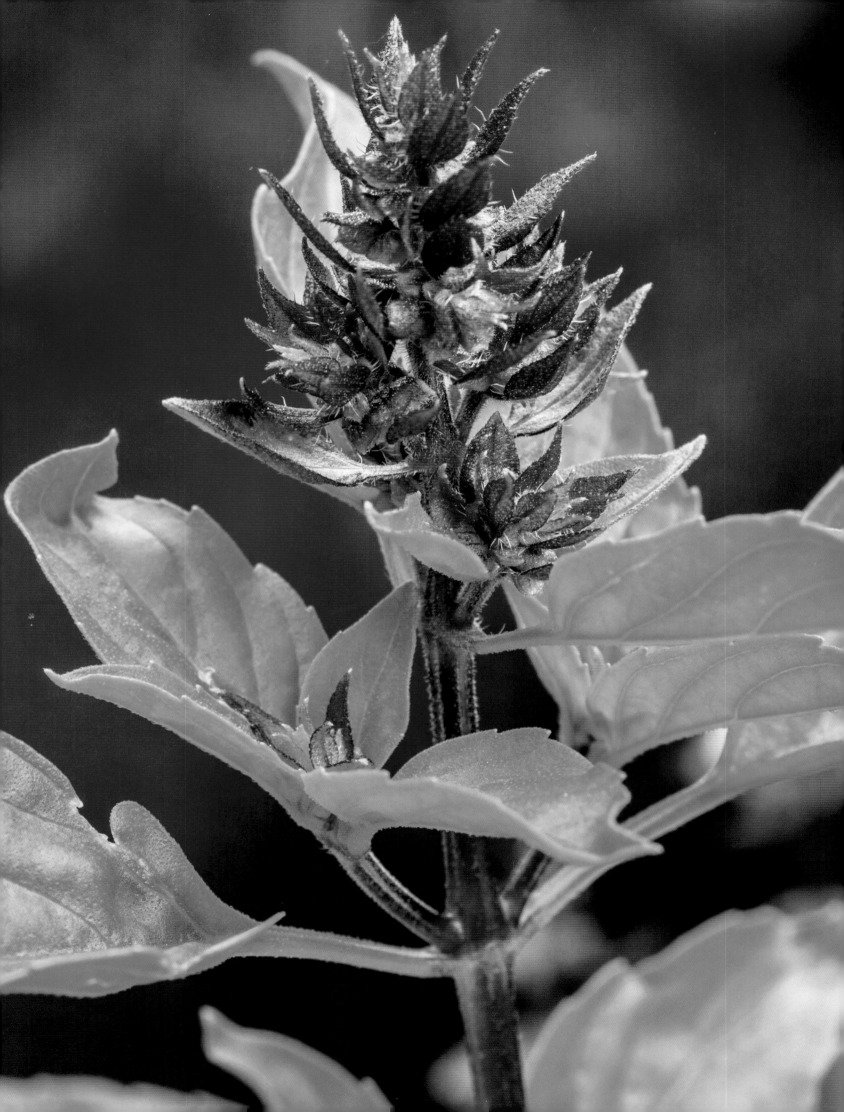

DETOXIFY AND SOOTHE INFLAMMATION WITH BALI'S SACRED HERB

All around me was the greenest green I'd ever imagined, spilling over with flowers, vines and herbs in every direction.

It was a perfect day — sunny and not too hot.

Westi and I were sitting in a kind of covered shelter with a big brown picnic table area after touring his incredible herb garden.

"You were telling me about holy basil," I said, "and you called it…"

"Tulsi. Also sacred basil," Westi said. "Tulsi is what they called it when I saw it in India, too."

Do you know holy basil?

It's a special type of detoxifying basil that can also boost your body's immune system and relieve pain.

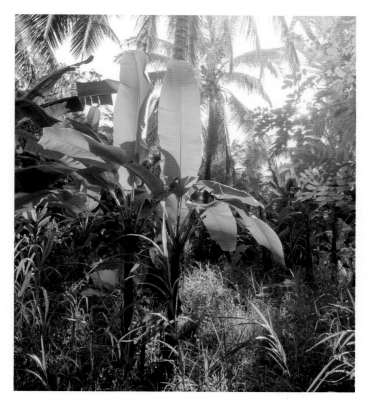

Bali is the lushest place I've ever been, with plants on top of plants, and flowers and herbs everywhere.

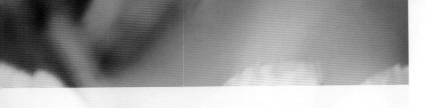

> "STUDIES HAVE FOUND THAT HOLY BASIL IS EFFECTIVE AGAINST BOTH ANXIETY AND DEPRESSION."

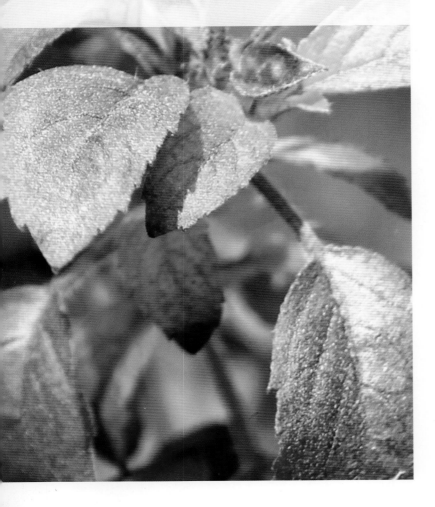

- In one study on immune health, researchers took a group of people and measured their normal levels of the immune markers interferon and interleukin-4, and their normal percentage of T-cells and natural killer (NK) cells.

  Then they gave them holy basil for four weeks and re-measured. Levels of all these immune-system defenders increased significantly, especially T-cells.[1]

- Holy basil is also anti-inflammatory. It contains dozens of inflammation-reducing nutrients, including one called *ursolic acid.*

  Ursolic acid inhibits the inflammatory COX-2 enzyme[2] that causes pain, but without the nasty side effects of pharmaceuticals.

- Holy basil also inhibits 5-lox, which is activated by cortisol, the stress hormone. 5-lox converts arachidonic acid (a bad fat made within the body from vegetable oils) to highly inflammatory leukotrienes, which promote arthritis.

- One animal study looked at holy basil's pain-relieving power. An extract was about 60% as effective as sodium salicylate (an aspirin-related compound) in reducing inflammation.[2]

- Holy basil also has other beneficial properties. Animal studies have found that holy basil is effective against anxiety and depression.[3]

- Holy Basil is also one of your best sources of the potent flavonoid, *apigenin.* The American Cancer Society sponsored a study which showed that apigenin was able to kill deadly brain cancer cells, while protecting healthy cells.[4]

- And in another study, apigenin protected animals against symptoms of Alzheimer's. Those given apigenin had improved learning

A Cornucopia of Cures

Westi grows three different kinds of basil. One is lemon basil, which smells exactly like its name — a combination of lemon and basil. Another is what he calls "fragrant" basil, which he and his wife Lelir use in their beauty formulas.

But the one with the most healing properties is holy basil. And science backs up the benefits of holy basil, which the Balinese have known for centuries.

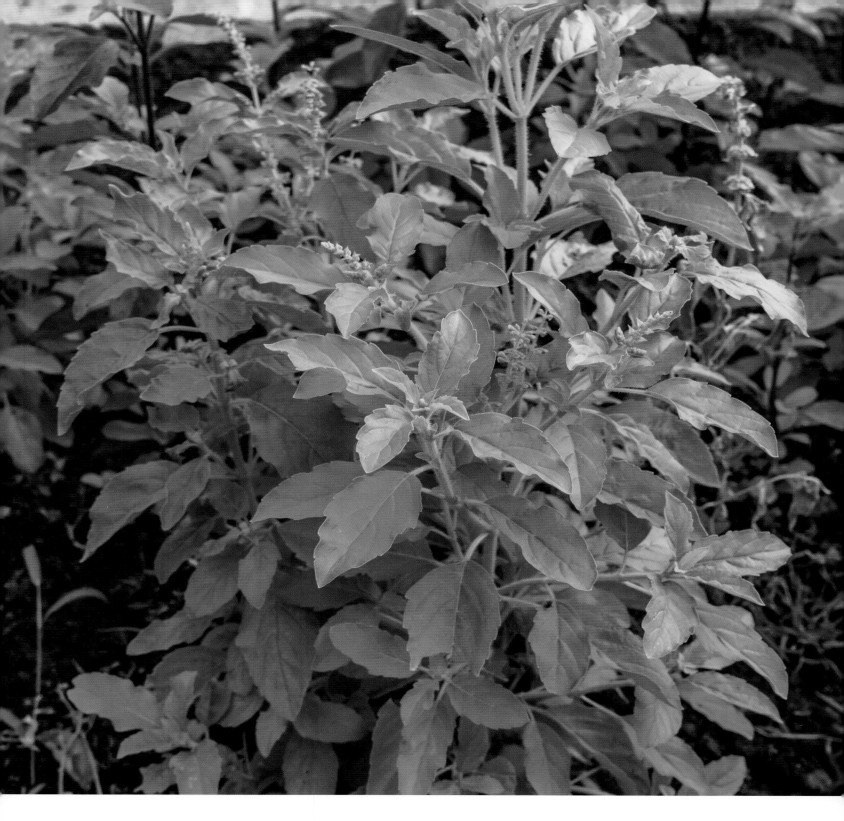

Holy basil, also known as sacred basil, is a natural immune system booster, an anti-inflammatory and recognized cancer killer.

and memory capabilities, maintained the integrity of their brain cells, had better brain blood flow, reduced free radical damage and improved brain-chemical transmission.[5]

• Holy basil is also detoxifying. In another study, a very small amount of holy basil extract reversed toxicity from the extremely poisonous industrial metal cadmium.[6]

• Westi also showed me how they use holy basil with citronella from lemongrass to repel mosquitoes and flies. Holy basil is toxic to mosquitoes, and especially to their larvae.

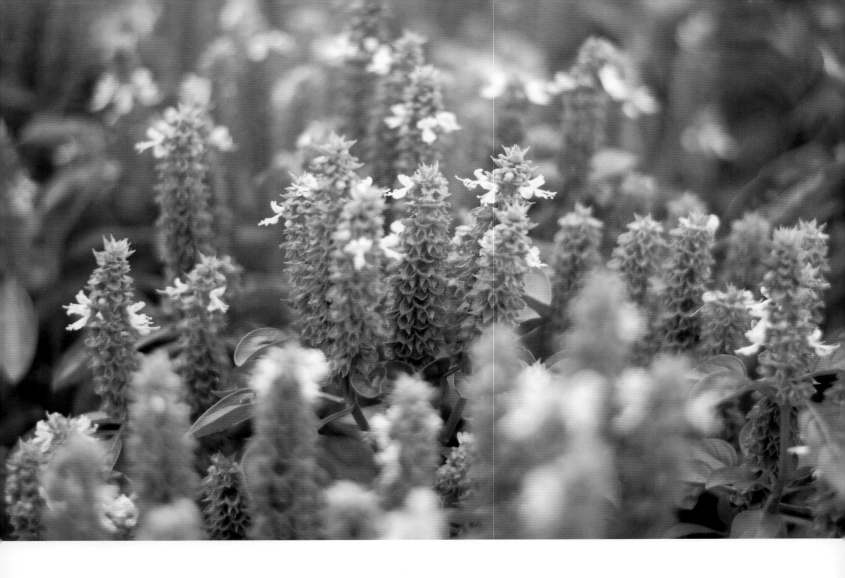

My Own Research and Discoveries

Plant holy basil around your door, in between your flowers, and around your patio. Even better, go for a full herb garden — rosemary and bay leaves repel bugs too.

You can also put basil leaves in your cabinets and pantry to keep bugs out of the kitchen. It works at my house.

You can get the dried plant at most health-food stores, and online at mountainroseherbs.com, taoofherbs.com, and indusorganics.com.

Holy basil extracts, leaves, roots, seeds and oil may be available from online wholesalers like naturalcosmeticsupplies.com.

You can also get an extract of holy basil to take as a supplement, in either liquid or capsule form.

Gaia Organics and Herb Pharm are two companies that sell the extract as a liquid. Take one dropper full two to three times a day between meals.

In a capsule, make sure the product you're buying has at least 2.5% ursolic acid to get the anti-inflammatory effect. I recommend 150 mg three times a day, but you can take as much as 800 mg.

OR YOU CAN DO WHAT I DO AND MAKE A DELICIOUS TEA. IT'S GREAT FOR COUGHS.

Holy Basil

Tulsi tea is easy to make, once you know how. All you need are a few leaves, dried or fresh, of the holy basil plant.

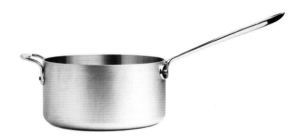

1. First, heat a quart of water.

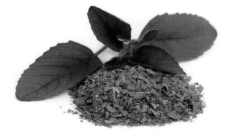

2. Put in 3 heaping teaspoons of leaves and let them decoct for about 5 minutes.

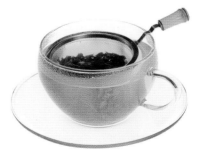

3. Strain into a cup or glass.

In Bali, they add lemongrass for flavor. Westi says they also put ginger in their holy basil tea for added effect. You can drink it warm, but I enjoy my holy basil tea over ice.

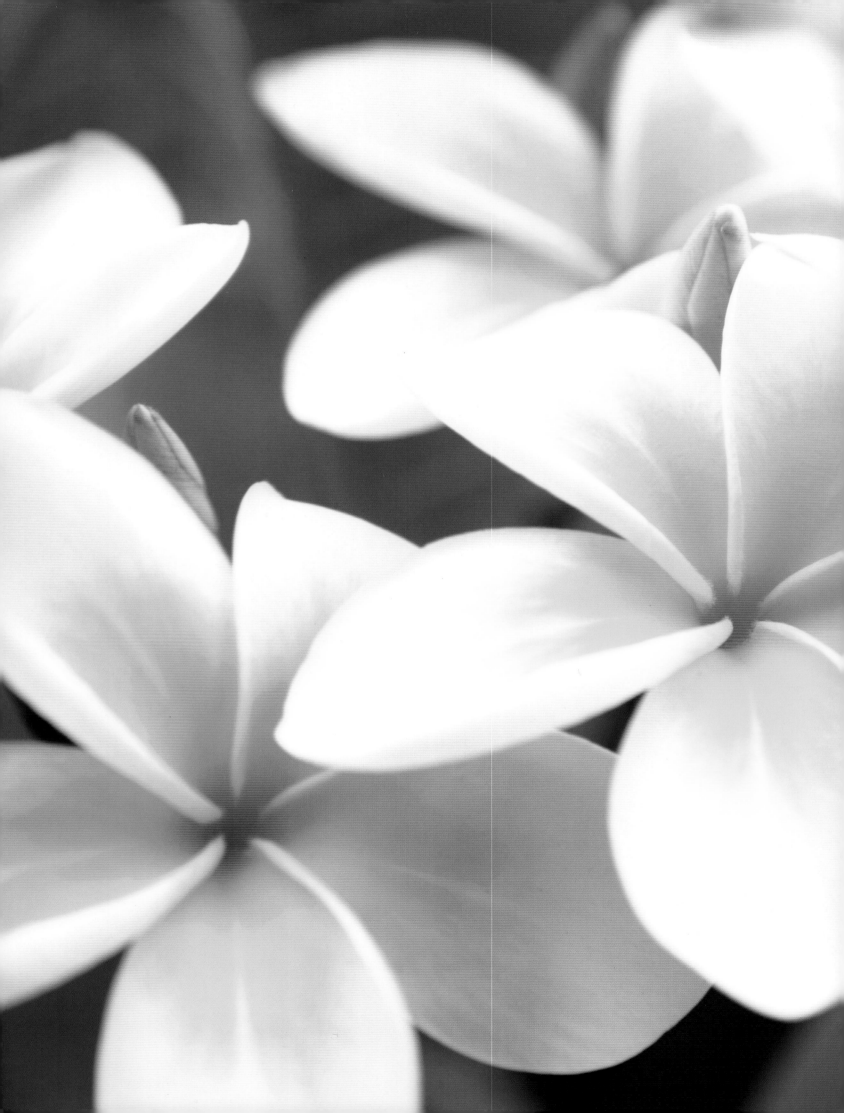

THE AROMATIC GARDEN HEALER AND... DRAGONFLY SOUP ANYONE?

All of the people I met in Bali were so sweet. They were genuine, untainted and simple people.

Most Balinese practice a form of Hinduism. They have three rules to live by. They're called the "Tri Hita Karana."

The first rule is to have good relationships with other people. Balians who follow this rule do their best to make sure their actions affect others in a positive way.

The second is to maintain your relationship with nature. Your work and day-to-day activities have to support and strengthen your relationship with the world around you.

And the third is your spiritual relationship. It's a more patient kind of approach. I like it because it's a very humble way of looking at things.

Instead of saying "Nature is wrong and we're going to fix it," like most Western doctors do, the Balinese Hindu respect nature and its healing power.

Balians have a sense of trust in the human body's abilities. They tend to trust Mother Nature first, and they are humble enough to use whatever Mother Nature provides for them.

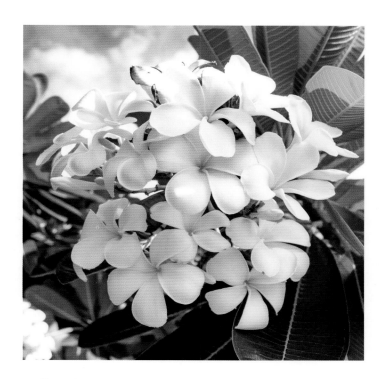

Frangipani grows wild all over Bali. Lelir showed me some of the most beautiful blooms I have ever seen.

For example, they don't eat much meat in Bali, in part because meat is relatively scarce, and in part because they practice Hinduism. But Westi told me they have an "alternative" source of protein: dragonflies.

Dragonflies get huge on Bali, and can even eat small fish for nutrition. And the Balinese children have a trick they use to catch the dragonflies, which involves the healing plant frangipani. I'll tell you more about frangipani in a minute. But first, here's what Westi told me...

First Aid From Your Garden

(Plumeria alba)

Balinese name: Jepun

When I was very young, I learned a trick that children in Bali have known for many generations. I learned to catch dragonflies.

We especially loved to catch them when we had holidays from school in June, July and August. Even during school, we would often not go to the playground. We spent most of our time playing in the fields. We would play with kites we brought from home, or catch dragonflies.

Dragonfly hunting may seem like a typical children's game... but in Bali, it's different. Catching dragonflies was fun, but it was also a treat. Because our mothers used the dragonflies we caught to make dragonfly soup.

You see, we don't eat a lot of meat in Bali. Most of us are Hindu, so we only eat meat on very special occasions. Balinese dragonflies grow very big. And they're not considered meat. So we often eat them.

If dragonfly soup sounds a little strange, the way we catch them will seem even stranger.

In Bali's tropical climate, water is everywhere. Rivers flow down from the mountains. We also grow a lot of rice. And dragonflies love the edges of rice paddies. It's the perfect place to hunt for the insects they eat.

To hunt dragonflies, you need a jepun tree – frangipani. Fortunately, frangipani grows in almost every Balinese garden, because we use its flowers for religious offerings.

Frangipani produces a sticky white sap. You take some of this sap and mix it with a little coconut oil to make a very strong glue. Then you head for the rice fields – or wherever water may attract dragonflies.

Once you've found your dragonflies, put a dab of your homemade glue on the end of a coconut leaf stem, and use it to snare dragonflies.

With a little practice, almost any child can master this. In no time, you're headed home with your catch for the day... and my mouth would water because I knew the delicious treat that would be for supper.

A Delicious Elixir

To make the soup, my mother would prepare the dragonflies. Meanwhile, she'd start the water boiling. Soon after she added the dragonflies, the aroma filled our little house.

Dragonfly soup smells very yummy and my mother would add turmeric leaf and make the aroma even better. It tastes a little like a cross between mushroom soup and chicken soup. Although we eat it often, we still think of it as a treat.

In fact, it's very rare to find it in a Balinese restaurant, but sometimes they will let you special order this really special Balinese food. It's so sought-after that people in Bali will barter a kilo of rice for just one large portion of dragonfly soup.

And, even though children all over Bali use the frangipani trick to catch dragonflies, we Balinese have another use for frangipani's sap. It makes an excellent emergency bandage.

Lelir and I have a couple of men who help us pick our herbs. They often use their Bali knives – like the one I gave Dr. Sears and used to carve a few coconuts for him – out in the fields. These men are experts at what they do. And they're very careful. But every once in a while, someone gets cut. Usually it's from a sharp leaf or stem – sort of like a bad paper cut. But once in a while a Bali knife slips.

The first time one of our workers got a bad cut, he was worried. But I knew exactly what to do. I went to a frangipani tree and sliced a branch with my knife.

I applied the sticky sap directly to his cut. The cut in his skin closed up quickly, and the bleeding stopped. You should have seen the relief on his face. It was a long way to the hospital.

— *Westi*

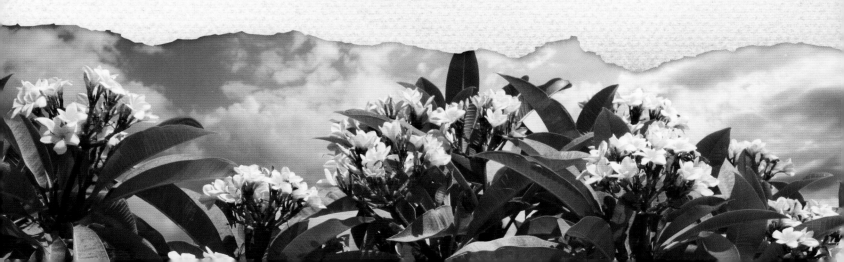

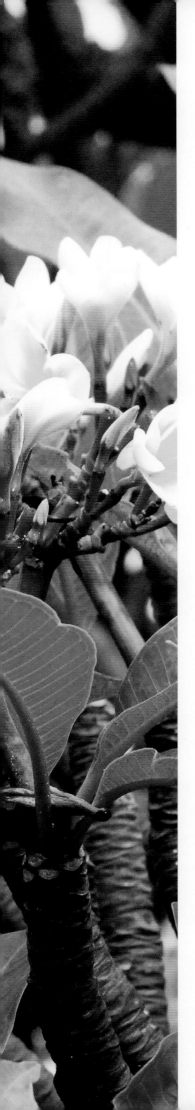

My Own Research and Discoveries

Frangipani does more than just seal a cut. Western science has revealed there's more going on with this ancient practice. The frangipani sap contains at least a dozen antibacterial and antifungal compounds.[1]

This explains why frangipani is so effective against infections when used on wounds.

This tropical tree thrives in a hot, humid climate. In the U.S., you can sometimes find frangipani growing in southern Florida. I don't have any in my yard, but I see it often, because it's been transplanted to South Florida because of its beauty.

Frangipani trees are fairly short — only about 20 feet high. But they can grow nearly as wide as they are tall. In spring, they burst with five-petaled blossoms, creamy white with a yellow center. They fill your garden with a heavenly perfume.

The Balinese people also put the petals behind their ears. Women beautify themselves by wearing the flowers in their hair. Often in Bali, the people wear frangipani as an accessory when they attend a temple festival or ceremony. One of the ceremonies where you'll find frangipanis in the U.S. is weddings. They are often in the bouquet or used for decor.

The scientific name *Plumeria* was derived from the French botanist and missionary Charles Plumier, who collected plants in the West Indies in the 1680s and 1690s. The Museum d'Histoire Naturelle in Paris houses his detailed manuscript, which contains his collection of 6,000 original sketches and drawings.

> "THE FRANGIPANI SAP CONTAINS AT LEAST A DOZEN ANTIBACTERIAL AND ANTIFUNGAL COMPOUNDS."

Because of its many species, the plumeria can range from a tall tree to a bushy shrub. The leaves can be wide and tapering, with pointed tips, or long thin leaves that are evergreen. The flowers can be petals so well joined that there are very few gaps, or very wide gaps and short petals, with colors ranging from white, pink, orange, red and all the shades in between.

There's a poster presentation in the *Journal of Infectious Diseases*. The presentation was about a compound using plumeria alba extract. It was applied three times a day to the skin of people with shingles, a condition linked with the herpes virus. After applying frangipani topically, the acute pain the people were suffering was gone in just ten minutes! Those using antiviral drugs continued to have pain. This shows that plumeria alba eliminated the virus that causes herpes and stopped the pain.[2] Plumeria alba has also been shown to stop the growth of, and shrink, tumors. And it helps you to have robust healthy red blood cells, too.[3]

Preparations

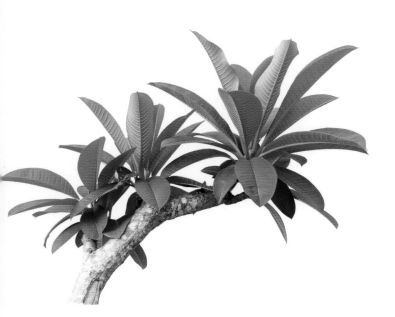

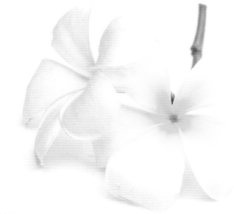

Treatment for Cuts and Scrapes

Parts Used: Sap (external use only)

Cut into the stem or bark and apply the sticky sap onto cut and scrape.

In Salads

Parts Used: Flower

Frangipani flowers are edible and can be used in a variety of recipes: salads, soups, and can even be consumed freshly picked. Of course, you'll want to get only organic flowers, not those that may have been exposed to pesticides.

Rinse the petals and simply add them to your salad.

Frangipani

Laxative Tea

Parts Used: Bark

Lelir has a recipe that makes a laxative tea from the frangipani bark. She learned it from her parents. She gave me this recipe, which has been handed down for years:

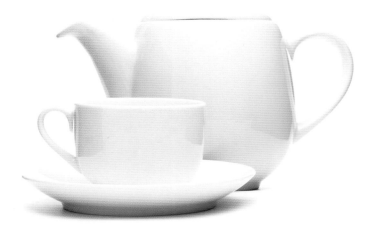

- Soak 2–3 grams of frangipani bark in water for several hours.

- Strain the bark out just before you go to bed.

- Drink the strained water, and you should feel relief by morning.

Make sure not to use more than 3 grams of frangipani bark. In larger amounts, it has a diuretic effect. You can drink this tea from frangipani bark. But only use frangipani sap externally. The sap can make you very sick if you drink it, and is poisonous to most animals that ingest it.

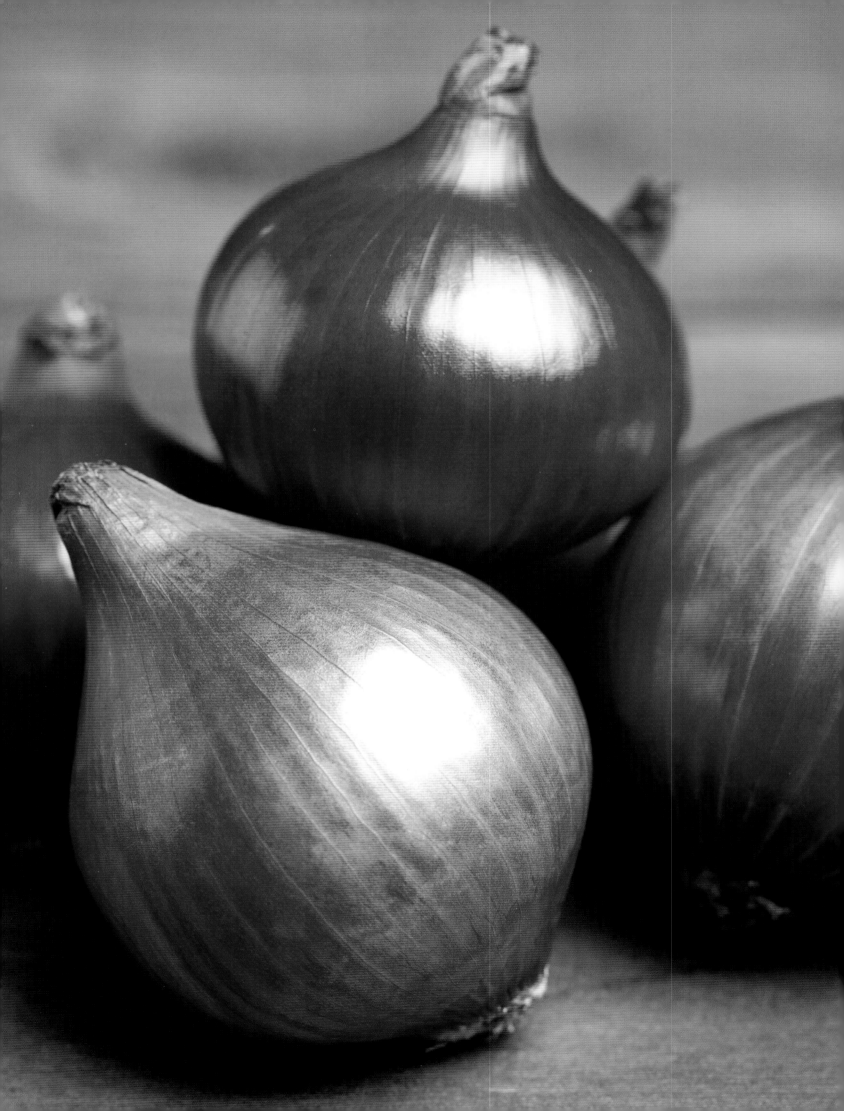

THE RED ONION HAS LAYERS OF HEALING TREASURES

When I worked the rice fields with Westi, not only was it hot, but there were also quite a few bugs. I don't get bitten by mosquitoes much, but those aren't the only critters that can get you in the rice fields. Fortunately, Lelir gave us a liquid she made from a base of onion to rub on any sting or bite.

As soon as you rub it in, the puffy skin around the bite would shrink rather quickly.

In traditional Balinese use, the red onion is used to ward off spirits. It also has anti-fever properties, and you can make a compress of it, which will relieve your high temperature.

Also, red onion has one of the highest food concentrations of the flavonoid quercetin. Flavonoids are a group of health-giving plant nutrients and antioxidants.

Quercetin is anti-inflammatory, a natural antihistamine and can increase your exercise performance.

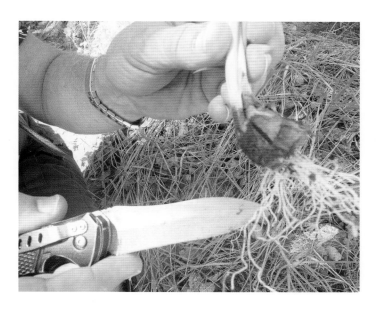

A closer look at the Balinese red onion from Westi's garden.

It also provides an energy boost for your cells. It increases the number of your mitochondria (the powerhouses inside every cell) in your muscles. That's good news for your body's hardest-working muscle, the heart.

But did you know...

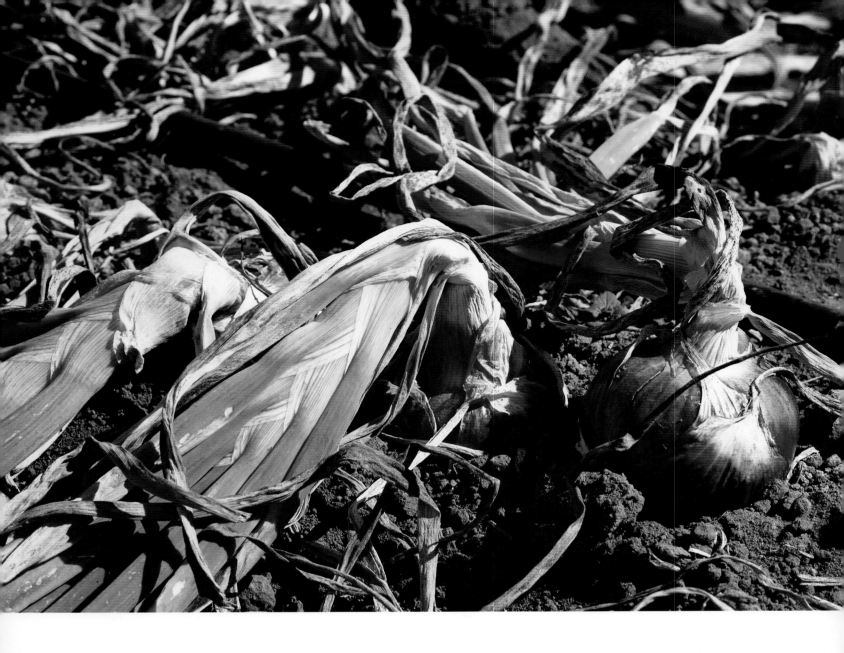

The Quercetin in Red Onion is also a Fierce Cancer Fighter

Quercetin can protect against lung, skin, pancreatic, ovarian, endocrine and cervical cancers.[1]

A study published in the journal *Carcinogenesis* found quercetin that could stop cancer-causing changes in prostate cells. It flushes away carcinogens and can block prostate tumor development and growth.

As healthy as onions are in general, red onions are the highest in total polyphenols and flavonoids, including quercetin and beta-sitosterol. They are also high in vitamin C, manganese, B vitamins and potassium.

Lelir showed me how the Balinese use the incredible health-giving power of red onions for many traditional uses.

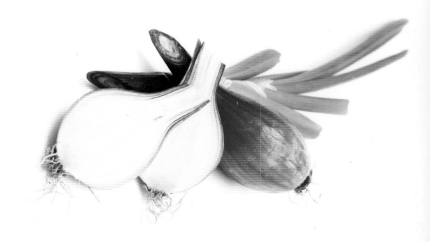

Soothe Itchy Bug Bites

(Alternanthera amoena)

Balinese name: Bawang Barak

In Bali, mothers begin teaching their daughters to cook from a young age. I can still remember my sisters and I taking turns in our home's little kitchen, helping our mother prepare meals.

Like most Balinese women, my mother used red onion in almost every meal. And I do, too.

In Balinese tradition, red onion was also used to ward off black magic. When I was a little girl, this belief was still very common.

I remember a friend's mother was about to have a baby, and the family called a "dukun bayi" – a traditional birth attendant or midwife.

It was a very difficult birth, and we could even hear my friend's mother straining and moaning as we waited outside in the yard. Finally, the baby came.

When the midwife came out to leave, my friend asked her if the birth had been hard for her mother.

"Oh, yes," the old woman answered. "Very hard. There were bad spirits keeping the baby from coming out. So I chewed some bawang barak and spit it on her stomach. Then the baby came right out."

In the old days, the Balinese believed demons loved the aroma of red onions. They thought the enticing aroma would distract the evil spirits away from the baby... making birth easier, and protect the infant.

I don't know about evil spirits, but red onions can certainly keep health problems from bothering you. They reduce inflammation. Red onion has anticancer properties, too.[2]

I've read that some people have trouble digesting onions. Here in Bali, we believe red onions aid digestion. And I can understand why they would.

Onions have a very high fiber content. Westi and I think that perhaps some people have trouble eating onions because they aren't used to so much fiber. Fiber is good for you, but when you eat a lot more than you're used to, it can create uncomfortable gas and other problems.

Red onions are good for more than digestion. They're also good for bug bites – especially mosquitoes.

If you get an itchy bug bite, just cut a thin slice of red onion and place it on the bite. In a few minutes, the swelling and itchiness should start to fade.

Red onion helps you avoid bug bites, too. Mosquitoes hate the smell of red onion. If you have to go outside in mosquito season and you don't have insect repellent, you can use red onion instead.

People here used to rub red onion on their babies. They believed babies were especially sensitive to black magic. So – like the dukun bayi – they'd use red onion to chase the evil spirits away from their baby.

I think this belief may have started because red onion repels mosquitoes. Babies rubbed with red onion probably aren't bitten by mosquitoes as often. So they're less likely to get sick from the diseases mosquitoes carry.

But many generations ago, people didn't understand about these diseases... so they thought they'd discovered that red onion chases away bad spirits.

— *Lelir*

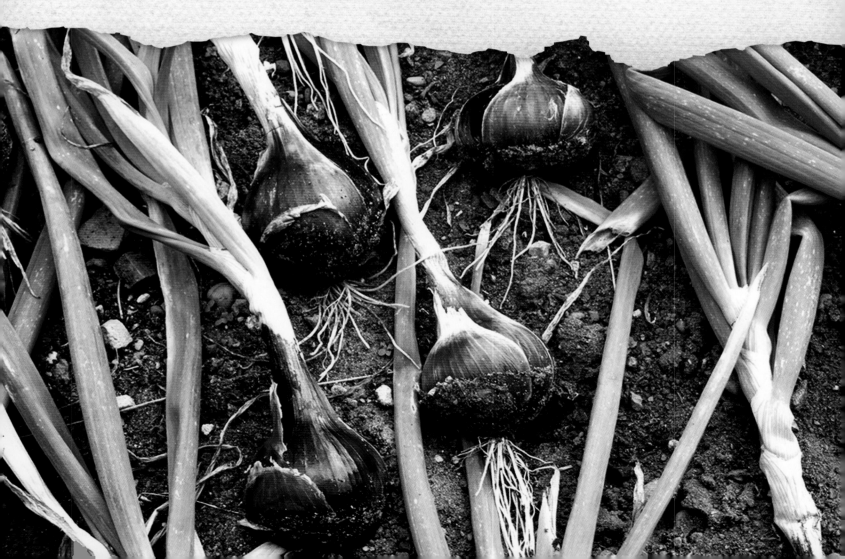

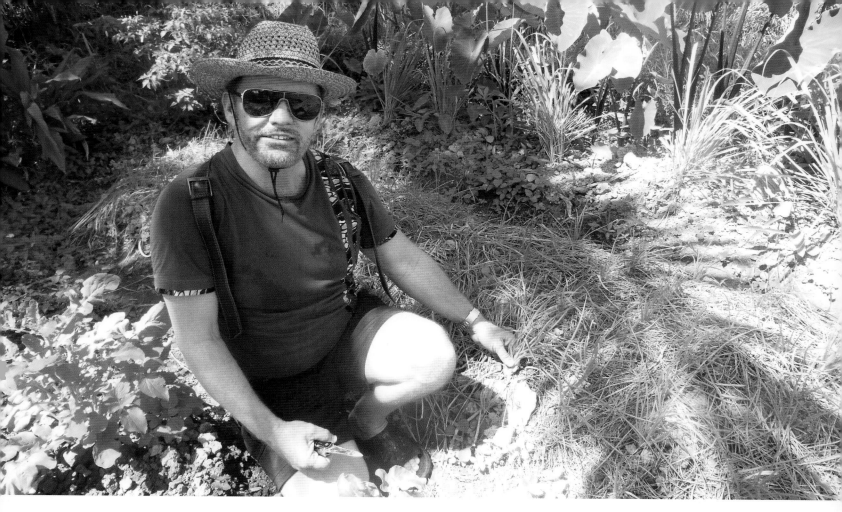

On my most recent visit with my friends Westi and Lelir in Bali I went back to the herb garden next to the rice paddies I worked during my first trip and dug up a red onion… they're small but powerful.

My Own Research and Discoveries

Soluble fiber is one of the hardest things to get in our Western diet. Red onions have a lot, and it's in a beneficial form called *fructans,* a special type of fiber that the good bacteria in your intestines eat.

Fructans are a prebiotic-like fiber that resists digestion from the small intestine and reaches the large intestine intact, where your microflora gets the most benefit from it.

Fructans are anti-inflammatory, and help you digest other foods and enhance immunity, because the beneficial bacteria in your intestines boost your immune system.[3]

So eating red onions keeps your digestive and immune systems toned and healthy.

Red onions are one of my favorite foods to add to any recipe. Once you've sautéed it, it adds a nice boost in flavor. I often add them to meals because they not only taste great, but they are very high in phytonutrients, vitamins and minerals.

That pungent aroma of the onion can be attributed to the many sulfur compounds within it. I bet those sulfur compounds are what keep bugs away.

The red onion contains a high content of quercetin and has twice the amount of antioxidants as other types of onions.[4, 5]

It also has a very high content of polyophenols, compared with many other vegetables, including tomatoes, carrots and red bell peppers.

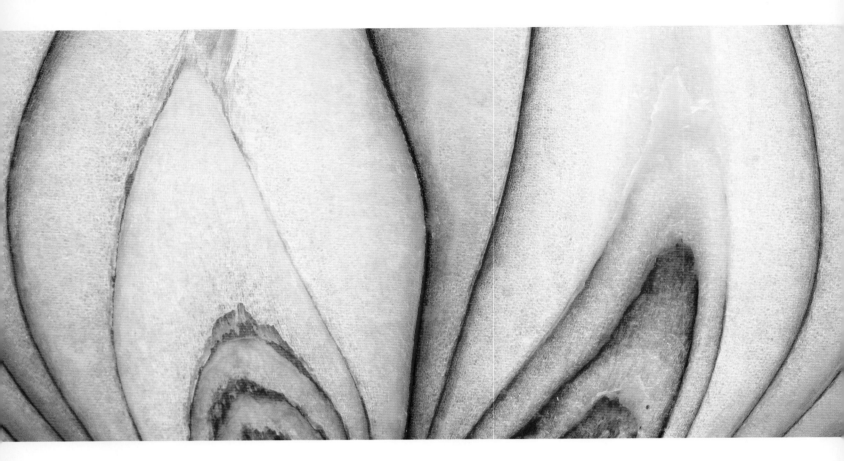

The Onion's Many Layers of Disease-Fighting Power

Red onions also have a multitude of health benefits. A recent study showed that women over 50, who are perimenopausal or menopausal, had less bone fractures when they included onion in their diet five times per week. Even as little as two times per week had some benefits.[6]

Other studies show benefits for diabetics and their blood sugar.[7, 8]

Red onions also benefit the cardiovascular system and anti-platelet activity. At the same, they are anti-inflammatory and anticarcinogenic, and they support bone and connective tissue health.[9, 10]

"SO EATING RED ONIONS KEEP YOUR DIGESTIVE AND IMMUNE SYSTEMS TONED AND HEALTHY."

In a recent study conducted with 1,268 people, red onion was used with two other ingredients. The researchers made a gel and applied it to wounds that could potentially scar. They found the gel to be effective in preventing excessive scarring and in promoting healing.[11]

Now researchers are taking an extract of the red onion peel and using it to fight obesity.[12, 13]

Red onions are great for just about everything, so eat them as often as you can.

Final Tips... So You Get Every Last Pungent Benefit

Remember when you peel a red onion that much of the quercetin is found in the outmost layers of the onion, so peel the outside layers minimally. When you remove too much of the edible outer portion you can lose 20% of its quercetin content and 75% of the anthocyanins, which have been shown to protect against a myriad of human diseases.[14]

Make sure that they don't have dark spots on their skin, or a lot of moisture to them. The dark spots indicate that they are getting older. If you can find them organic, you are doing even better.

You can sauté an onion, by cutting it into ¼-inch thick slices. Then add them to either broth or oil and cook for five minutes on a medium heat. Let them stand for five more minutes and serve. Quercetin is not lost during cooking.

Here is a meal that is loaded with red onion; it's one of my favorite recipes from my *Doctor's Heart Cure* book.

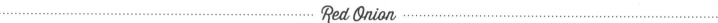

Red Onion

Dr. Sears' Baked Alaskan Salmon Salad with Red Onion

Salad Ingredients:

1 bag of mixed spring greens

½ cup of sliced mushrooms

1 red onion chopped

1 avocado peeled and chopped

¾ cup of chopped walnuts

1 cup of crumbled goat cheese

1 lemon and 1 lime

Black pepper

Fresh basil

2 lbs of Alaskan salmon *(1/2 lb. per person)*

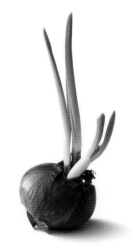

Dressing Ingredients:

2 tablespoons of cold pressed olive oil

2 tablespoons of balsamic vinegar

2 tablespoons of water

1 tablespoon of apple cider vinegar

½ teaspoon of honey

½ teaspoon of gourmet mustard

Black Pepper and Basil to taste

Directions:

In a large bowl, add *salad dressing ingredients* and whisk.
Add the red onion and mushrooms. Put aside.

Drizzle olive oil in a glass baking dish. Place fish in, skin side down. Squeeze lemon and lime over fish. Season with basil, black pepper and red pepper flakes to taste. Add a 1/3 cup of burgundy wine. Bake at 350 degrees for 20 to 30 minutes.

Mix salad dressing into the greens and toss to distribute dressing. Add avocado, walnuts and toss again. Serve greens on plate, top with fish and goat cheese. Garnish with lemon and lime.

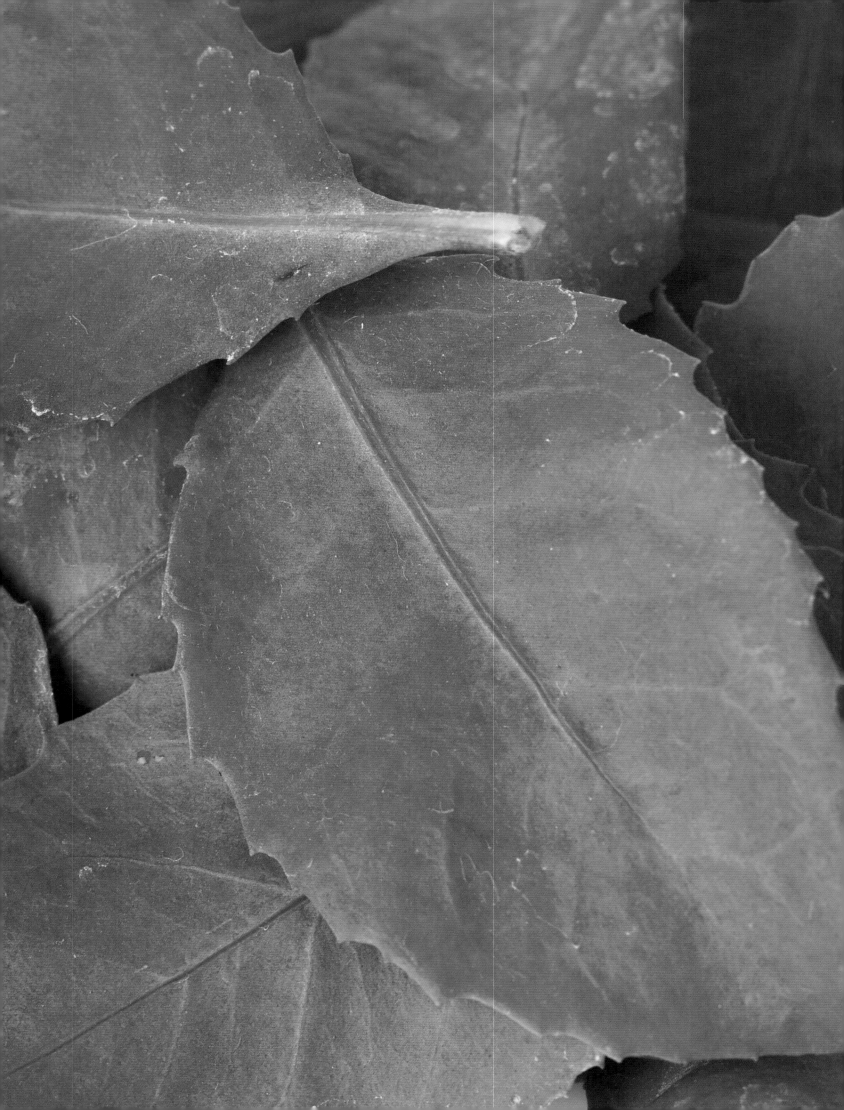

BALI'S PROSTATE-PROTECTING, CANCER-KILLING SUPER LEAVES

I've never been to China... but my clothes have.

The first time I visited Bali, that's where the airline sent my bags.

But you know me... I just went with it and bought clothes at a little local flea market in the town of Ubud. Except that it's very humid in Bali and I didn't have any personal items, either.

I don't use commercial deodorants because they have aluminum and other toxins in them. I asked Westi and Lelir if they had any herbs I could use.

Westi opened a cabinet full of herbs and grabbed a handful of these little serrated leaves. Then he washed them, and started to mash them up in a bowl with some water.

He added a little salt and tamarind for flavor, and told me to drink it. I was skeptical but I drank it anyway.

Well, I drank that every morning, and I had no body odor... even after working in the rice paddies and Westi's herb garden in the hot sun for hours.

They call the plant he used, *daun beluntas.* Westi told me the local healers use fresh beluntas to help relieve coughs, digestive problems and reduce back pain.

Beluntas is just one of the herbs and plants I found in Bali that almost no one in the West knows about. I discovered so many, I knew I had to put them in a book so you could use them yourself.

But when I went to do research on daun beluntas, there wasn't much to find... in English.

If you look up its English name, "Indian camphorweed," you'll find a lot of botanical references, but not much else.

I had to go digging into research from the Far East to learn that the extract from the leaves and roots is a strong antioxidant.[1]

It's so strong that beluntas has a powerful secret...

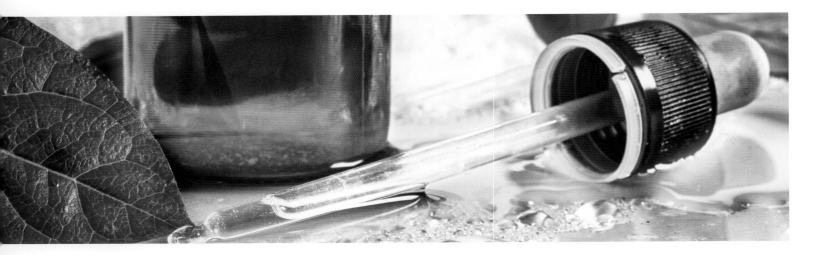

Beluntas Extract Suffocates Cancer Cells at their Source

In a study that has been completely overlooked by Western medicine, researchers from Kaohsiung Medical University in Taiwan looked at beluntas extracts and tested them for their cancer-killing power.

They treated cells with differing amounts of beluntas extract. After 10 days, the more beluntas extract they used, the more cancer cells died off. Just a 200 µg/ml of the root extract decreased the cancers' ability to survive to nearly *zero*.

Beluntas destroyed and stopped the spread of 75% of brain cancer cells (glioma) and 70% of cervical cancer cells.[2]

Extracts have also been shown to strongly inhibit leukemia, liver cancer, gastric cancer and other tumor cells.[3]

Why does beluntas work so well against cancer?

Chronic inflammation caused by oxidation can help tumors form. But powerful antioxidant components found in beluntas help prevent tumors from forming in the first place.[4]

Also, the antioxidants found in beluntas get rid of prostaglandins, which cause inflammation in your body and can promote cancer.[5]

Beluntas has several known antioxidants, like rutin, quercetin and beta-sitosterol, both of which can protect you from cancer.

Quercetin and beta-sitosterol are two of the most powerful natural healing compounds we know of.

Quercetin has been shown to protect against lung, skin, pancreatic, ovarian, endocrine and cervical cancers.[6]

Beta-sitosterol protects your prostate from enlarging, and can both treat and kill prostate cancer cells as well. In Bali, the *Balians* (traditional Balinese healers) use beluntas in men with a loss of urinary flow. Science and tradition backs them up on this.

The use of simple plant formulas to promote health in this way goes back to the beginning of civilization. It's called *phytotherapy* ("phyto" is the Greek word for plant). And that's what you get with beta-sitosterol from beluntas.

> "POWERFUL ANTIOXIDANT COMPONENTS FOUND IN BELUNTAS HELP STOP TUMORS FROM FORMING."

One randomized, double-blind, placebo-controlled, multicenter study — the gold standard in clinical trials — looked at 200 men with benign prostatic hyperplasia (BPH), or enlarged prostate, which can make you have trouble urinating. Half the group received 180 mg of beta-sitosterol daily, while the other half received placebo.

After six months, the beta-sitosterol group saw improvement in the International Prostate Symptom Score, the measurement of urine flow (QMax), and the amount of residual urine remaining in the bladder (PUR).[7]

Bali's Beluntas Deals a Double Dose of Prostate Defense

I always have faith that something works when I see the same tradition of using it spring up in unrelated places around the world.

When I visited South America, I found that traditional herbal healers use Sacha Inchi seeds to help restore urinary flow in men. Turns out, every 100 grams of Sacha Inchi seed has more than 75 mg of beta-sitosterol.[8]

In Africa, my friend Dr. Josiah Kizito showed me how they use the African potato, called *hypoxis*, to treat urinary tract infections and prostate problems like BPH. Hypoxis is full of beta-sitosterol. Hypoxis is so powerful that

it's traditionally used as a tonic in African medicine known as "muthi," which simply means "medicine."

Besides quercetin and beta-sitosterol, beluntas has two unique components, plucheiosides A and B. Researchers in India and China, almost the only places where beluntas itself is studied, have found these to be very potent antioxidants as well.

Westi told me how they use beluntas in traditional Balinese medicine to relieve and cure many illnesses.

Soothe Coughs, Nausea... and Snakebite

(Pluchea Indica)

Balinese name: Daun Beluntas

Visitors to Bali are often surprised by our varied landscape. Many people seem to think that most tropical islands are patches of low-lying jungle surrounded by white sand beaches.

But Bali is a very large island. And it lies along what most of the world calls the "Ring of Fire" – an active volcanic "ring" that encircles the Pacific Ocean. So Bali has mountains and many different habitats.

One of the most beautiful areas of Bali is in the northwest of the island, about a four hour drive from our city of Ubud. Here you will find West Bali National Park.

The park takes up almost 5% of the island, and is home to one of the world's rarest and most beautiful birds, the Bali mynah – or "Jalak Bali," as we call it.

Bali mynahs are about the same size as an American robin. But they're pure white, except for black wingtips and patches of brilliant blue skin around their eyes. On their heads, they have a long, white crest.

West Bali National Park is the last stronghold of the Bali mynah. Large parts of the park are closed to visitors to protect these beautiful birds. But you can hike through parts of the park – and even visit a Bali mynah breeding station.

One of the open areas of the park includes a thick mangrove swamp. These swamps are the "nurseries of the sea." Many creatures lay their eggs in the swamps, because the mangrove roots and other plants provide lots of places for young fish to hide from predators.

The mangrove swamps are also home to a special healing plant – daun Beluntas, or Indian fleabane, sometimes called "camphorweed." This plant grows best in low, wet places, and it grows along streams near our home in Ubud.

When someone has a bad cough in Bali, we don't run to the drug store to buy cough medicine. We walk down to the stream and pick beluntas. We then have a recipe that turns the leaves into a liquid.

When you drink it, it calms the cough quickly. And you can drink the liquid several times a day.

We also use this same liquid for bad body odor. If you have an unpleasant body odor, the same recipe will help your body to smell better. Drink a glassful every morning, and the bad odor usually fades away within a few days.

The leaves of Indian fleabane are also good for lowering a fever and easing an upset stomach. It's very effective against nausea.

— Westi

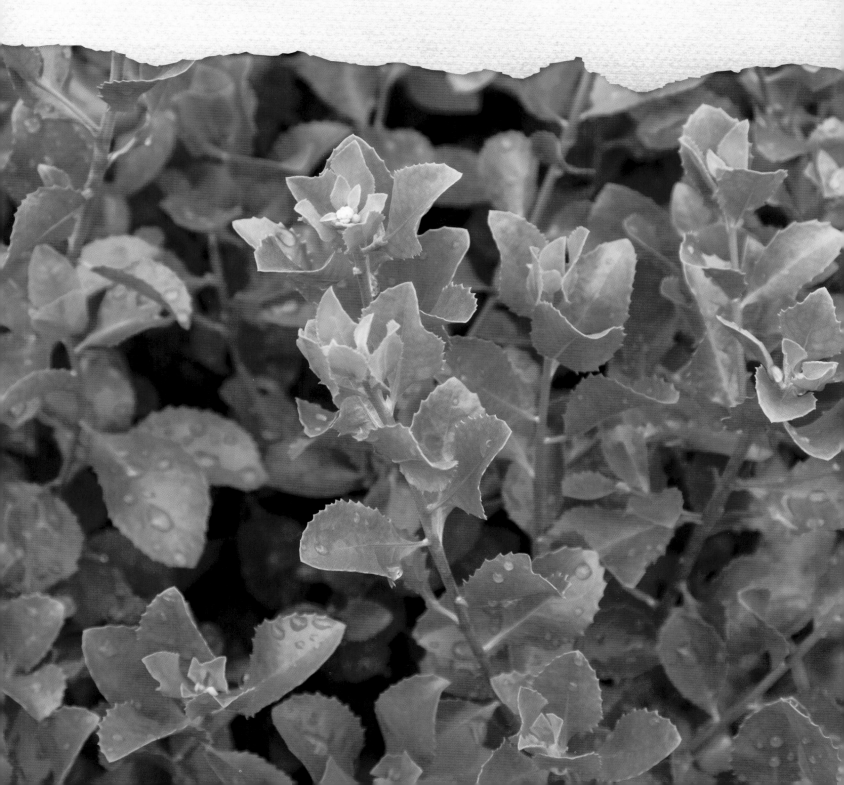

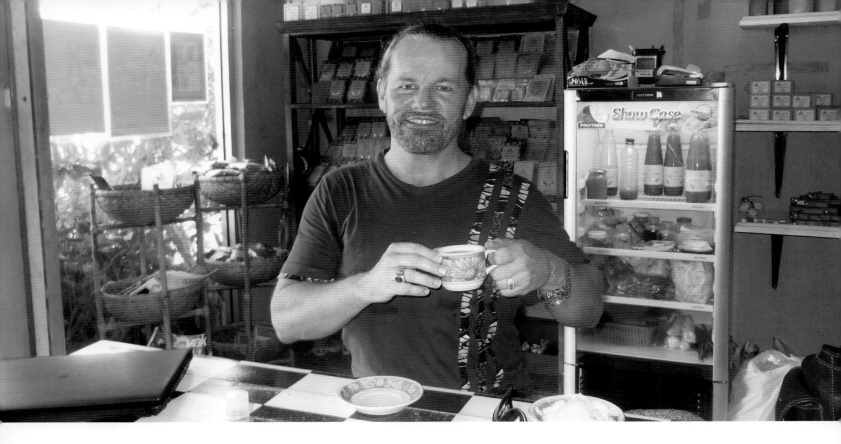

I drank my beluntas tea every morning in Westi and Lelir's shop in Ubud.

My Own Research and Discoveries

I have read several studies about Indian fleabane and stomach trouble. Studies show it eases inflammation[9] and has strong anti-ulcer activity. It appears to lower acidity while strengthening the mucous lining of the stomach.[10]

Researchers in Malaysia recently tested 78 traditional herbs for anti-tuberculosis[11] activity. They discovered that Indian fleabane is one of only six of these plants that may have a powerful effect against tuberculosis. This is important, because so many Western drugs are no longer effective against the disease.

Recent studies also back up the traditional use of beluntas as a cure for snakebites. A group at the University of Calcutta in India extracted beta-sitosterol and stigmasterol from beluntas.

They discovered these natural chemicals acted as a sort of anti-venom against bites from certain cobras and vipers.[12]

Traditional anti-venoms are hard to make (you must "milk" the venom from a live snake) and are very expensive. So this could lead to a safer, more accessible alternative.

It's rare to find beluntas in the West, and if you'd like to use it yourself, you can sometimes buy beluntas leaves (the scientific name is "pluchea indica") at Indian specialty stores online. But it's not widely available.

Where you do find it, the leaves are often dried and ready to use for tea. But it also tastes excellent raw, and the Balinese pick it fresh and use it as a raw vegetable.

I recommend growing it yourself. It grows fast in sandy soil that's wet and shady. Places like myfolia.com and davesgarden.com have information on where to buy seeds and how to grow the plant.

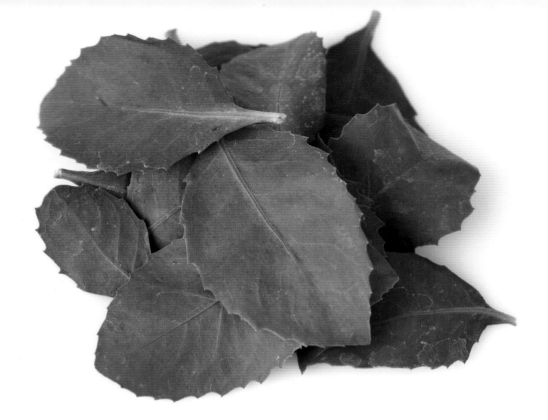

Preparations

··· *Beluntas* ···

Bali Cough Relief

Gather a small handful of beluntas leaves and wash them thoroughly.

Place the leaves in a bowl with one or two cups of cool, clean water and gently mash by hand.

Add a little salt and tamarind for flavor and strain the liquid into a glass.

··

Beluntas Body Odor Cure

It's very simple. All you have to do is rinse 10g of fresh beluntas leaves and boil them in just enough water to cover the leaves.

Then allow to cool, strain out the water into your teacup and enjoy!

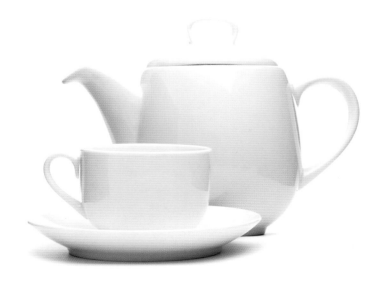

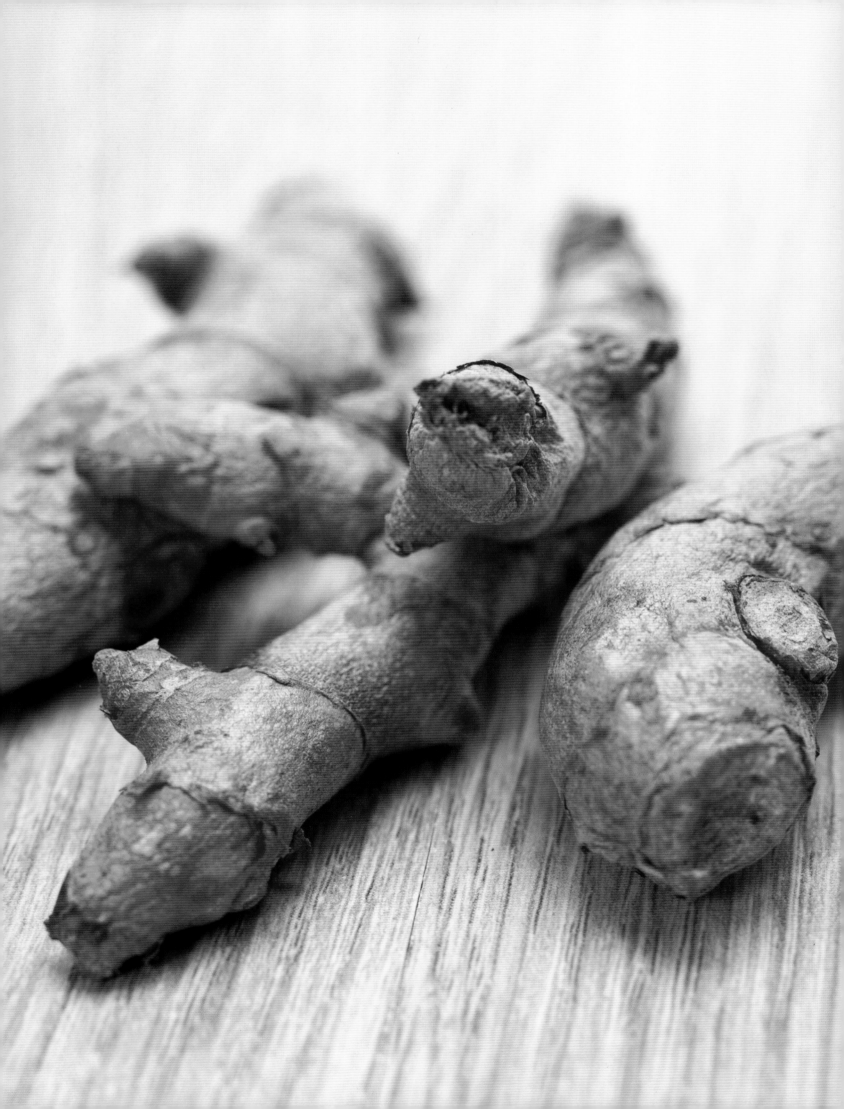

BALI'S MOST IMPRESSIVE TONIC ROOT

Westi walked under the soursop tree and past the lemon basil, and dug up the root of a tall plant with his knife. "This is white turmeric."

Instead of the orange color that I was used to seeing with turmeric I encountered in Peru, this was a curiously yellowish white.

"What do you use that for?"

"It's antibiotic." He looked to his right, cleared some grass and dug up another root. "Different type of turmeric. This is for the liver."

An even taller plant was next. Westi hauled it up to show me. The root grew in a huge bulb. "One root is half a kilo of turmeric," Westi said.

Past the aloe and the tapioca, he pulled up another kind of turmeric. "This is curcumin pandurata." He shook the dirt off and broke one open. Lelir said, "It's more fragrant. We use it for anti-aging."

"Anti-aging? I'd be very interested to use that in my new center. How are you using it? Do you make it into a powder and put it in a capsule?"

"A facial scrub," Lelir said. "But I also make it into a powder and add it to sugar cane juice. I'll show you in the shop. It's anti-aging, but sweet."

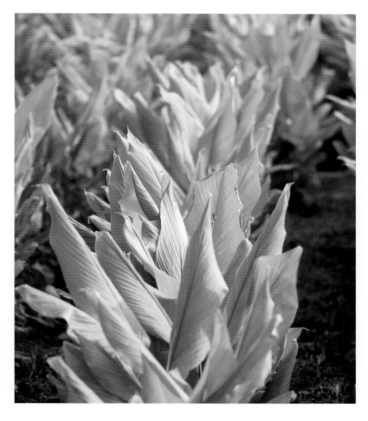

Westi's turmeric plantation in his garden near Ubud was so large, I couldn't see where it ended.

"You grow a lot of this kind of turmeric. Look at that field!" I couldn't see the end of it even with the zoom in my video camera. They must have had half a mile of turmeric growing...

When we got back to Lelir's shop in Ubud, she gave me a "Jamu" class. Jamu is the daily herbal tonic used by many Balinese.

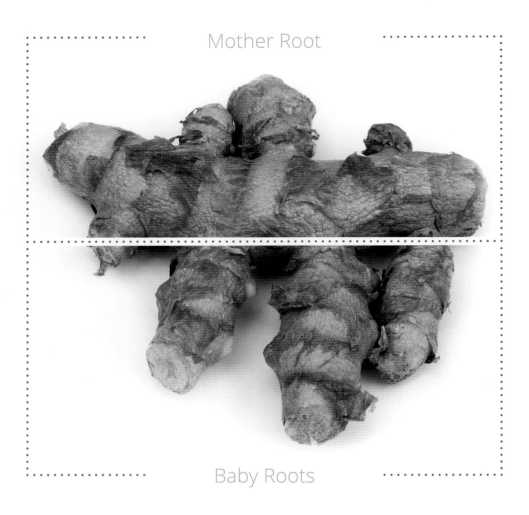

Mother Root

Baby Roots

She pulled out another kind of turmeric called *curcuma longa.*

"We don't like to go to doctors. We don't need chemicals. For everyone in the fields, we still use herbal medicine. We use the herbs surrounding us. Like for immune health, we use turmeric.

"This big part is the 'mother' root, and these are the 'babies.' We use the mother for medicine and the babies for cooking. Why? Because they taste different. And the medicinal properties of the baby roots are less.

"Also, after so long, if we use the mother root for cooking, it will taste like medicine to us!"

Westi has at least six different kinds of turmeric growing in his garden. It's the single root that they're most impressed with. And it's a whole science. They know exactly how

old the root is supposed to be and what to mix it with... and it's central to a lot of the things they do.

"TURMERIC AND ITS MAJOR COMPOUND, CURCUMIN, ARE WELL KNOWN ANTI-INFLAMMATORIES."

Turmeric and its major compound, curcumin, are well known anti-inflammatories. The journal *Family Practice* did a study on turmeric and the researchers wrote simply: "Does turmeric relieve inflammatory conditions? Yes."[1]

It has a combination of curcuminoids, volatile oils and proteins that give it its powerful anticancer properties, and it's being looked at as a treatment for other inflammatory conditions, like asthma, arthritis and high LDL cholesterol.

The Anti-Alzheimer's Spice

(Curcuma longa)

Balinese name: Kunyit

When I was a boy, most of my family's friends were farmers — just like us. We didn't think of ourselves as poor, but none of our families earned much more than we needed to make end meet.

With friends and family around us, we were happy. We grew plenty of rice, vegetables and spices... and, of course, we lived on the most beautiful island in the world. All of Nature was our playground.

Nature was also our pharmacy. When we cut ourselves while playing, or fell and scraped ourselves up, my parents knew just what to do. They headed straight to the kitchen for a common spice. We call this spice "kunyit," but you probably know it as Indian saffron or turmeric.

When we had a cut or scrape, our mothers would wash it off. Then they'd grate some fresh turmeric root and apply it to the cut. The turmeric acted as a natural antiseptic and helped the cut heal faster.

In Bali, turmeric is well known for its healing properties. You can even buy it in local stores as an ingredient in topical medications. We still use turmeric this same way. And modern studies show Bali's herbal healers made a good choice. Studies from India and the University of North Carolina show that curcumin — an active ingredient in turmeric — is antibacterial[2] and promotes wound healing.[3]

These properties also show the wisdom of another Balinese tradition. For generations, the "mangkus" — priests and priestesses — here would have newborn babies washed in warm water infused with grated turmeric root. They said this would "seal the baby's skin."

These spiritual leaders may not have understood the science. But they were right. This tradition was tremendously effective, because it helped protect the baby from bacteria and fungi.

Lelir and I also make an effective compress for earache using turmeric. We grate some fresh turmeric root and mix it with coconut oil. Then we wrap the mixture in a banana leaf and toast it in a fire. Holding the warm compress against your ear is very soothing. And within a few days, the earache should be gone. Of course, bananas don't grow in most of the United States. So this may not be a convenient use for you. But you can put turmeric's healing powers to work in other ways.

— *Westi*

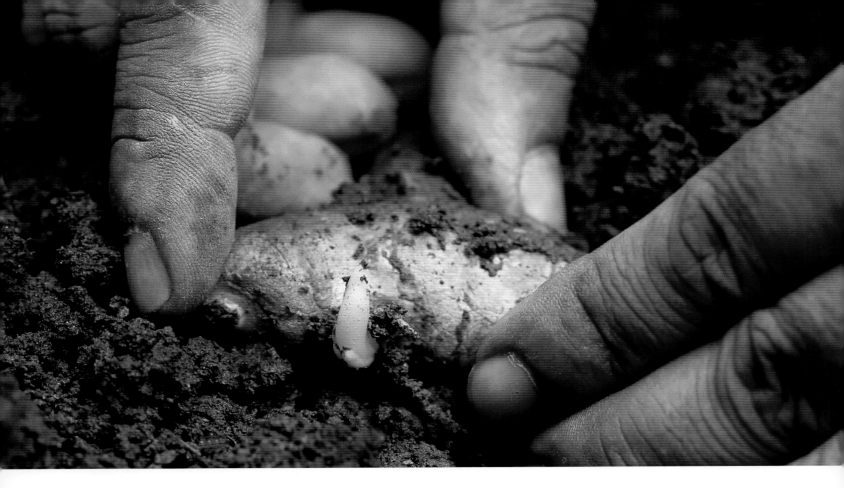

The Balinese have a tradition of growing turmeric, and they know exactly when to harvest the carrot-like roots at the right stage of growth. Even this young one I dug up had a very pleasant aroma. The leaves are also aromatic, and used to make "dragonfly" soup.

My Own Research and Discoveries

Turmeric is an excellent example of how different cultures can come to use the same plants for the same purposes, independent of one another. Something I look for in my travels...

As the world becomes more connected, this process is rapidly being replaced by a process of sharing and copying success. And because 80% of the world still uses herbs for healing, when word gets around that a plant is valuable as a healing agent, I start seeing it in more places.

Turmeric is one of the main spices in curries. In fact, in India, where curries are eaten regularly, there is an extremely low incidence of Alzheimer's — thanks to the use of turmeric.

Turmeric has remarkable properties. It looks like a stubby, ugly carrot wrapped in a brownish wrapper. When you cut it open, the flesh of the root is a bright orange. It's aromatic and so are the leaves.

A local tradition in Bali is to use the leaves to make dragonfly soup. In Uganda, Africa, they grind the dried root into a fine powder for their tonics, and it fights inflammation everywhere in your body.[4]

One of the reasons turmeric is so good at fighting inflammation is that its major constituent, curcumin, suppresses two of the major causes of inflammatory activity in your body.

In one study from India, one of the few places in the world where they have intensely studied turmeric, they found that people who took 1200 mg a day had less joint swelling, less joint stiffness and could walk much better than those who consumed no turmeric.[5]

An animal study I read from the University of South Carolina looked at the effects of turmeric's major component, curcumin, on athletic performance.

They divided male mice into four groups and had them run. The placebo mice got very tired very quickly running downhill. But the curcumin-fed mice had improved performance. Curcumin also offset inflammation created by the downhill running.[6]

I also discovered that turmeric may suppress the growth of fat cells. When I got back to the States, I found supporting evidence from a Tufts University study.

Researchers at the Jean Mayer USDA Human Nutrition Research Center on Aging at Tufts University discovered that curcumin prevented the growth of fat cells in mice.[7]

That means turmeric soothes your joints, gives you better muscle function and even helps you lose weight.

According to various studies, turmeric — or the curcumin it contains — may be effective against a host of problems...

Arthritis	Inflammatory bowel disease[8]	Prostate cancer[9]	Nerve damage[10]	Skin conditions[11]

But the biggest benefit this little root may deliver to us is...

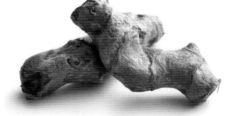

Turmeric's Mighty Brain-Bolstering Abilities
— Even against Parkinson's, Alzheimer's and Brain Tumors

Turmeric has a unique ability to reduce the inflammation common to all of these diseases, where free radicals do damage to the fats, genetic material and proteins that make up the brain.[12]

In an animal study, researchers were able to use turmeric to reduce the beta-amyloid plaque that builds up on the brain by 40%. The turmeric also reduced buildup of a harmful protein by 80%.[13] That means curcumin could help you keep your memory longer.

How does it work so well?

A team of biotech researchers at Sastra University in India discovered that the curcuminoids in turmeric help break apart the plaque that disrupts the brains of Alzheimer's patients.[14]

And in a study on mice, researchers discovered that turmeric can also clear away the enzymes that help make up the plaque in the first place.[15]

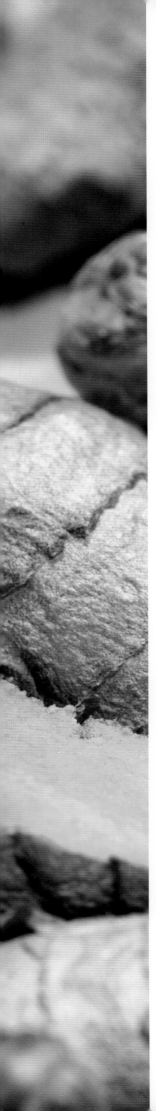

Preparations

Adding curried foods to your diet may help boost the health of your skin, joints, nerves... and help protect your memory.

If you're not fond of spicy curries, you can get some of turmeric's benefits by eating an American favorite: mustard.

Turmeric is used to color most yellow mustards. So using bright yellow mustard to flavor your foods can give you some of turmeric's benefit, too.

You can also buy the root in conventional ground form or whole. I prefer to get whole turmeric root because it's delicious in soups and stir fry. If you're going to buy it ground, make sure it's all turmeric and not just some of the root ground up with curry.

One of the easiest things you can do is cook with turmeric. I mix up different combinations of turmeric, ginger, cinnamon, paprika, cumin and garlic and use it as a dry rub for lamb and chicken. You can also throw a teaspoon of turmeric into your pan when you're sautéing vegetables to give them a little kick.

Turmeric is also available as a supplement. Studies use up to 3 grams of extracted root daily. But there are some who believe that turmeric supplements aren't as effective because they either aren't absorbed very well or pass through your system too quickly.

Look for either a curcumin supplement that contains piperine, a black pepper extract that increases the absorbency of other compounds, or the optimized form of turmeric that is more absorbable. I recommend you get about a gram of turmeric's major compound, curcumin, each day to get the most benefit.

Remember that the curcumin is the main beneficial component of turmeric root, so look for at least 90% or greater curcuminoids, whichever formula you use.

"Jamu" tonic with turmeric

Lelir was nice enough to give me a Jamu class to teach me how to make her daily "internal medicine." Here's what she taught me:

Turmeric

Start with two pieces of turmeric root (about 50 grams), one bulb of alpinia galangal root (from the ginger family), 30 grams of fresh, raw tamarind pulp, 50 grams of raw palm sugar (you can substitute cane juice) and a teaspoon of salt.

- Peel the turmeric root and cut it up into small pieces.

- Take the skin off of one bulb of galangal root and cut into small pieces.

- Add the roots together with about two cups of water in a blender or chopper of your choice and blend for about a minute and a half.

- Pour the mixture into a 5-quart saucepan.

- Add the palm sugar, tamarind, a teaspoon of salt and mix with a spoon.

- Put the saucepan on high heat and boil for 15 minutes.

- Stir again and strain into a glass container. Cool and drink.

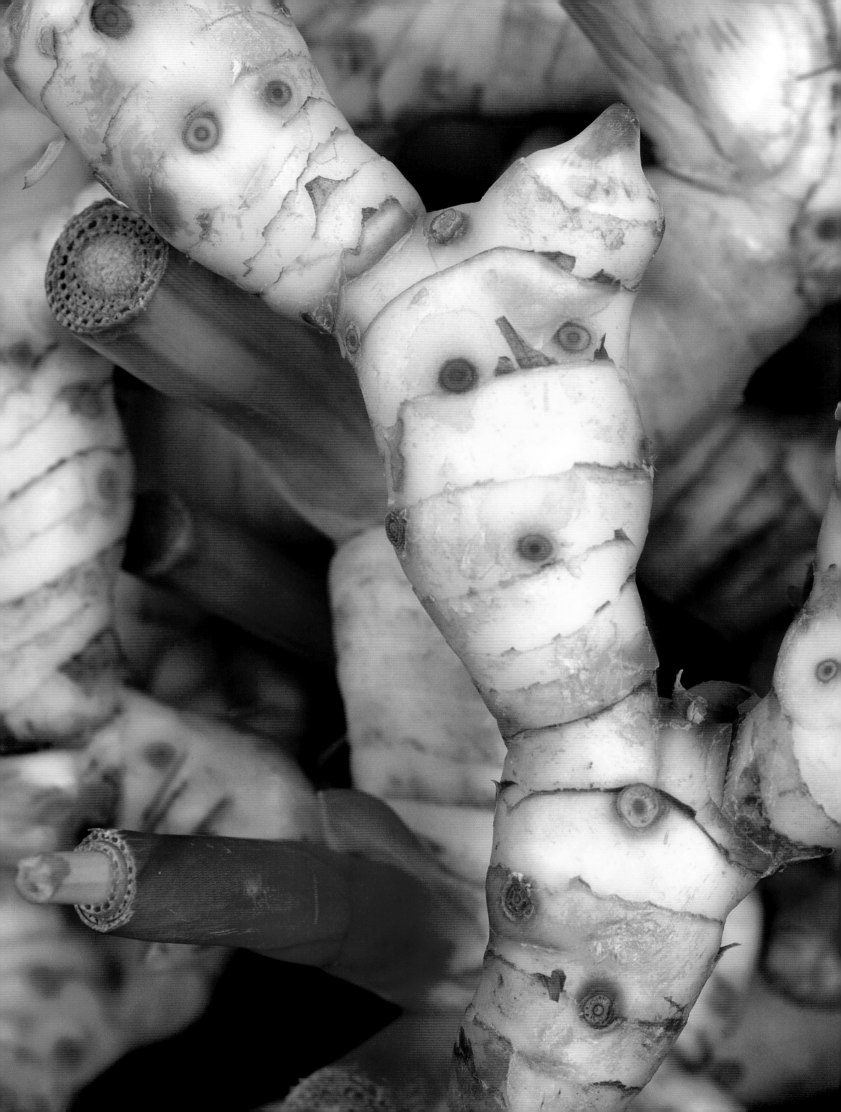

BALI'S "BIG" ROOT IS A MINIATURE DRUG STORE

Dinnertime... sunsets are beautiful and peaceful in Bali.

As I looked out the window of Westi and Lelir's home, I had the thought that being away from the fast-paced American life made it all the more serene.

Lelir came over to the dinner table and placed our plates in front of us. The vegetables smelled delicious and I was happy because they were sprinkled with a *basa gede*, the Balinese sauce that's spicy and delicious.

One of the main ingredients in basa gede is a root called "greater galangal."

In Bali, they use galangal to boost the immune system, treat flu and colds, and reduce fever. But the components also have anticancer, antibacterial, anti-inflammatory and antiviral qualities.[1, 2]

That's quite a healing combination. And galangal turns out to be like a whole drugstore in one incredible plant.

Galangal root is very aromatic. You can make an essential oil from the root. It's called "essence d'Amali." In India and China, this

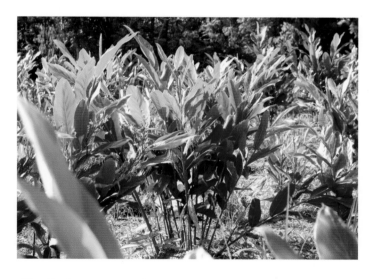

The Balinese use galangal root as an expectorant, and it improves breathing and lung problems. It's very fragrant, and also spicy, so they use it in a lot of their cooking.

essential oil has many uses, especially for treating children's respiratory problems.

Essence d'Amali is also an effective natural insecticide. Scientists at Kasetsart University, in Thailand, proved it's even effective against oriental fruit flies.[3] These little flies cause a lot of damage to fruit crops... and I've read they've spread into the U.S.

Other research shows greater galangal effectively kills many dangerous bacteria — including E. coli, salmonella, staph and strep.[4]

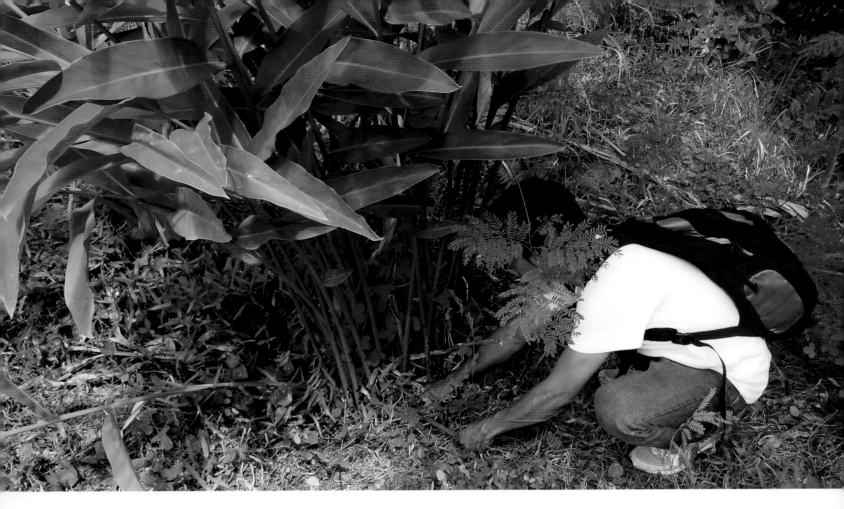

*Westi and his family use greater galangal root as a spice in their meals
and also for inflammatory and other medical conditions.*

More Uses for Galangal are Surfacing Every Day

In the last few years, scientists have found brand new uses for greater galangal.

Researchers working in Malaysia discovered that galangal kills the malaria parasite in mice.[5] Another animal study in China recently proved that greater galangal also acts as a pain reliever.[6]

Perhaps most exciting of all, greater galangal may hold one key to stopping Alzheimer's disease.

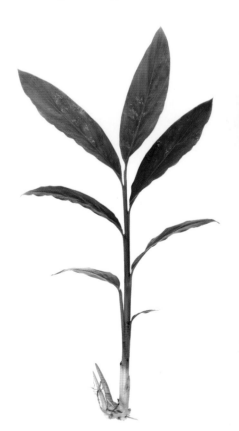

Indian scientists caused Alzheimer's-type amnesia in mice. Treating mice with an extract from greater galangal greatly reduced the effect. The treated mice had lower levels of free radicals and they showed better performance in remembering their way through a maze.[7]

Perhaps this is another reason why Alzheimer's disease has never been very common in Bali. They use a lot of greater galangal in their food and herbal medicine.

Westi told me a story about what he did for his mother...

Warming the Bone

(Alpinia (Lengkuas) galanga)

Balinese name: Isen

Did you ever notice how when we get older, it becomes harder to stay warm? Temperatures that feel comfortable to you are just too chilly for your parents or grandparents.

That even happens here in tropical Bali. When my mother reached her 60s, she began to wake up feeling chilled every morning.

Greater galangal — what we call "Isen" — has warming properties. So Lelir and I gave my mother a cup of galangal tea in the morning. Since she began drinking this tea, she feels much better every day.

Of course, a cup of hot tea will help you feel warm. But the galangal tea gradually warms the body over a few weeks so that you no longer wake up feeling so chilled.

Many herbs work this way. Their gradual effect can help you prevent or gently recover from all sorts of sickness.

Greater galangal does this both inside and outside. We use the root in our "boreh" — a Balinese body scrub.

Bali is home to thousands of rice farmers. These farmers work in hot, wet paddies. These conditions are perfect for growing fungus. Even on people's skin.

Galangal has an antifungal action. So it helps kill the fungus that might otherwise take hold on the farmers' skin. So the boreh is doing more than warming and relaxing the farmers' tired muscles. It's also helping keep their skin healthy.

Some galangal root is red and some is white. The red root helps clear out congestion when you have a dry cough.

Greater galangal has lovely white blossoms with pink veins. These flowers — along with the plant's young shoots — are often eaten as a vegetable.

— *Westi*

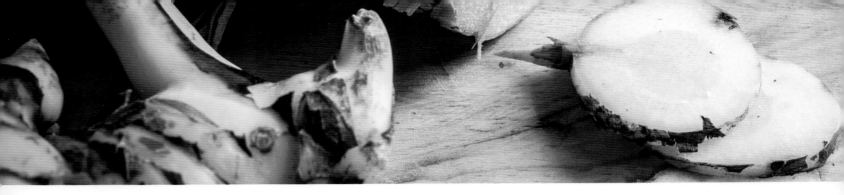

Galangal root is related to ginger... and it has multiple ancient medicinal uses — from treating deafness to heart disease to indigestion.

My Own Research and Discoveries

Galangal is one of the most ancient remedies in the world. The history books will tell you that it was called "the spice of life" by one of the most famous early herbalists, St. Hildegard of Bingen. She used it to treat everything from deafness to heart disease to indigestion.

Of course, neither she nor the ancient Balinese healers — Balians — knew why galangal worked, but modern science gives us a clue.

The root is an excellent source of iron, vitamins A and C, and it has a lot of flavonoids and phytonutrients that act as antioxidant protectors.

For example, it has beta-sitosterol, a natural prostate protector that's not on modern medicine's radar at all.

What makes it so potent? For one, it helps protect your prostate gland's cell membranes,[8] allowing your prostate continue to function normally. Phytonutrients are also potent antioxidants. They can reduce inflammation and improve blood flow. So beta-sitosterol improves the health of your prostate and urinary tract.

In one review of many clinical trials, beta-sitosterol helped men with benign prostatic hyperplasia improve urinary flow and volume *in every study.*[9] It also has quercetin, which protects against lung, skin and prostate cancers.

Two More Cancer Fighters in "Nature's Drug Store"

Galangal also has two unique components that are very potent cancer cures. The first is galangin. In one study, galangin killed off human colon cancer cells.

Emodin is another component of galangal. In clinical trials, it was shown to suppress tumors and improves immunity. Aloe and kiwi fruit also have emodin.

Numerous studies also show that galangal kills off strep bacteria, and even helps cure tuberculosis. Although Western medicine doesn't believe in using natural cures, scientists from other countries do. I found a study carried out by a team at Thammasat University in Thailand, which found that galangal can be used to help treat different kinds of throat cancer. So the ancients were right: galangal is very effective for the throat and lungs.

Here is What I Recommend

Asian specialty stores around the world offer fresh galangal root. Fresh galangal will keep in your refrigerator for three or four days, but after that it starts to break down. That's why I recommend the dried root.

Galangal is also available as an immune-boosting supplement. You can get capsules and the root powder, and you can often find it in tinctures mixed with ginger.

.... *Galangal* ....

For Sore Throat: Cut a small piece of the root and chew.

For a Cough: Take 20 grams of grated red galangal root (about ¾-ounce) and squeeze out the juice. Mix it with one teaspoon of honey and drink. This makes a great expectorant. On Bali, Lelir uses this simple recipe for children all the time.

For Headache and Fever: Grind an equal amount of sugar and rootstock together. Pour 3 grams in hot milk and drink before going to bed.

For Nausea: Cut a piece of root and dip in castor oil and then roast it over a flame. Turn it into powder and eat 3 grams with honey daily.

The white galangal root is used in cooking. It's especially popular in Thailand.

The root — called "laos" — gives Thai soups their distinctive flavor.

Fish Dishes: Crush the dried root and use it as a spice, or cut up the dried root and add it to fish. It tastes great and will help reduce any "fishy" taste.

Galangal Vodka: Take chunks of galangal root and put in vodka. Let it sit for two months.

Balinese Galangal Tea: The tea is very easy to make.

- Grate a small piece of greater galangal root and a small piece of red ginger root.

- Place the grated roots in the bottom of a cup and fill the cup with boiling water.

- Let the tea steep until it's cool enough to drink.

- Strain out the root, add honey to taste and enjoy!

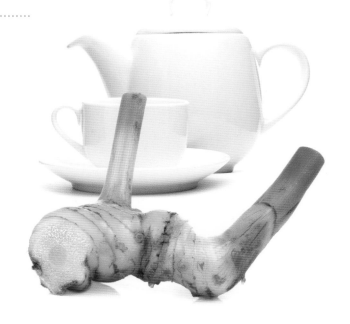

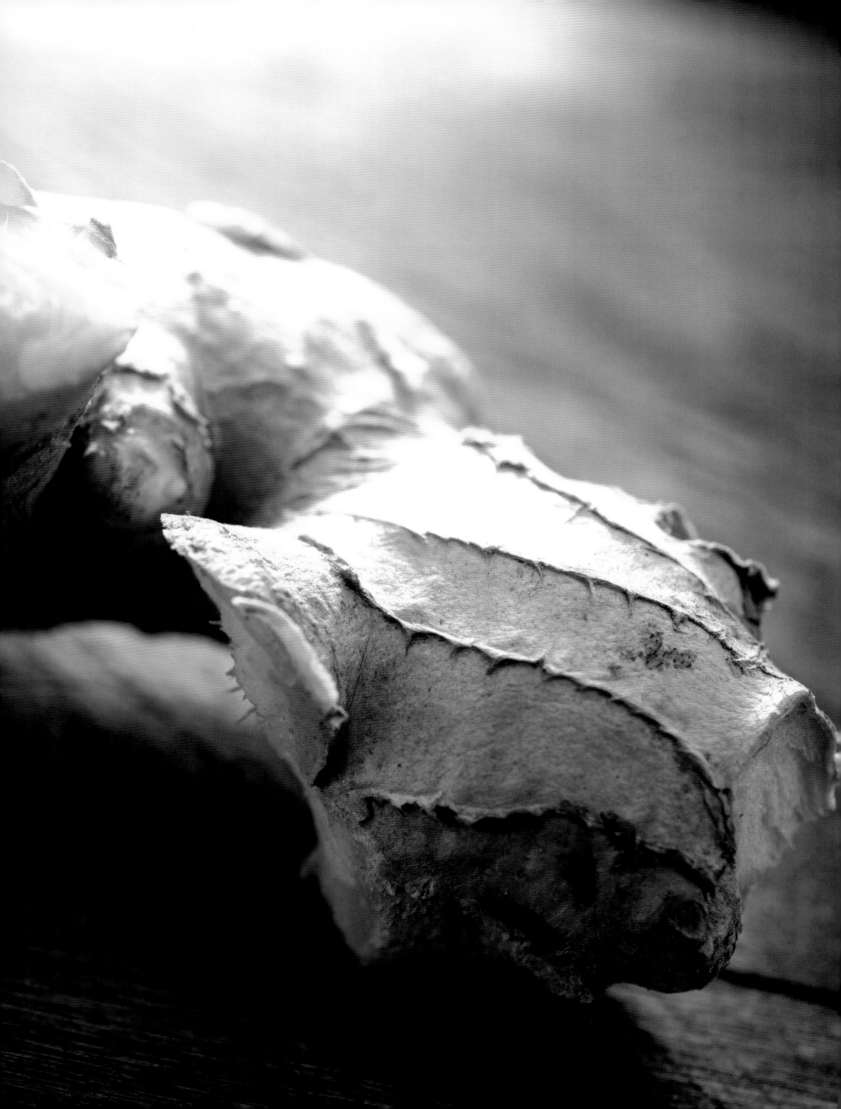

NATURE'S BEST TOOL FOR CURING PAIN, STOMACH ACHE, HEADACHE, MORNING SICKNESS, HEARTBURN, VIRUSES...

"Can you introduce yourself? Tell us who you are?"

The camera was rolling and I quickly set it down on the counter in front of her.

"Can you stop for one moment please? I'm sorry!" She looked straight into the camera and doubled over from shy, anxious laughter.

"Does the camera make you nervous?" I pushed the little red stop button.

"Yes!" She covered her smiling face with the Jamu class schedule in her left hand. Now we both busted out laughing.

It's no wonder she was nervous. She had just met me not 10 minutes ago, and here I was putting her on film.

"Let me start the recording over. Go ahead when you're ready."

"Hello, good afternoon. My name is Lelir. In today's Jamu class I will show you how to make 'daily medicine.' Jamu is very important for our life in Bali..."

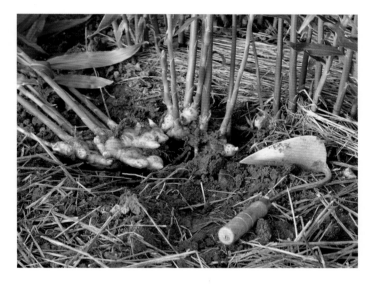

Ginger root has medicinal value and immense health benefits.

Lelir, a fifth generation Balian healer, is only about four and a half feet tall, and a bundle of sweetness and energy.

She was taught by her mother and grandmother. We'll be working with her to develop some formulas you can't get anywhere else, so that we can regain and preserve some of the wisdom of the Balinese healers that's unknown in the West.

In fact, when I visited her in her workshop, she gave me a 50-minute presentation on how to make your own formulas. She was so excited to have me there that she started right in with almost no introduction, and I almost forgot to turn my video camera on.

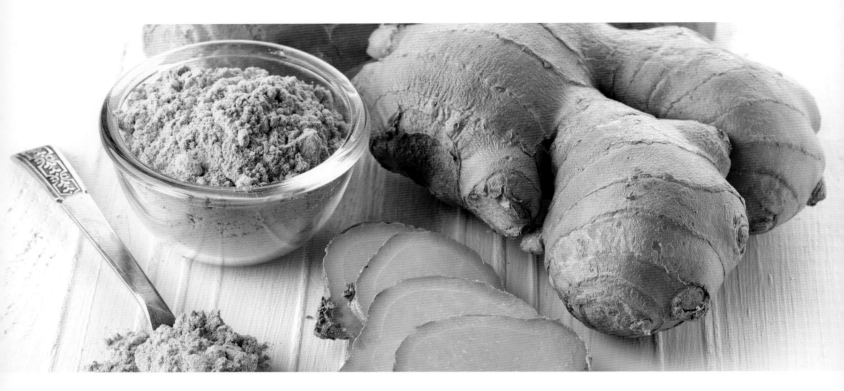

Wisdom from a Jamu Expert

Lelir used herbs that she grows in her garden. But she talks about substitutions you can use if you don't have access to the same herbs and other ingredients she uses. Some of the herbs are available now in the U.S. and Europe, like turmeric and coconut oil.

Lelir and Westi buy everything else from local farmers, and try to help the farmers by coming up with ways to use their products. Lelir buys from cocoa farmers and makes a lot of cocoa butter and powder. Restaurants buy the powder from her, and she sells the cocoa butter as a base for white chocolate and cosmetics. She gets cinnamon from farmers, too, and makes cinnamon powder, which she sells to bakeries.

At her workshop, she makes many different kinds of teas. She also makes a daily tonic — kind of a detoxifying, immune strengthening tonic that you drink every day, which contains ginger and turmeric. She makes them from scratch. She puts the herbs in a stone pestle and grinds them up, boils them down, and makes the tonic. It was very nice. I had it every day I stayed with them.

The exfoliating body scrub she makes has rice and a whole bunch of herbs in it. It felt fantastic just rubbing it on my hands. She makes an anti-aging facial cream and clay masks made from volcanic clay. And she makes moisturizing oil they call "Sweet Dream." It's coconut oil-based and takes an entire month to brew. She makes Ayurvedic oil that takes six weeks for the base to distill.

Feeding and Healing Bodies with the Same Plants

Lelir makes everything by pressing fresh ingredients. Sweet Dream has pressed vanilla, cinnamon and cocoa butter, all of which are very good for dry skin. You can even eat Sweet Dream. She told me you can put it on bread and cookies, and it's part of traditional Balinese pancake batter.

For her lip balm, she uses Balinese bitter orange leaves and she infuses them with coconut oil.

All her formulas are part of the Indonesian tradition of "Jamu," which means "herbal healing" in Javanese. Lelir told me that Jamu is very important for life in Bali, because they treat illnesses mostly with herbal medicine. Most Balinese don't go to Western-style doctors because they don't want to take chemical medicines. There is only one hospital near Ubud.

To help prevent infection, soothe muscles, and help people who have respiratory problems, she makes what she calls "internal medicine" — a kind of juice made with roots and herbs — for a daily tonic.

One of the roots I saw Lelir use the most is ginger. She puts it in her Jamu tonics, and she uses it in her scrubs and anti-aging formulas, too. She told me they use ginger for almost everything in Bali.

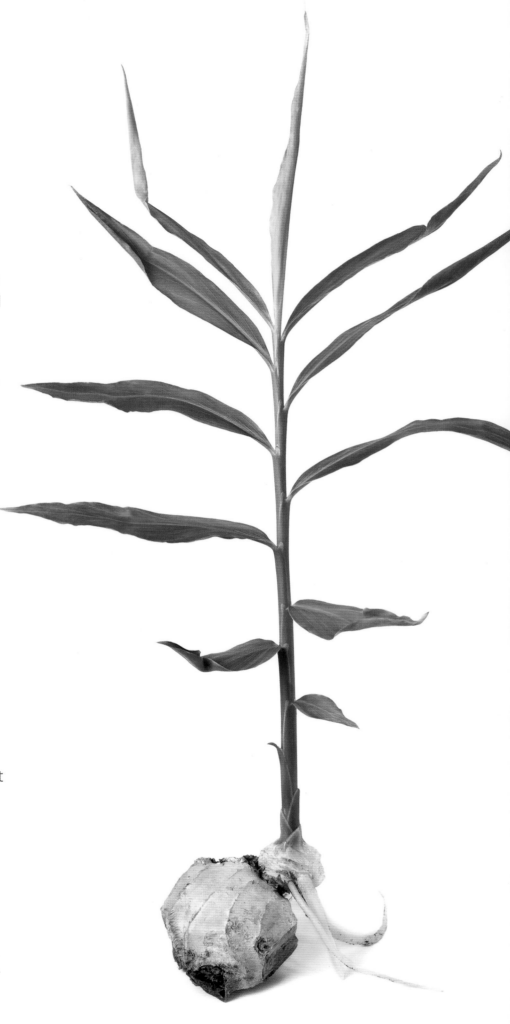

Our Amazing Cure-all

(Zingiber officinale)

Balinese name: Jahe

Westi and I have a little shop on a busy street in Ubud. The front opens out right onto the street and people wander in and out all day. Motorbikes and mini-trucks zoom by. Conversations and the scent of food cooking in nearby shops drift in all day.

Locals drop in looking for a particular remedy or favorite incense. Tourists are fascinated with our natural cosmetics, candles and other items they can bring home to family and friends.

I love chatting with our customers, so I'll often bring work out to the front where I can answer questions, but still keep working.

You can often find me working with a tool that may be quite familiar.

Here in Bali, we call it a "lesung." But you probably know it as a mortar and pestle.

I use my lesung often. In fact, we have several here in the shop. We work with so many herbs and seeds... and we spend a lot of time crushing them for our recipes.

One herb that keeps our mortars and pestles busy is jahe – what you call ginger.

Ginger grows throughout Bali. You'll find it growing in almost every garden. And it's common in the jungle, too. It may be the most-used herb in all of Indonesia.

There must be hundreds of recipes using ginger in Indonesia alone. You could eat ginger with practically every meal for months and never have the same dish twice.

Ginger is certainly delicious. But we don't use it just for its flavor. Ginger is one of Nature's great cure-alls. It provides relief for so many health issues...

We use ginger to help people with diabetes lower their blood sugar. And ginger relieves people's soreness and pain, and arthritis. Ginger root relieves heartburn very quickly, too.

And here in Bali, we use ginger not only on the inside, but on the outside. You can try it yourself.

The next time you have an ache in the front of your head, mash some peeled ginger root into a paste and apply it to your forehead. We find it eases most headaches in just a few minutes.

— *Lelir*

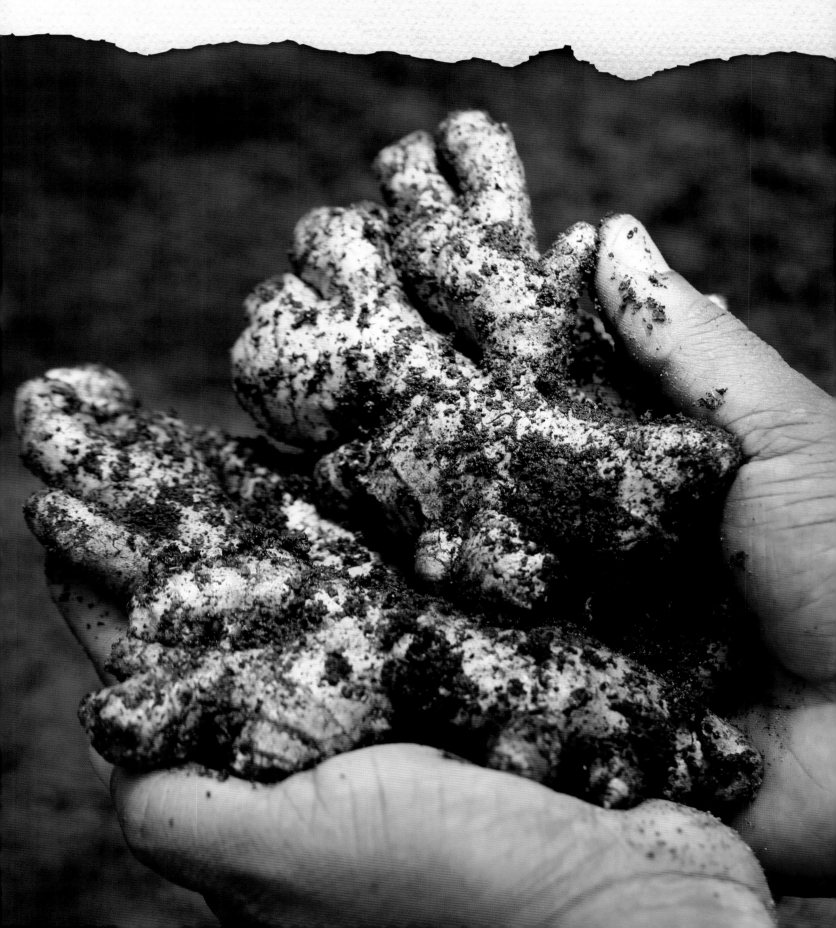

My Own Research and Discoveries

Traditional Eastern herbalists often suggest one multi-purpose herb for several different problems. But Western medicine seems stuck on "one problem, one solution." Chances are, if you visit a clinic with six different complaints, you'll wind up taking six different pills.

That's never struck me as the best way to approach overall health. Like traditional herbalists, I prefer natural remedies that support multiple health goals.

That's why ginger is one of my favorites. Lelir and Balinese herbalists call it their "cure all" and I call it "Nature's multi-tool."

First of all, ginger lowers triglycerides, one of the main indicators of heart-related disorders, like type 2 diabetes.[12] And here's another way that ginger boosts heart health...

Taking a little ginger every day can give your heart a real antioxidant boost. That's because ginger contains 12 antioxidant compounds more powerful than vitamin E.[1]

Plus, studies show that ginger lowers inflammation.[2] Ginger has many anti-inflammatory compounds. Some block inflammatory COX-2. Some lower pain-receptor and nerve-ending sensitivity. In one trial, over 75% had relief from pain and swelling after taking ginger.[3]

A study in the *Journal of Alternative and Complementary Medicine* looked at ginger along with traditional pain medications. They found that ginger can reduce pain in the muscles and joints by as much as 25%.[4]

You may have heard about ginger for "morning sickness," but did you know it also

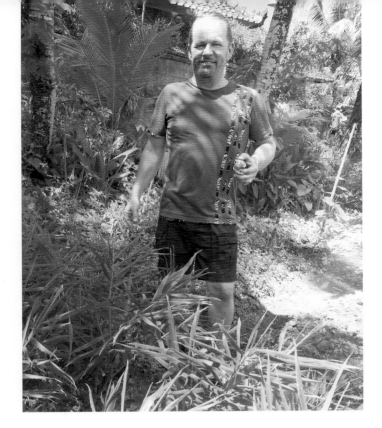

Like traditional herbalists, I prefer natural remedies that support multiple health goals — that's why ginger root is one of my favorites.

helps settle many other types of queasiness[5] − Like stomach upset from motion. A German team echoed this finding, calling ginger's effectiveness "proved beyond doubt."[6] I agree, and I like to keep it handy when I travel... just in case.

Ginger can get your digestion moving, too. When researchers tested it with a group of healthy volunteers, their stomach contractions increased... and food moved through more quickly.[7]

And here's another good reason to keep ginger on hand...

In one study, a group of 50 female nursing school students suffering serious "monthly discomfort" tried ginger for relief. Researchers compared this group to two similar groups using more conventional approaches. They found discomfort levels dropped equally in all three groups.[8]

Here is What I Recommend

Ginger

Here are some ways to get your daily doses:

- **Stir fry food with it:** It'll add an invigorating taste to any meat and vegetable dish. Sprinkle some grated ginger on top for even more great flavor.

- **Supplement:** Most pharmacies or health food stores sell ginger powder in pills or capsules. Look for an extract with 5% gingerols.

  I like to take my ginger supplement in liquid form.

You can also:

- **Use a ginger compress on painful areas:** It'll stimulate blood flow and ease achy joints.

- **Use it to relieve heartburn:** Add one-half teaspoon of freshly grated ginger root to a cup of hot water. Let the ginger steep for 10 minutes. Strain the ginger and drink.

- **Soothe a stomach ache:** Drink ginger tea, or ginger ale (made with real ginger), to sooth an upset stomach.

- **Antiviral:** Ginger is also an antiviral and can help you recover from viral infections.

Lelir makes a simple tea from ginger that's helpful for your stomach and to cure a headache. It's refreshing and easy to prepare.

- For each serving, peel about 1 inch of fresh ginger root.
- Crush the peeled root with a mortar and pestle.
- Place the crushed root in a cup and add 8 oz of hot water.
- Steep until cool enough to drink, then strain off the liquid.
- Drink hot or cold, adding honey to taste.

Here's a ginger tea recipe I use:

- Boil 4 cups of water in a saucepan.
- Peel a 2-inch piece of fresh ginger root and slice it into thin slices.
- Add the ginger to the boiling water.
- Cover it, reduce the heat, and let it simmer for 15-20 minutes.
- Strain the tea. Add honey and lemon.

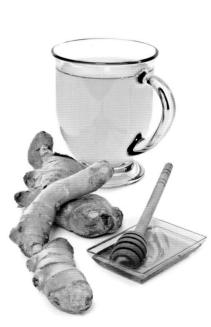

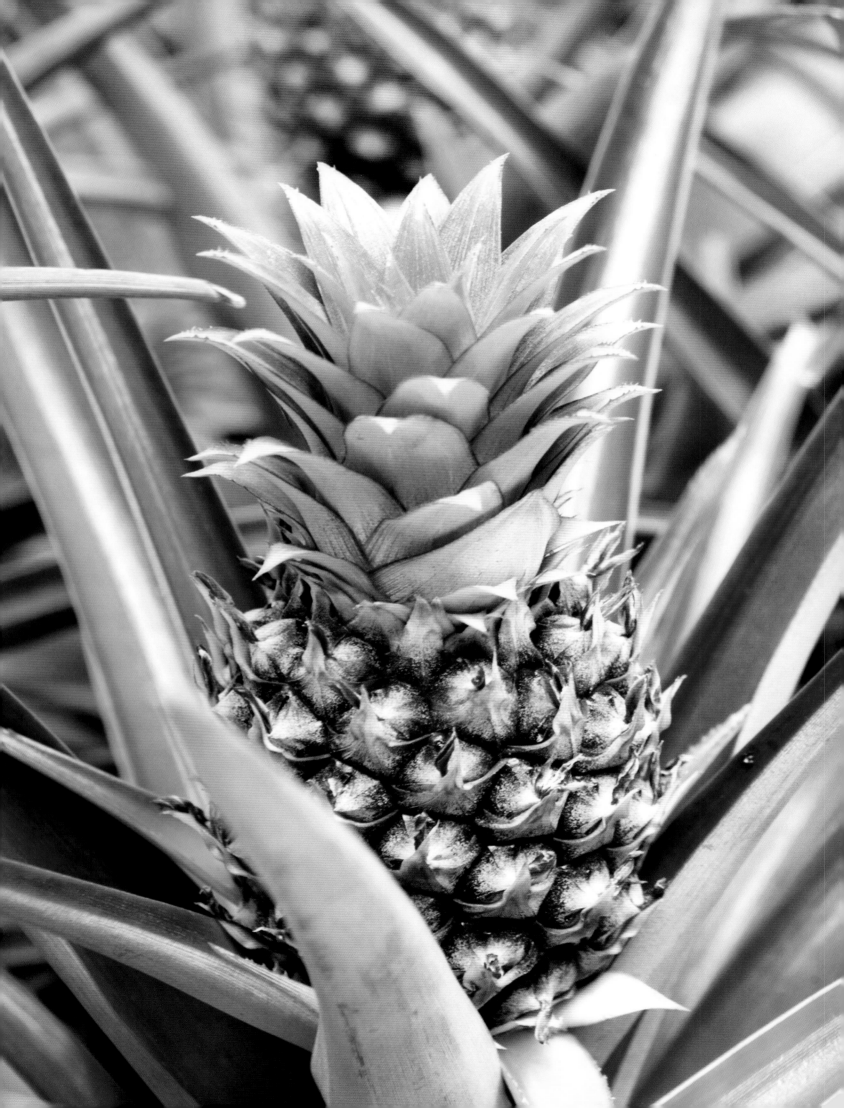

WILD FRUIT IS A DELICIOUS STOMACH AND JOINT PAIN CURE

"Did I tell you Westi gave me a Bali knife?"

My friend C.S. knew I'd just come home from hacking my way through the jungles of Bali. She said, "What is that? Like, some kind of a machete?"

"It's called a Bali knife. It's cooler than a machete. It's like half-knife, half-hatchet. It's got a big thick blade and a heavy handle to balance it out."

"How'd you get that home?" She kind of chuckled at me.

"I just put it in my suitcase and checked it on the plane."

Now that I think about it, I'm sure glad I didn't put it in my carry-on and forget it was in there. They'd probably still have me detained in Bali.

But I made it home just fine and now I have my Bali knife. I love to use it on coconuts, but there's another fruit I grow that it comes in handy for too — pineapples.

I'm now eating more pineapples, because I can cut them up so easily with my Bali knife. And that's a good thing. Eating pineapples helps with digestion, boosts immunity, lowers inflammation and relieves pain.

I had always thought of pineapples growing in groves, like they do them in Hawaii. But on Bali, pineapples grow wild in people's yards. I grow pineapples all over my yard, too. I love them and not just because they taste good.

"EATING PINEAPPLES HELPS WITH DIGESTION, BOOSTS IMMUNITY, LOWERS INFLAMMATION AND RELIEVES PAIN."

They have a wide range of health benefits. Science backs up many traditional uses of pineapple, but Lelir showed me even more uses I had never heard of before.

Help for Digestion and Women's Troubles

(Ananas comosus)

Balinese name: Manas

On Bali, we make rice paper by hand. The traditional craft probably traveled here from China, where paper was first made.

Some of the best handmade papers come from right here in our city of Ubud. You can still find traditional rice paper, but the most popular fiber we use today is from manas leaves. You know it as pineapple.

Many people grow pineapple in their gardens, but it also grows wild all over the island. So we have plenty of pineapple leaves to make into paper.

Workers chop the leaves into pieces then soak them for a while before cooking them until the fibers begin to loosen and come apart. Then they mash the fibers into pulp.

The pulp goes into a big tub. The papermaker then draws out a sheet of wet mash using a wooden frame with a fine mesh screen. The thin sheet of mash is transferred to a cloth base and then pressed to remove most of the moisture.

During the dry season, the paper can be laid out in the sun to dry. When the weather is rainy, the sheets are hung to dry in a shed. After drying, they're pressed one more time to flatten them.

This process produces a fairly heavy paper. But each sheet is unique. And the use of natural coloring agents means you can buy pineapple paper in many unusual colors. Sometimes, the papermaker even presses spices or flower petals into the paper, giving the sheets an unusual look or alluring scent.

Pineapple fibers also make a sturdy cloth. Traditionally, women would bury pineapple leaves deep in mud for about two months — to break down and soften the fibers. Then it can be washed, spun and woven into cloth.

This cloth is famous in the Philippines, where they sometimes use it to make men's formal shirts. These intricately embroidered shirts are called "Barong Tagalog."

Here in Bali, we don't use pineapple for fabric much anymore, but we have many uses for the pineapple fruit.

We enjoy the delicious fruit just as it is. It's one of our sweetest traditional foods, so we often think of it as a treat. But it's also very useful.

You'll rarely find a Balinese kitchen without pineapple. We juice the fruit or add it to salads and cooked dishes. If we have a tough piece of meat, we'll wrap the meat for a couple of days with a slice of young pineapple. The enzymes in the pineapple make an effective tenderizer.

Sometimes, women would come to my parents because their menstrual cycles were irregular. My parents would have them eat pineapple to help regulate their menstrual cycles.

The enzymes in pineapple can also trigger miscarriage. This knowledge has been passed down from mother to daughter for countless generations. That's why no pregnant woman in Bali will eat pineapple.

But these enzymes also aid digestion. If proteins seem to upset your stomach, try eating a little pineapple with your meal. The bromelain in the pineapple will help your stomach digest the protein.

Pineapple is also helpful for urinary tract problems. It's sort of the cranberry of Asia in that way. I remember my parents would give it to my sisters, brothers and me if we had a urinary tract infection. The pineapple would clear things up quickly.

— *Lelir*

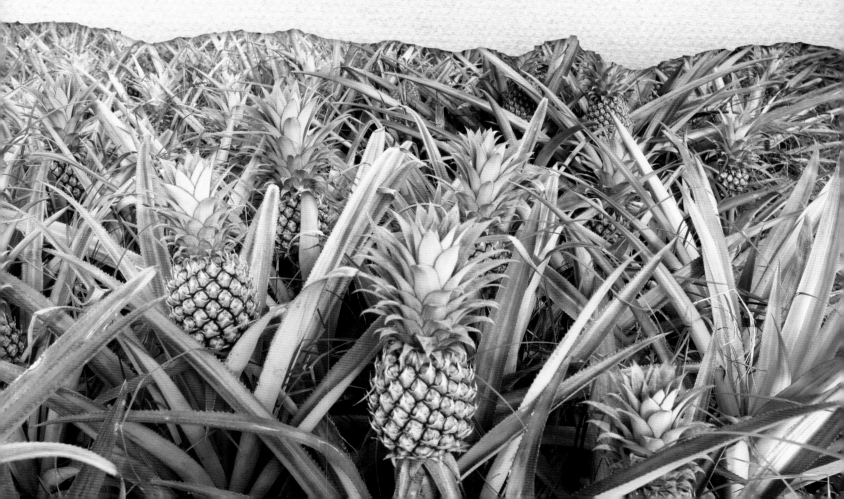

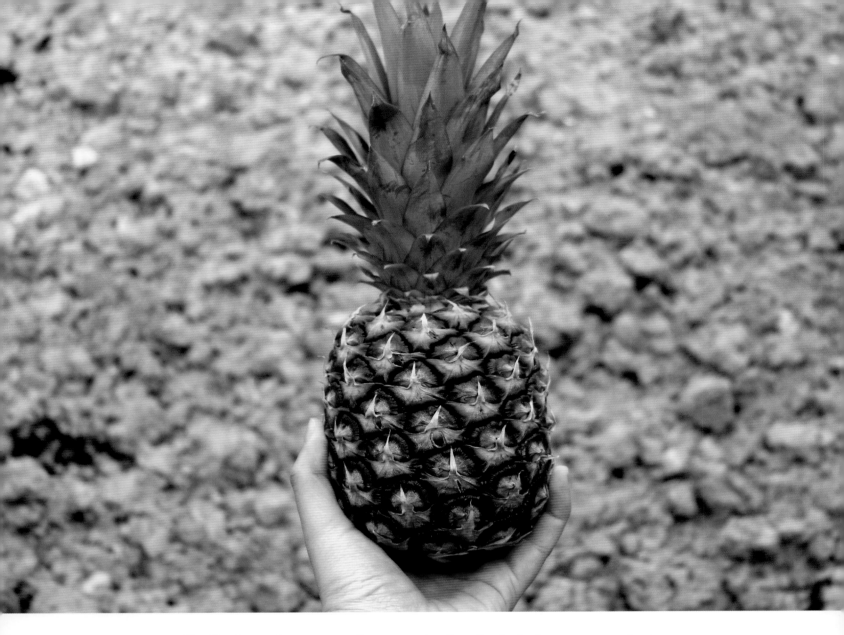

Westi's pineapples are sometimes rounder than the typical ones you see in stores.

My Own Research and Discoveries

On my last birthday, I celebrated with my staff, family and friends at my house.

We had pig roast, Hula chicken and teriyaki steak. We also had a huge fruit buffet with pineapples, and pineapple upside-down cake for dessert.

I supplied the pineapples from my own yard.

One of the reasons pineapple is so versatile is a secret ingredient — an enzyme called *bromelain.* It's a protease, which means it helps break down proteins. That's why it helps with digestion, especially if you eat a lot of protein like I do.

Bromelain from pineapple also promotes wound healing and discourages dangerous blood clots. There's bromelain in the fruit, and even more in the root.

Scientists are researching this pineapple extract because there is evidence that it prevents and treats some cancers.

More Than a Tropical Treat — A Cure for Cancer?

Researchers have found that pineapple can kill off stomach cancer cells,[1] colon cancer,[2] breast cancer[3] and other cancer cells. It has also been shown to stop the spread of some cancers.[4]

Bromelain is also good for preventing sickness. It boosts the activity of many different kinds of immune cells. This could be why extracts can fight problems as diverse as asthma and cancer tumors.[5]

But bromelain has another benefit. It can stop everyday aches and pains, as well as the pain from sports injuries.

One study showed bromelain was as effective as some commonly used nonsteroidal anti-inflammatory (NSAID) drugs for reducing pain associated with osteoarthritis.

Athletes like bromelain because it speeds up healing when they get cut, scraped, bruised and wounded. It also speeds up healing time and decreases pain following injury to soft tissue. Bromelain is especially good for sprains and strains, bruising and tenderness from those muscle injuries.

ONE OF THE REASONS PINEAPPLE IS SO VERSATILE IS AN ENZYME CALLED BROMELAIN.

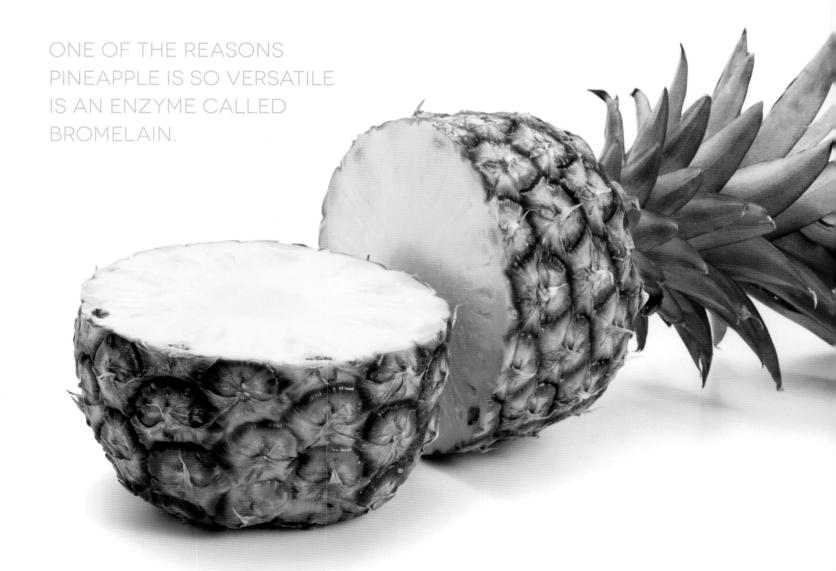

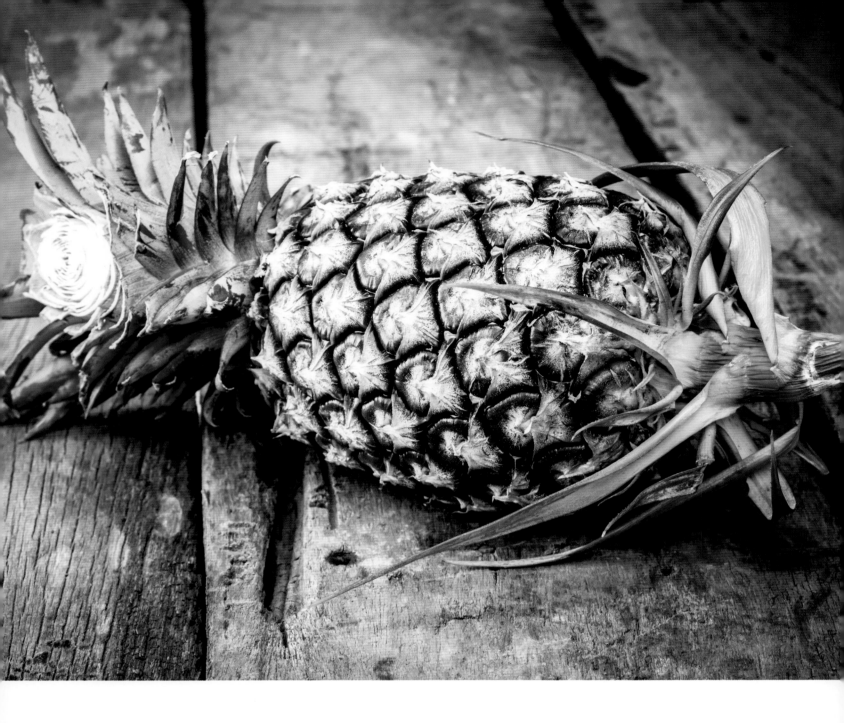

Mainstream Medicine is Using Bromelain.

Hospitals even use it to relieve post-surgical pain. But even though it works after inflammation and injury, it works even better if you take it prior to a traumatic event like surgery. Or before an intense workout or playing a sport that's physically demanding on your soft tissue or joints.

One study looked at how bromelain helps people who do intense exercise. They had a group of people do a workout consisting of some very strenuous leg exercises. Then they gave half the group a placebo and the other half a supplement containing bromelain for 21 days.

When researchers had the people work out again, they found that the bromelain group performed better. Their legs produced greater force, their running times improved and they had almost no inflammation.[6]

Here is What I Recommend

Pineapple is nutritious. It's a very good source of vitamin C, manganese and fiber. It also contains B vitamins, copper and a little protein.

And with only 3 grams of sugar per ounce, it's a sweet treat you can enjoy in moderation without spiking your blood sugar.

Besides eating a lot of pineapple, I often put pineapple in water to make a naturally sweetened and healthy drink.

Just cut up pineapple and put it into a pitcher of water and leave it overnight. When you wake up, you have yourself a refreshing glass of flavored water.

To get bromelain's effects a little faster and more consistently than eating pineapple, you can take a supplement. Bromelain is very bioactive, which means your body will absorb it well. But some extracts are stronger than others.

Bromelain potency is measured in GDU (Gelatin Digesting Units). Try to get a capsule that is at or near 2,400 GDU, the highest standardized potency you can get. I recommend you take 400-500 mg a day.

Pineapple extract helps heal a diverse number of problems, including:

Angina	Arthritis	Athletic and skeletal Injuries
Bacterial infections	Bronchitis	Cancer lesions and tumors
Cellulitis	Staphylococcus infection	Burns
Asthma	Thrombophlebitis	Sinusitis
Dysmenorrhea	Edema	Inflammation
Poor digestion	Steatorrhea	Platelet aggregations
Pneumonia	Rectal abscesses	Surgical trauma

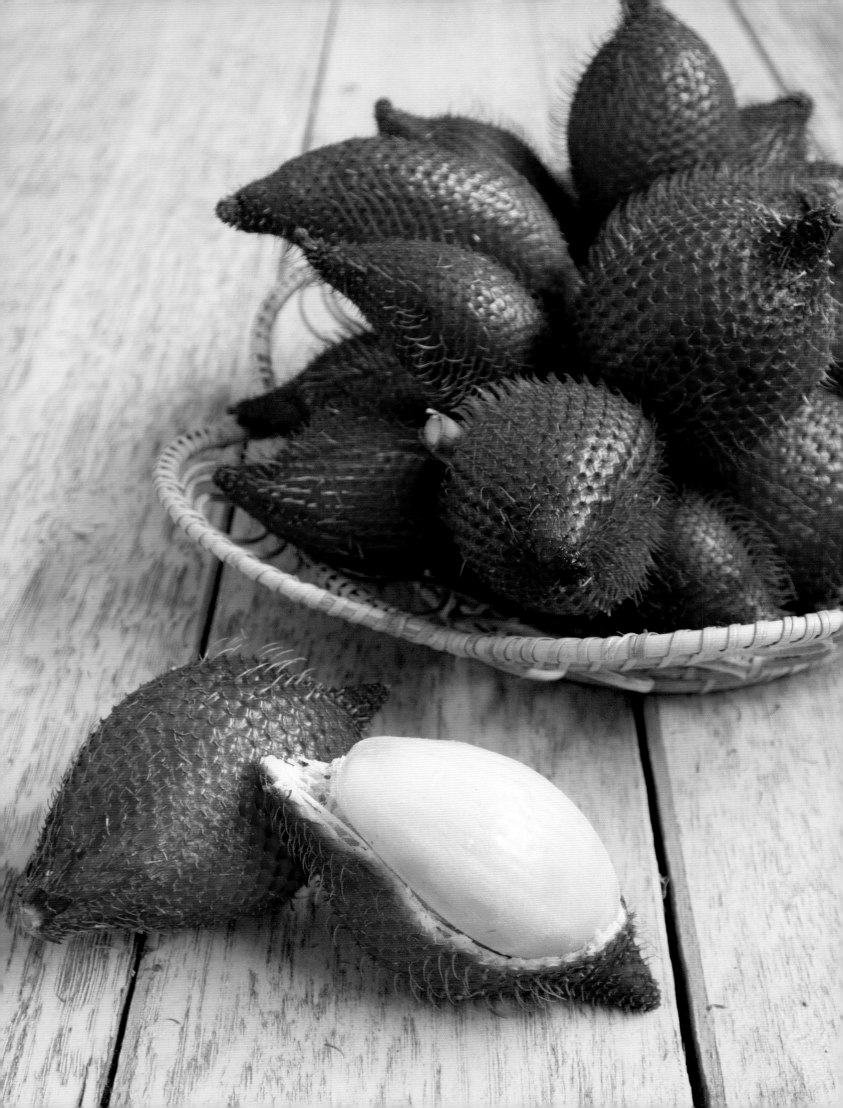

BALI'S HIDDEN ANTIOXIDANT SUPER–FOOD

I"I didn't know you had cacti in Bali."

I had never seen anything like it. I looked down at my bleeding leg.

The "cactus" had almost torn a hole in my only pair of shorts.

I hadn't meant to walk into it, but I swear, you step off the sidewalk in Bali and you're in the jungle.

I live in Florida, where plants grow like weeds. But this was different. It was plants on top of plants. The thickest, densest green I have ever seen. When you're in it, you know you're on the other side of the world.

And here I was without almost any clothes.

It had taken me more than a day and a half to fly to Bali, and long flights like that are grueling. I was tired, grabbed my pack and got off the plane. I followed the signs to baggage claim and waited... and waited. No luggage.

I went to the airline's baggage office and they kept me there while they searched for it.

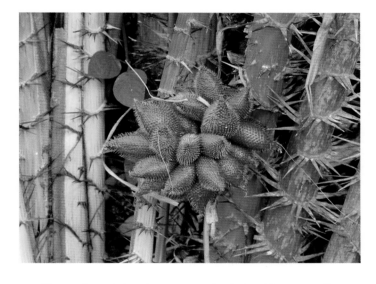

The spiky salak palm protects its fruit with cactus-like needles. A big spike I didn't even see stabbed me on the leg.

After three more hours, they told me they had found my bags. As I mentioned to you earlier, they found my bags in China.

It wasn't until the day before I was leaving Bali that I got my luggage back. Luckily, I had my camera and a few other things with me.

For the first two days I was in Bali, I wore the same shirt, shorts and sandals I wore on the plane. So I was happy I had cut my leg and not one of the few pieces of clothing I had bought at the flea market in Ubud.

Westi chuckled and shook his head.

"This is not a cactus. It's a palm tree. "Salak," it is called."

I remember thinking that this spiky cactus couldn't be a palm tree. Then Westi showed me some others like it, with long leaves — palm fronds — growing out of them. I looked a little closer.

Inside the tangle of spikes were some brown pods with pineapple-like scales on them.

I asked him: "Are those some kind of seeds?"

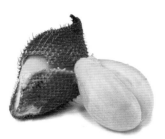

"Salak fruit," Westi said. "Thorns protect them from animals. The sweetest salak are found here in the mountains."

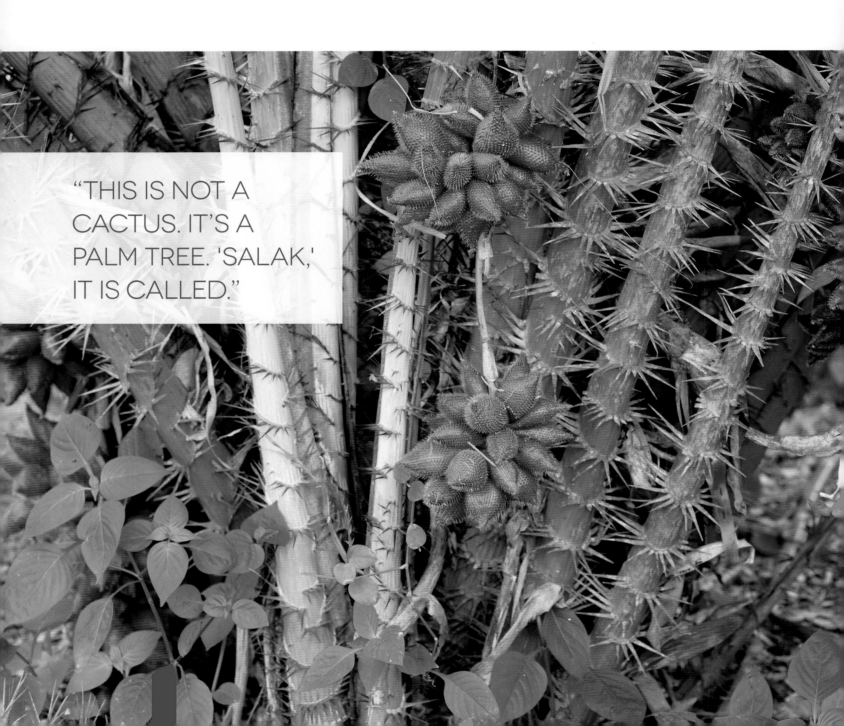

"THIS IS NOT A CACTUS. IT'S A PALM TREE. 'SALAK,' IT IS CALLED."

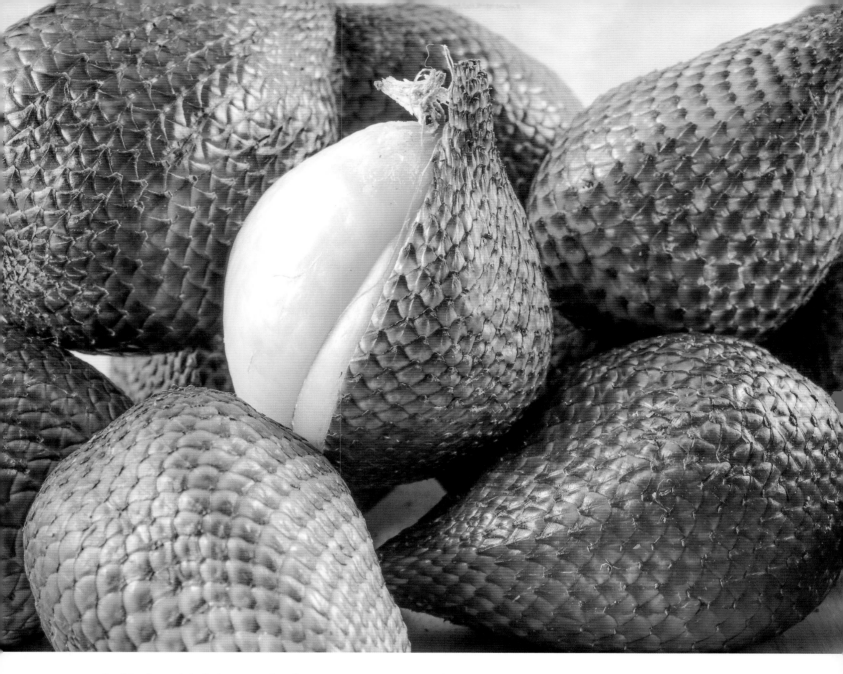

Inside the salak fruit are pods of white, juicy pulp. The sweetest salak are found in the mountains of Bali.

The Missing Nutrient You Need

He reached his hand carefully in between the spiky branches and pulled out one of the small brown pods. I peeled it open and took a bite.

It was delicious. Salak is full of the kind of fiber, micronutrients and minerals we're missing from so many of our fruits and vegetables in the corporate-farmed Western world.

When researchers tested salak, they found it had significantly more antioxidant power then the so-called "superfruit" you may have heard of called *mangosteen*.[1] These antioxidants — called *polyphenols* — are also cancer-fighting. Research has shown that Salak extract is able to stop lung and gastric cancers from growing.[2]

Balinese salak fruit *(salacca edulis)*, have what are called "neo-fatty acids," a small group of beneficial fats that are anticancer and antifungal.

A Natural Balinese Skin Softener

(Salacca edulis)

Balinese name: Salak hed

We call Salak fruit "snake skin fruit" because... well, it looks like snake skin!

The fruit tastes a bit sweet and sour at the same time, because it's astringent. So you don't want to eat it if you are constipated. But also, that means it's good if you have diarrhea.

You can remove the sour taste by boiling the fruit for 30 minutes. Then only the sweetness will remain.

When you open the skin of the salak fruit, it's very soft inside and white. In our Balinese culture, it's very desirable for women to have soft light brown skin... if you have it, it's the first thing Balinese women will mention if they see you.

This is why most Balinese women do not walk in open spaces like rice fields without large hats to cover their facial skin because they don't want to be too tanned.

There are a lot of spa treatments in Bali that lighten women's skin and the inside of the salak fruit is a natural skin softener and lightener.

— Westi

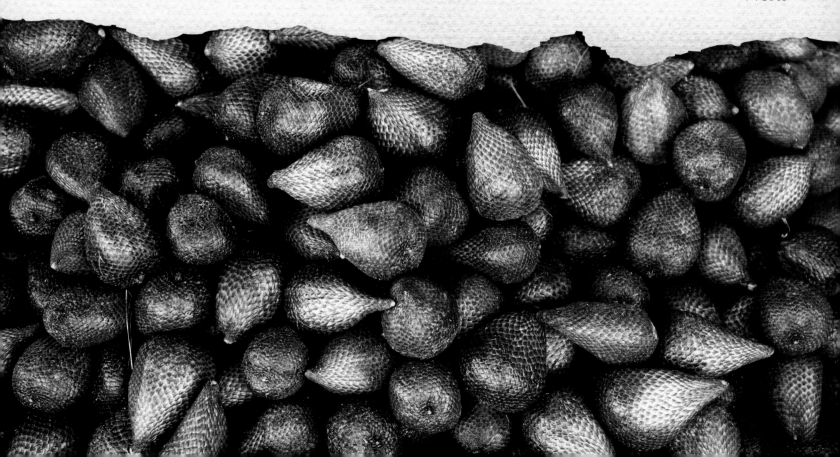

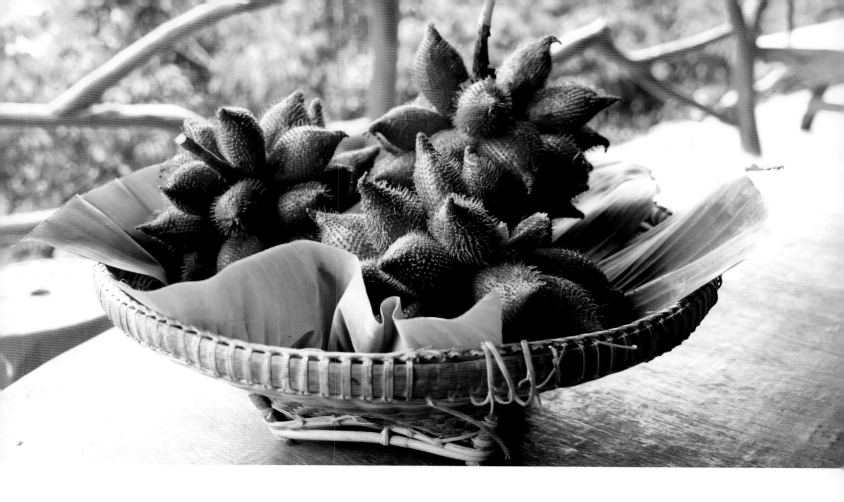

My Own Research and Discoveries

Most salak fruits from other parts of Indonesia are a little like apples, because they're often crunchy and tart. And not too juicy.

In Bali, it's a different story. The salak fruit that grows in the mountains near Ubud have a richer, deeper skin coloring. The fruit inside is tender and tasted incredibly sweet.

Salak is called "snake fruit" because it's thin skin kind of looks like a snake's skin. I think it looks more like a flattened pineapple hide.

They're easy to peel open, and inside are these pods of white, juicy sweet pulp.

The Balinese ferment the pulp and make homemade wine from the juice. I do not recommend drinking more than about two cups with dinner. I didn't discover that little secret until the next day, unfortunately.

If you live in the south like I do, you can grow salak yourself. The palms have to be planted in moist, well-draining soil... and, of course, be careful of the thorns.

The seeds and seedlings are available online at seedwonder.com, kadasgarden.com and the Australian seed seller daleysfruit.com.au.

There are also marketplaces like alibaba.com and ecrater.com that have salak for sale. I've even seen salak fruit chips at 21food.com.

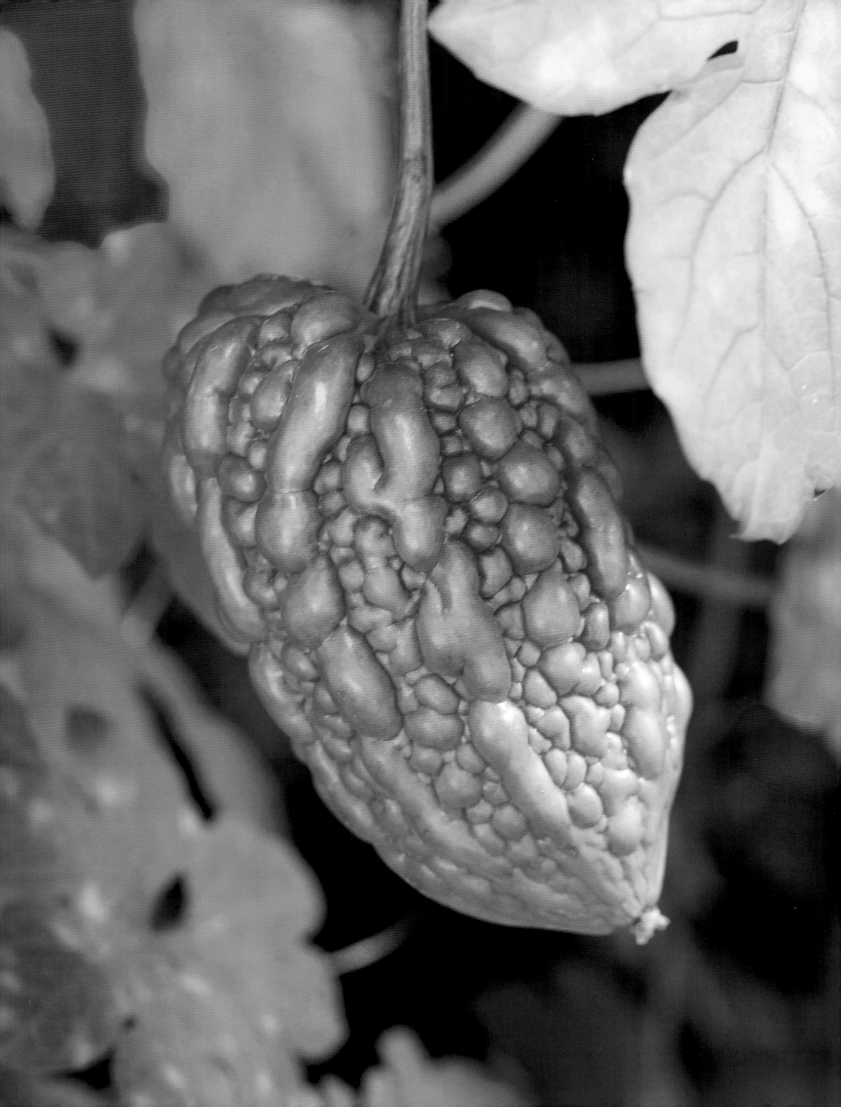

TROPICAL VINE
THAT STOPS CANCER COLD

*I*t took a couple of years to re-grow all the bitter cucumber in my yard.

It used to grow naturally along my fence. Until my neighbor read that it was a weed and killed it all with Roundup.

I like bitter cucumber, because it produces a flower that we use for detoxification. So I replanted, and now I have a nice, healthy hedge again.

I'm waiting for the flowers to bloom and for some ripe fruit, too ... because bitter cucumber is no weed.

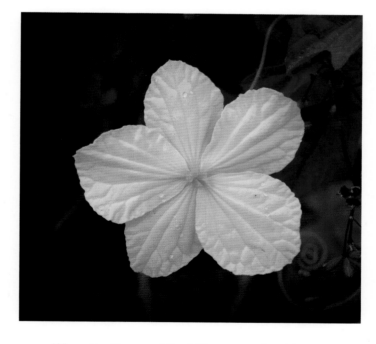

When the flower of the bitter cucumber blooms, it means the fruit is getting ripe.

"BITTER CUCUMBER HAS POWERFUL ANTIVIRAL PROPERTIES."

True, it's not very well known in the West. Apparently, not even by the botanists at the University of Florida where my neighbor got his information.

But this lime-green vine that grows wild on Bali and now at my house again deserves more respect.

Especially since it fights cancer. I'll tell you all about that in just a bit, but Westi tells me bitter cucumber is an important herb in the day-to-day lives of the Balinese, as well.

Baby's Best Friend and Great for Diabetics

(Momordica charantia)

Balinese name: Paye

I think babies everywhere must come down with "thrush." This is a yeast infection in the mouth and throat. And it's pretty common.

But when our son was very young, the appearance of a whitish coating in the back of his mouth and throat had me pretty worried. At least until Lelir reassured me. Once I knew it was thrush, we both knew what to do.

We took some paye leaves – bitter cucumber – and kneaded them thoroughly in water. Then we strained out the leaves. We painted our little boy's mouth and throat with the liquid every few hours. Within a couple of days, the infection had cleared up.

This is the same remedy Lelir's parents used when she was little. And their parents before them, for as long as anyone can remember.

Grandparents and sickly folks also get thrush. They can gargle with the same liquid to clear it up. And so can diabetics, who also frequently suffer with thrush. (This is because the extra sugar in their saliva feeds the yeast in their mouth, causing it to overgrow.)

We do use the fruit of the bitter cucumber in our cooking. It's one of those foods you either love or hate, because it really is quite bitter. But if you like arugula or other bitter vegetables, you may like bitter cucumber.

— Westi

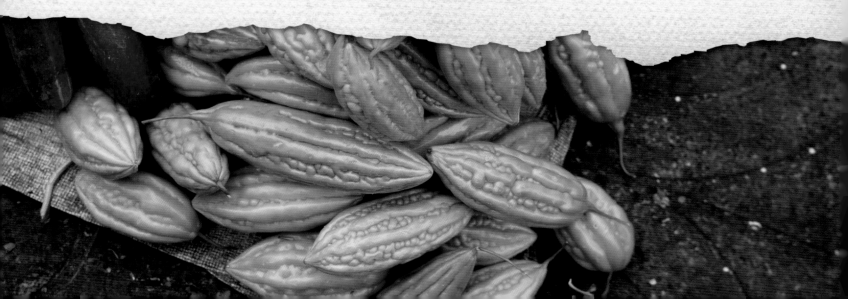

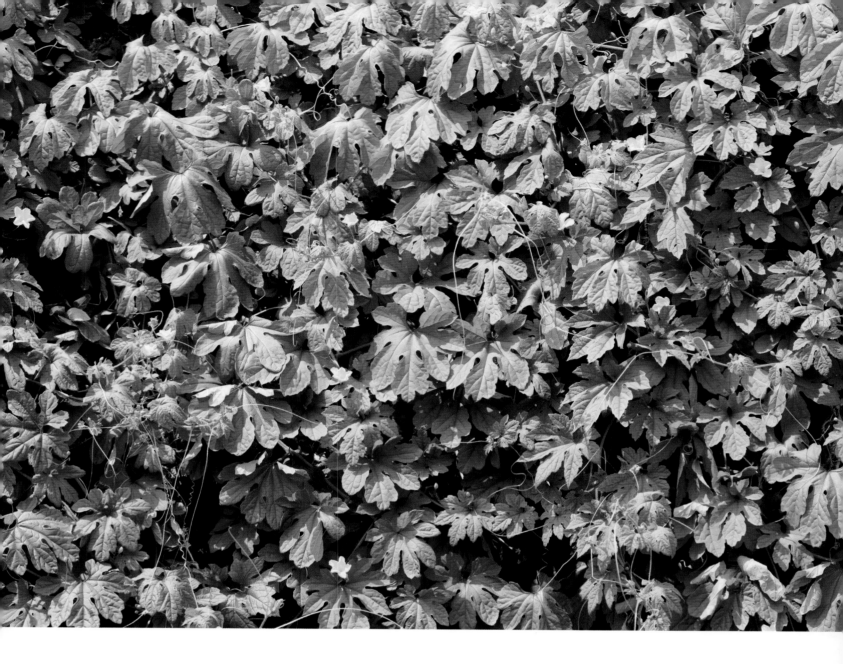

My Own Research and Discoveries

Bitter cucumber has so many healing properties that researchers brought it to the University of Miami to study it. They discovered that an enzyme in the ripe fruit can inhibit the growth of cancer cells.

A recent study looked at a compound called "kuguaglycoside C" that's in the leaves of bitter cucumber. They found that the extract killed off cancer cells of the nerve tissue (neuroblastoma) in just 48 hours.[1]

One of the ways it works is by increasing "apoptosis-inducing factor" inside the cancer cells.[2] This stops the cancer cells from making energy and tells them to shut down and die off.[3]

Another compound in bitter cucumber, DMC, works to kill breast cancer tumor cells. Extracts of bitter cucumber also fight hepatitis B and kill off liver cancer cells.

And a fatty acid that's in both the fruit and the seeds called *alpha-eleostearic acid* kills off leukemia cells and colon cancer cells.[4]

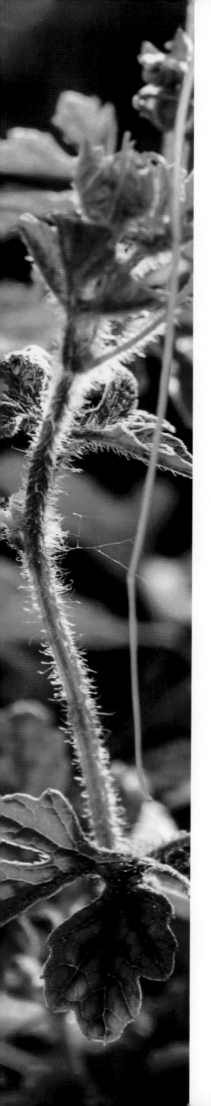

The leaves are also an excellent choice for skin problems. Researchers have discovered that bitter cucumber interferes with an enzyme that's been linked to psoriasis, a skin condition that causes skin cells to grow ten times faster. It may sound like a good thing, but these skin cells are not shed off, so they build up quickly, causing raised red patches of skin.

For many skin problems, or even just to have naturally healthier and cleaner skin, traditional herbalists from around the world crush bitter cucumber leaves and add them to their baths. It also works on skin tumors and wound healing when they use it to heal animals.[5,6]

An Immune System Powerhouse

It always boosts my faith in plants when I see the same traditional use spring up in totally unrelated places around the world.

For instance, the Maroon healers of Jamaica traditionally used bitter cucumber for diabetes — although they didn't understand the causes or progression of the disease. Still, they made a good choice, because bitter cucumber contains a compound that helps normalize blood sugar[7] — a major problem for diabetics.

When I traveled to India I found bitter melon there, too. Although Ayurvedic medicine, the oldest system of medicine in the world, calls it "karela."

Ayurveda treats diabetes with it as well.

Science backs up this use. In 2011, at the Patil Institute of Pharmaceutical Sciences and Research, researchers developed a patch with bitter cucumber for reducing blood sugar in diabetics and they found it worked very well.[8]

One study showed that less than an ounce of bitter cucumber a day lowered blood sugar in diabetics. In fact, it worked almost as well as a dose of Metformin, a drug commonly used to lower blood sugar, for type 2 diabetics.[9]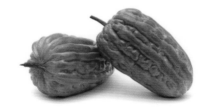

Bitter cucumber also has antiviral properties that are active against a number of types of flu.[10] One of the reasons might be that it stimulates the immune system. Bitter cucumber boosts natural killer (NK) cell activity.[11]

The leaves have been used by many cultures as an antimicrobial. One study showed antibacterial activity against H. pylori, the bacteria that is linked to ulcers.[12]

Here is What I Recommend

The fruit looks a bit different in India, with pointier ends, and they use it in their cooking when it's still green.

I sometimes use bitter cucumber in my cooking, too. I cut the green fruit open lengthwise without peeling. Then I remove the seeds and the unripe fruit from inside and chop it like a green pepper. Then I boil the pieces until they are tender, and add them to my stir-fry.

.... *Bitter Cucumber* ....

I also like bitter cucumber because you can use the leaves and the flower to make a detoxifying and purging daily tonic or tea. Use the young leaves to make the tea, then drink it for breakfast.

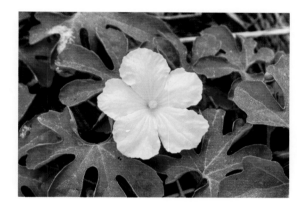

All you have to do to make it is:

1. Add 10 grams of dried or fresh bitter cucumber leaves to ¼ liter of boiling water.
2. Simmer on low for 5 minutes.
3. Turn off the heat and steep for 10 minutes.
4. Strain off the tea into a cup.

To make it sweeter, add a bit of brown sugar and ginger.

....

I also want to give you a recipe for one of the healthiest, most anti-inflammatory juices that I had in Bali, taught to Lelir by her family.

It's best to put all the ingredients in a blender. The drink will be bitter and a little sour (so you can sweeten with honey if you like), but also extremely healthy and anti-inflammatory:

- Labu (calabash fruit) – 1/2
- Paye (bitter cucumber) – 1
- Mint leaves – 10
- Tomato – 1
- Kunyit (Raw Turmeric) – as much or little as you like
- Jahe (Raw Ginger) – small amount
- Lemon – squeeze juice in, for flavor

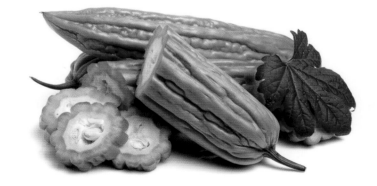

Now, if you already have low blood sugar, stay away from bitter cucumber. Also, it has antifertility properties, so if you want to get pregnant, do not use this plant.

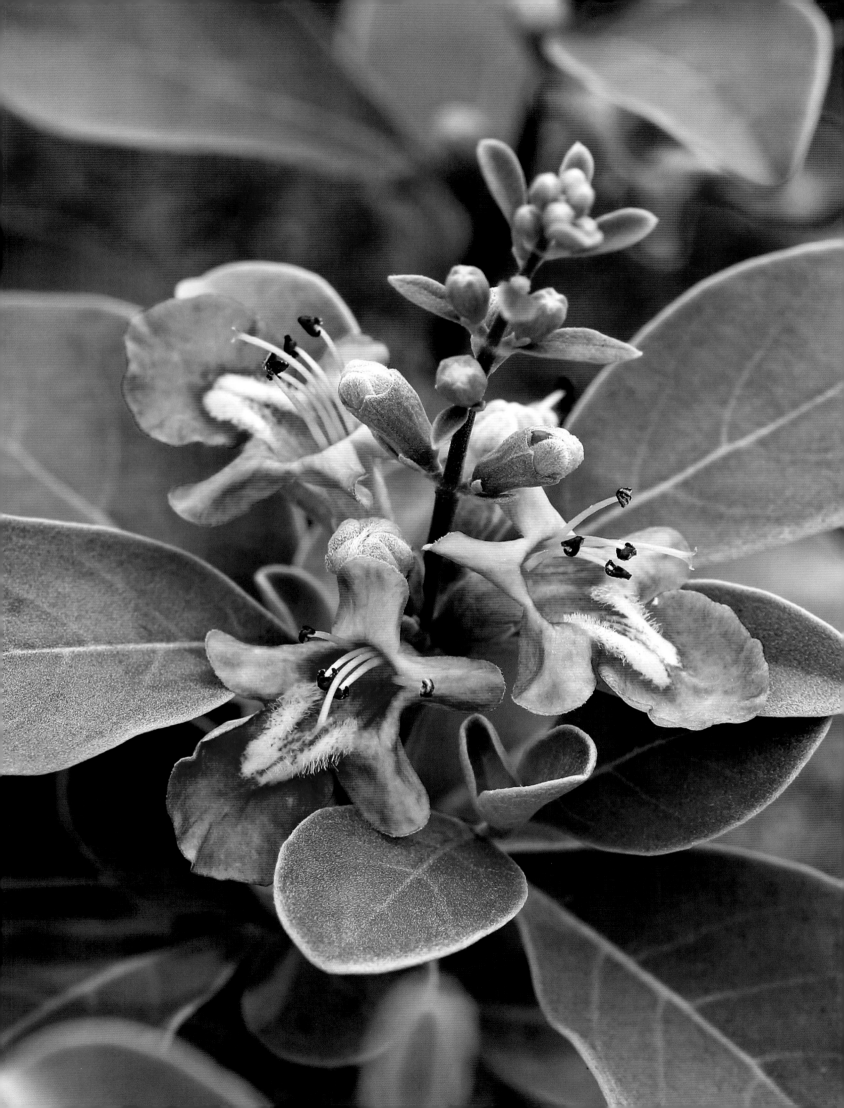

TROPICAL PLANT CAN PREVENT PARKINSON'S CAUSED BY PESTICIDES

When the summer comes to South Florida, so do the mosquitoes. I kind of forget about them for a couple of months during the winter. Then I get reminded that we're still in the thick of the Everglades. Even my house used to be a swamp.

I've been lucky not to have many problems with mosquitoes, even when I travel. In parts of the world known for swarms of insects, they still don't bite me much. There's one called "The Assassin" in the Amazon rainforest. It makes the bugs in Florida look small.

Every culture I've visited has its own way of dealing with pests. The most common mosquito repellent in the West is a chemical called *DEET*. It's known to scientists as "N,N-Diethyl-m-toluamide" or "N,N-Diethyl-3-methylbenzamide." All of the popular brands use it.

The U.S. Army developed it in the 1940s and it's been on the market since the '50s. The Environmental Protection Agency says

DEET is okay for you to use, and that it doesn't cause any "unreasonable risk to human health." But in my opinion, it's just another man-made poison.

"IN BALI, THEY HAVE ONE OF THE BEST NATURAL REPELLENTS."

Scientists used to think DEET worked by confusing mosquitoes and interfering with their sense of smell. But recent research shows that DEET is a neurotoxin to insects and mammals. That means it attacks the central nervous system, like nerve gas does. If it does that to rats, I don't want it on my skin.

I recommend natural bug repellents instead. And when I went to Bali, they had one of the best natural repellents I've ever come across.

Simpleleaf Chastetree, World's Best Mosquito Repellent

(Vitex trifolia)

Balinese name: Legundi

Mosquitoes are one of the biggest challenges of living in the tropics. Their constant buzzing is annoying... their bites are itchy... and they carry disease. But when I was growing up, mosquitoes weren't as big a problem as you might think.

I can remember walking to the rice fields with my father back when I was only 5 or 6. As we walked, sometimes he'd tell me about the many trees and bushes that lined the dirt lane.

My father knew more names and uses for these plants than most other farmers. He may have been a rice farmer, but he was an herbalist at heart. And he loved sharing his knowledge with me.

But when we arrived at our family's rice fields, he got right to work. And the first thing he often did was cut a small branch or some leaves from a particular bush.

These bushes grew wild along the edges of rice fields. This was the best place to find the sun they seem to love.

My father would take the branch of leaves he'd cut and lay them out where they'd be in the sun all day. By late afternoon, when we were ready to go home for supper, they'd be almost dried out.

On our way out of the rice field, I'd gather up the leaves or grab the branch, and carry our prize home to my mother.

One of us would bring home these little treasures almost every day. And after they'd dried for a couple more days, they were ready for use.

Mother would take a small bowl, place a leaf in the center and light it on fire. A wisp of smoke would curl up and fill the room as the leaf slowly smoldered. Before long, the room would be full of the pungent smell of the smoke... and cleared of mosquitoes.

In Bali the plant is called "legundi" – from our word for mosquito, "legu." In the West, it's called "simpleleaf chastetree." And it's probably the world's original mosquito oil.

Chastetree isn't well known in the West, but it grows across much of Asia, Polynesia and even parts of Africa. And almost every culture that knows it, uses chastetree as a natural mosquito repellent.

Lelir and I make an essential oil from the leaves. You can rub this oil on your skin to repel mosquitoes. It's very aromatic, but most people don't think the smell is unpleasant. But mosquitoes sure do!

We've also used the dried leaf in incense. This incense also repels mosquitoes. We've found that even the fresh leaves can chase mosquitoes out of a room.

I have learned that scientists are studying making chastetree extract into a natural alternative to the chemical sprays used against mosquitoes today. This would be very good for Bali, and much of the rest of the world.

In some parts of the Pacific, chastetree is also used for "women's problems." Here in Bali, we sometimes make a sort of strong tea from chastetree.

We'll brew the tea in a large tub, and then strain out the leaves. Then a woman who's recently had a baby soaks in this "tea" bath to ease postpartum discomfort.

— Lelir

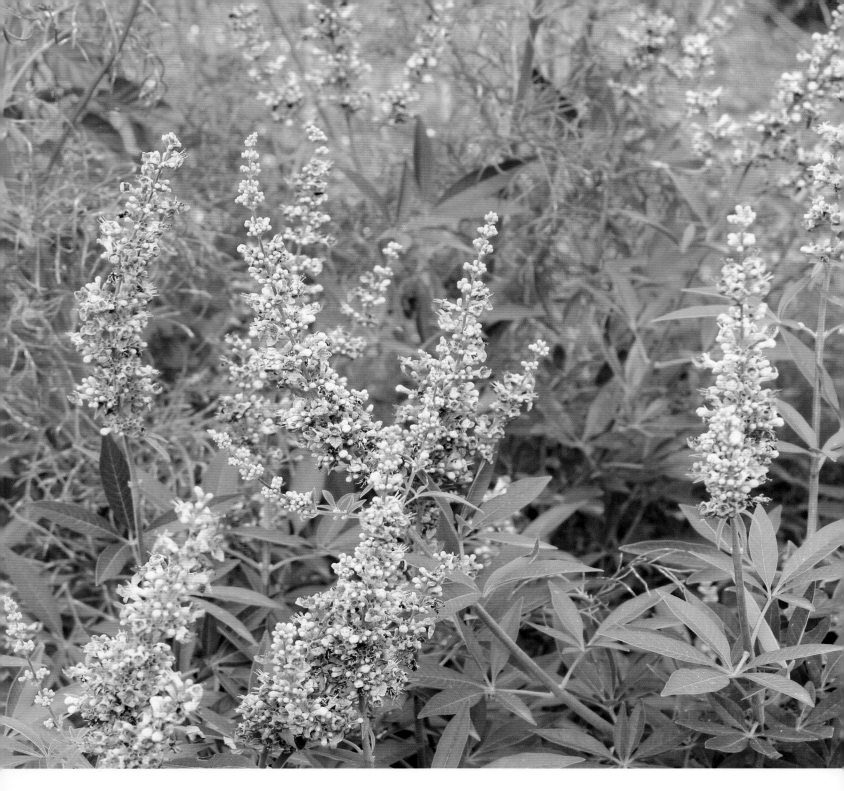

Chastetree is a natural mosquito repellent used in many parts of the world — but it's virtually unknown in the west.

My Own Research and Discoveries

I want you to know about organic pesticides, because chemical pesticides have been linked again and again to Parkinson's disease.

In a study published by the journal, *Archives of Neurology*, researchers looked at people's occupations and how likely they were to get Parkinson's disease.

What they found shocked them.

There was almost no increased risk for Parkinson's, regardless of what kind of work people did. But they did find that anyone who used at least one of eight different kinds of pesticides was more than twice as likely to get Parkinson's.

And if you used the insecticide permethrin, you were *three* times more likely to develop the disease.[1]

Permethrin is a common insect killer that's widely sold for use on clothing. It's also put in a pharmaceutical cream meant to be rubbed on the skin to kill mites.

Another study by the University of California at Berkeley found that people exposed to maneb, a common pesticide used in gardens, were 75% likelier to develop Parkinson's.[2]

Then there are the findings of the huge Agricultural Health Study.

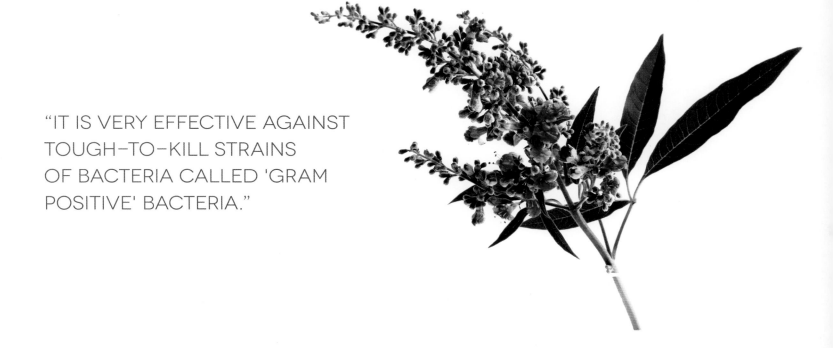

"IT IS VERY EFFECTIVE AGAINST TOUGH-TO-KILL STRAINS OF BACTERIA CALLED 'GRAM POSITIVE' BACTERIA."

Researchers followed about 90,000 licensed pesticide applicators and their spouses and monitor them for illnesses.

The results revealed that people who used commercial herbicides/pesticides like rotenone or paraquat developed Parkinson's disease 250% more often than non-users.[3]

These pesticides damage your cells. Rotenone, for example, impairs the ability of your mitochondria to make energy. And paraquat increases oxygen-induced damage to cells.

Some of the cells hardest hit by these pesticides are in an area of the brain that is also damaged by Parkinson's.

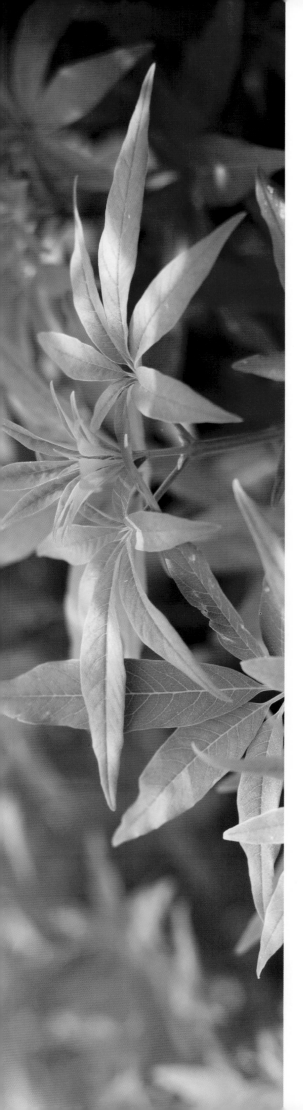

A Natural Insecticide

If you'd like to avoid this kind of damage from pesticides and keep your brain working just as well as it does right now, here's what I recommend:

- Stay away from products that claim to be "eco-friendly" or "natural," when they clearly are not. For example, avoid synthetic pyrethroids. They're similar to pyrethrins, which are natural insect-killing extracts from the flower chrysanthemum. But pyrethroids are created in a lab. Permethrin, which I mentioned earlier, is one of them.

- Also, stay away from "geraniol." It's billed as natural, because it's made from roses, lemons and geraniums, but it's been banned in Europe because of its toxicity to humans.

This is why I believe natural alternatives like chastetree are so important. It's completely safe and natural.

Studies show chastetree is the perfect choice for getting rid of insects. Scientists at India's Annamalai University discovered it also kills mosquito larvae. In their experiments, chastetree extract proved very powerful. A solution of just 9.25 parts per million was enough to kill half the larvae in their tests.[4]

The leaves also have antibacterial properties.[5] Chastetree is very effective against tough-to-kill strains of bacteria called "gram positive" bacteria.[6] For example, staph and strep, two bacteria you may know of, and which cause damaging infections, can't stand up to chastetree extracts.[7]

One research team discovered the plant's extract has anti-inflammatory effects, too.[8]

Animal studies from India show chastetree can even speed the healing of wounds.[9]

Science also backs up the traditional use of chastetree to treat cancer. Like many components of herbs and plants, chastetree can kill many different kinds of cancer cells.[10] The Chinese Academy of Sciences found that vitetrifolin from chastetree kills tumor cells.[11]

Westi combines lemongrass, holy basil
and chastetree to repel mosquitoes and flies.
Basil is toxic to mosquitoes as well.

Chastetree

You can also put chastetree leaves in your cabinets and pantry
to keep bugs out of the kitchen. It works at my house.

Remember that the simpleleaf chastetree *(Vitex trifolia)* is not the same
as the chaste berry tree *(Vitex agnus-castus)*.

The fruit powder is available as a supplement...
you'll often see it in Asian specialty stores as "Man Jing Zi."

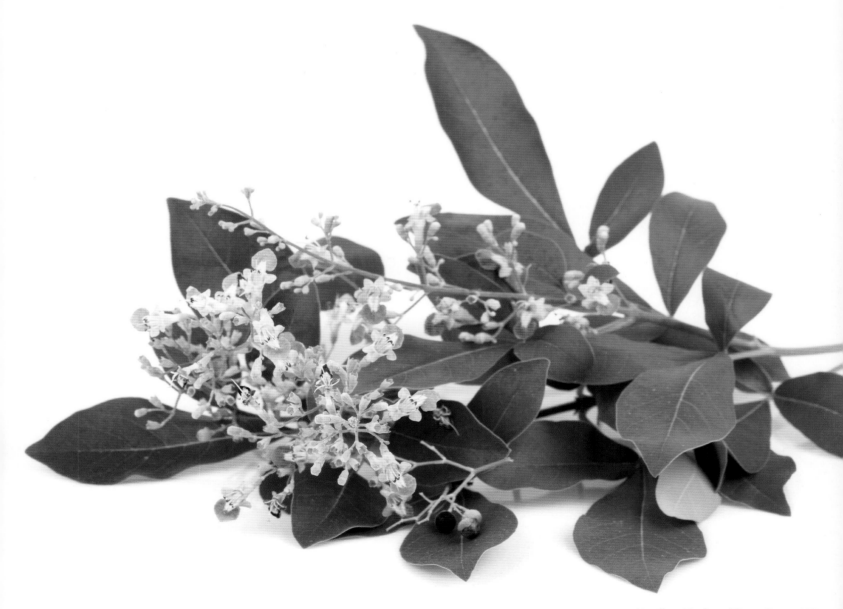

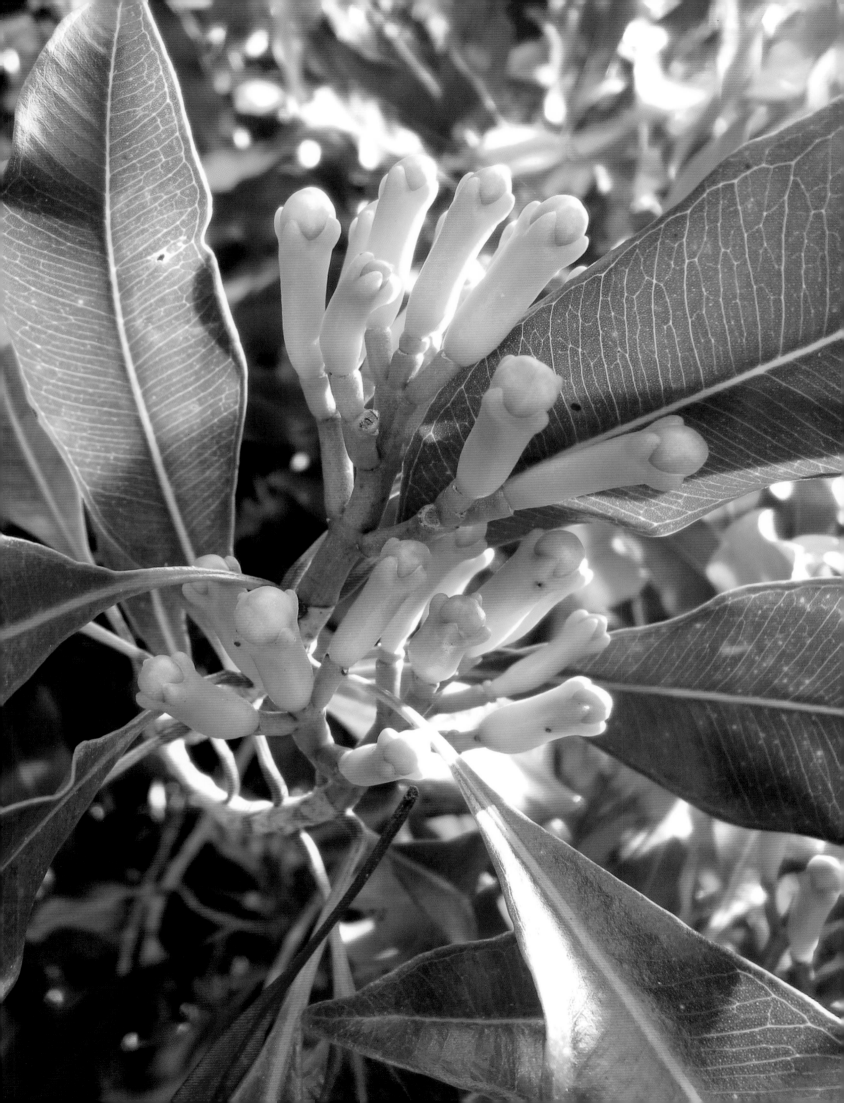

USE BALI'S ESTROGEN-ZAPPING HERB TO KNOCK OUT PAIN... AND PREVENT CANCER

Westi and Lelir often cook with cengkeh. Most of us know this spice as "cloves."

When I returned to the states after my first trip to Bali, I started doing research on the local plants and herbs they use there.

"CLOVES CAN KEEP MOSQUITOES AWAY FOR FOUR HOURS"

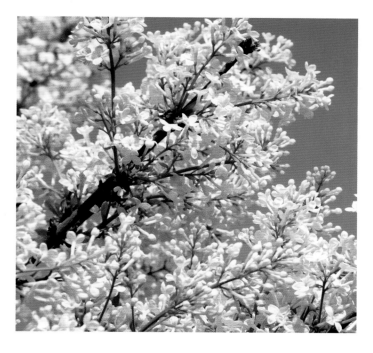

Cloves are a natural antidote to the mass of excess estrogen in our modern world.

I found out about some new benefits of cloves that I'll tell you about in a minute. But it was while doing research on a completely unrelated subject that I stumbled on something else I hadn't known before.

I discovered that cloves can lower estrogen — something modern medicine has overlooked.

This is extremely important in today's world. Nearly every chemical we encounter, from pollution to pesticides to the ingredients in cosmetics, acts like estrogen when it gets into your body.

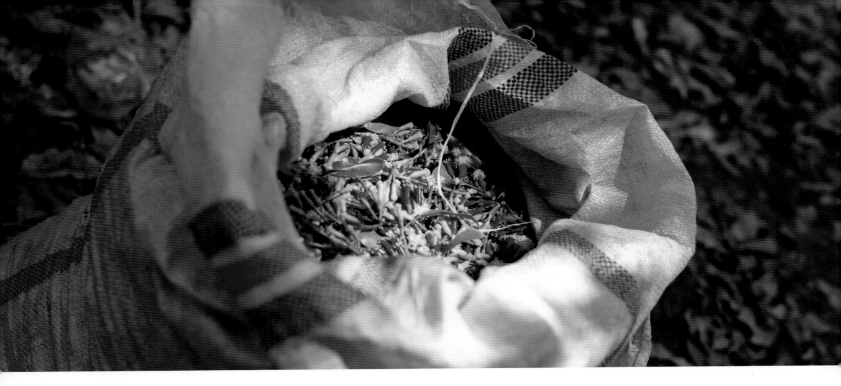

Balians harvest cloves by hand. They anchor very simple pole ladders to the ground with wires and then climb the trees to pluck the clove buds from the branches.

A Natural Antidote to Fake Estrogens

Too many fake estrogens have numerous negative consequences for the health of both men and women health.

Low libido, loss of muscle tone, fat gain and fatigue are just the start. At higher levels, estrogen is a known cancer-causing agent. It acts like radiation, producing extremely destructive free radicals and causes your DNA to "misfire." It produces the defects that are the beginnings of cancer. After certain estrogens break down, the quinines produced can also cause DNA errors.

Too much estrogen also decreases one of your body's "master" antioxidants, glutathione. This raises oxidative stress in your cells and can be an early step in cancer-cell formation.

Cloves are a natural antidote to the mess that excess estrogen can cause. Cloves have an important fake estrogen-zapping nutrient I want to tell you about, called *eugenol.*

Eugenol helps keep your body from absorbing estrogens, including the fake estrogens that seep into your body from our chemically polluted world. The eugenol in cloves helps your stomach convert these fake estrogens into harmless compounds and eliminates them from your body.

Clinical studies on how your stomach gets rid of toxins like synthetic drugs and fake estrogens show how eugenol helps. It stimulates an enzyme in your stomach that converts chemicals and foreign substances — especially fake estrogens — to a water-soluble form that your body quickly flushes out.[1]

This is one of the most important health benefits of cloves... but not the only one. Westi told me a bit about traditional Balinese uses for cloves, one of which his father showed him when he was very young.

Sweet-Smelling Insect Repellent Also Eases Back Pain

(Syzygium aromaticum)

Balinese name: Cengkeh

The water was halfway up my father's shins... which means it came almost to the top of my legs. It was cold – bone-chilling cold. All around us rose young rice shoots.

Father was bent over, carefully tending the rice plants... finding weeds and pulling them by hand, careful not to disturb his crop. He stood up slowly, painfully, pushing up on his thighs with his palms to take some of the burden off his back.

He looked at me as I "helped" him, now and then pulling a weed here or there. I was too young to be much real help, but at least I was some company.

"Westi," he said as he gazed up at the terraced hills above us, "it used to be much harder to grow rice." He swept his hand towards the seemingly endless green terraces. "Once, all these paddies gave us just one harvest each year. But since the government gave us fertilizers and insecticides, we can grow two crops."

He winced and placed his hand on his lower back. "Now we have much more rice to sell," he continued, "but our backs never get a rest. I'll be glad to get home tonight. I need your mother's boreh."

Then he went back to his weeding.

"Boreh" is what we call our traditional mixtures of herbs and spices that we use externally. Balinese women apply boreh to their husbands' backs and joints to ease the aches caused by working in the rice fields all day. Its natural heat soothes sore joints and muscles, headaches and rheumatism.

One of the most important spices Lelir uses in her boreh is cengkeh – cloves.

You wouldn't know it to look at the cloves you buy in a store, but they actually come from a tree. It's an evergreen, but it doesn't have needles like a fir tree. Instead, it has dark green, tapered leaves, tinged with red.

Clove trees smell heavenly. Like so many of our neighbors, Lelir and I have clove trees in our garden at home.

But the scent of our clove trees is nothing compared to the scent in the northeast of Bali. Entire jungles of clove trees grow there... along with cinnamon, candlenut, nutmeg and vanilla. I don't think anywhere else on earth smells quite so lovely as this corner of Bali.

Long ago, European empires battled over the spices grown in Bali and the surrounding "Spice Islands." Great Dutch and Portuguese sailing fleets loaded up with the spices grown here and took them back to Europe, where they were in great demand.

Today, Indonesia is independent, and farmers on Bali can grow and sell spices to support their own families, just as Lelir and I do.

Lelir and I grow many of our own spices. But we also buy spices from small farmers all over Bali. Some we use to make the cosmetics and other products we sell in our shops. But much of what we buy, we combine and sell to restaurants and other companies.

Each small farmer doesn't grow enough spices to sell commercially. But when we combine the output of many small farmers, we have enough. So we can help our neighbors by finding a market for their crops this way.

Here is how cloves go from flowering trees on Bali to your table...

When the cream-colored flowers of the clove tree lose their stamens (the pollen-producing rods in the center), purple berries develop. These berries eventually dry and turn brown. What is left are the familiar cloves you find in your supermarket.

Balinese herbalists value cloves highly because they have so many uses. We extract the essential oil from the flowers, leaves and stems. This oil is a safe and effective antiseptic. You can also soak a piece of cotton in the oil and apply it to a tooth to stop a toothache.

Sometimes neighbors come to us when their children are sick. If the child has a stomach ache with spasms, we tell the parents to use clove oil. We have them heat a little of the oil and gently massage it on the child's belly. Pretty soon, the spasms stop.

Of course, we use cloves in cooking, too. It not only has a delicious flavor, it also aids digestion. Lelir and I use cloves to protect against ulcers.

Here in Bali, the rainy season lasts about two-thirds of the year – from September to April. With all the rain – and all the rice paddies – mosquitoes can be a real problem.

But clove oil makes an effective insect repellent. Just spread a little of the aromatic oil on your skin, and it will keep mosquitoes away for a couple of hours. And because it's an oil, it clings to your skin when you get wet.

— Westi

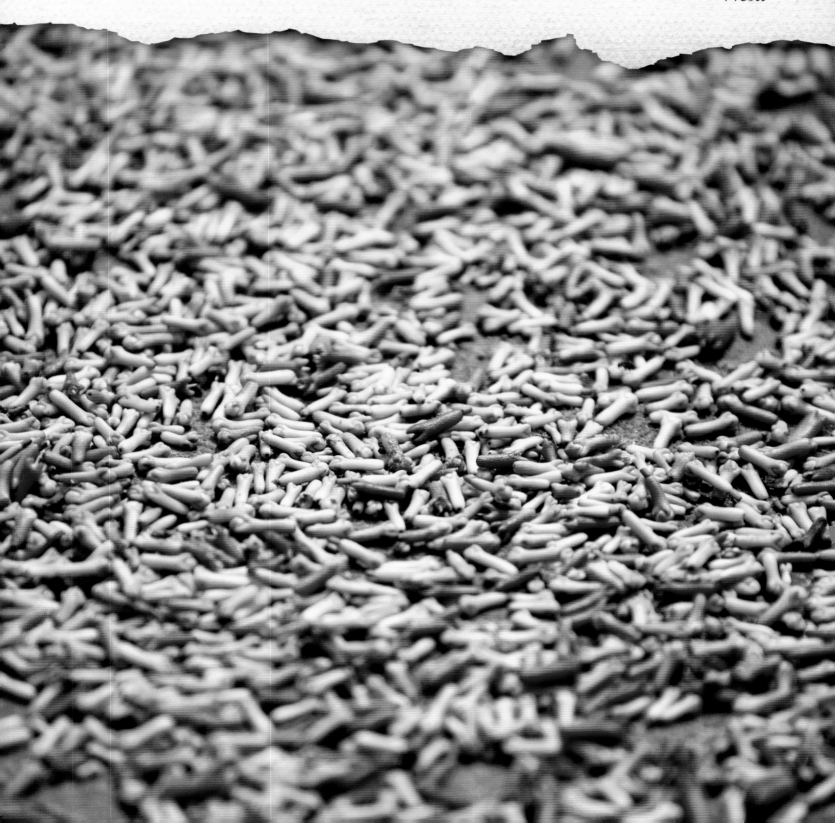

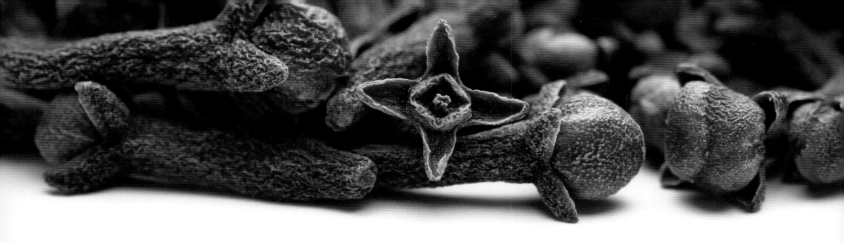

My Own Research and Discoveries

Scientists in Thailand tested several essential oils as insect repellents and discovered that clove oil worked best. In their experiments, it kept mosquitoes away for up to four hours.[2]

Studies have also shown that Balinese wives are smart to include cloves in their boreh. Animal tests at the University of Florence in Italy revealed that a compound in clove oil has an anesthetic effect.[3] In other words, it dulls the feeling of pain.

The eugenol in clove oil also stimulates the stomach lining to produce more protective mucous, helping to relieve ulcers, just as the Balinese have known for hundreds of years.

Cloves don't have much in the way of vitamins, with the exception of one: vitamin K.

Most doctors overlook the critical role vitamin K plays in your body.

It can help prevent liver cancer.[4] And in a study published in the *Journal of Cancer Research and Clinical Oncology*, vitamin K killed leukemia, pancreatic and ovarian cancer cells.[5,6] It does this by programming cancer to "self-destruct."

Cloves can also help keep your blood sugar under control. As part of the Framingham Heart Study, researchers found that people with the highest levels of vitamin K had better insulin sensitivity and lower blood sugar than people with the least vitamin K.[7]

Better than Most Multivitamins

Cloves are also filled with fiber and minerals like potassium, calcium, magnesium and iron. Just a couple of tablespoons will give you 10% of what you need every day.[8] That's more than what you get with many big-name multivitamins!

In our westernized world, antioxidants are still the best way to guard against disease.

That's because any time you increase your intake of antioxidants, you're saving your healthy cells from damage.

Spices, herbs and teas are surprisingly powerful antioxidants. And cloves are the most powerful antioxidant food ever measured.

Cloves have an ORAC value (Oxygen Radical Absorbance Capacity, a measure of how well a food can clean up free radicals) that is through the roof, at over 315,000.[9] That's the highest of any food in the world. For comparison, garlic is around 6,000 and broccoli is around 3,000.

Here is What I Recommend

The best way to use cloves is to add them for flavor to one of the many teas I describe in this book, add them to mulled apple cider or wine, or make clove tea.

You can buy culinary cloves whole, as they are the dried flower buds of the clove tree, or you can get them in the ground form.

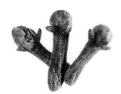 I like whole cloves, because they have more flavor... and I can grind them myself on the spot if I want. I don't recommend clove powder, because it doesn't stay fresh for very long. I just put the whole buds in my portable coffee grinder and make only as much as I need at a time.

I also use clove buds and flowers the way I was taught by Lelir. Every month or so, I make a body scrub that's very invigorating and detoxifying. In Bali, the traditional herbalists call these kinds of mixtures "boreh."

The original boreh recipes came to Bali many centuries ago. Like many traditions on Bali, they arrived through the many wars and refugees from the surrounding islands. These recipes have been handed down through the generations of Lelir's family, and they have added to the recipes with unique Balinese herbs, and subtracted those that did not grow locally.

Lelir's Boreh Recipe

Lelir makes her own boreh recipe just as a good ol' fashioned cook would: she does it "by eye." A pinch here and a handful there... so I can't tell you exact amounts.

But what you do is:

- Chop a medium ginger root and a medium galangal into pieces small enough to crush.
- Using a large mortar and pestle, crush the chopped roots with 3 pieces of cardamom.
- Add and crush together some coriander, nutmeg and clove bud and flowers.
- Add rice (Lelir uses a mixture of red and white rice) and crush with spices.
- When all ingredients are thoroughly crushed, mix in a little water.

Lelir's unique Balinese body scrub is mostly used for sore muscles and joints. You should not use boreh on your face or internally, but it has many other uses...

- For headache, apply a little scrub to the center of the forehead and on the temples.
- For flu, apply behind the ear lobes and along the base of the back of the neck.
- For chest coughs, apply to the center of the chest.
- For backache and to soothe sore muscles and joints, apply to shoulders, back or wherever soreness occurs. This is especially effective with acupressure or after deep massage.

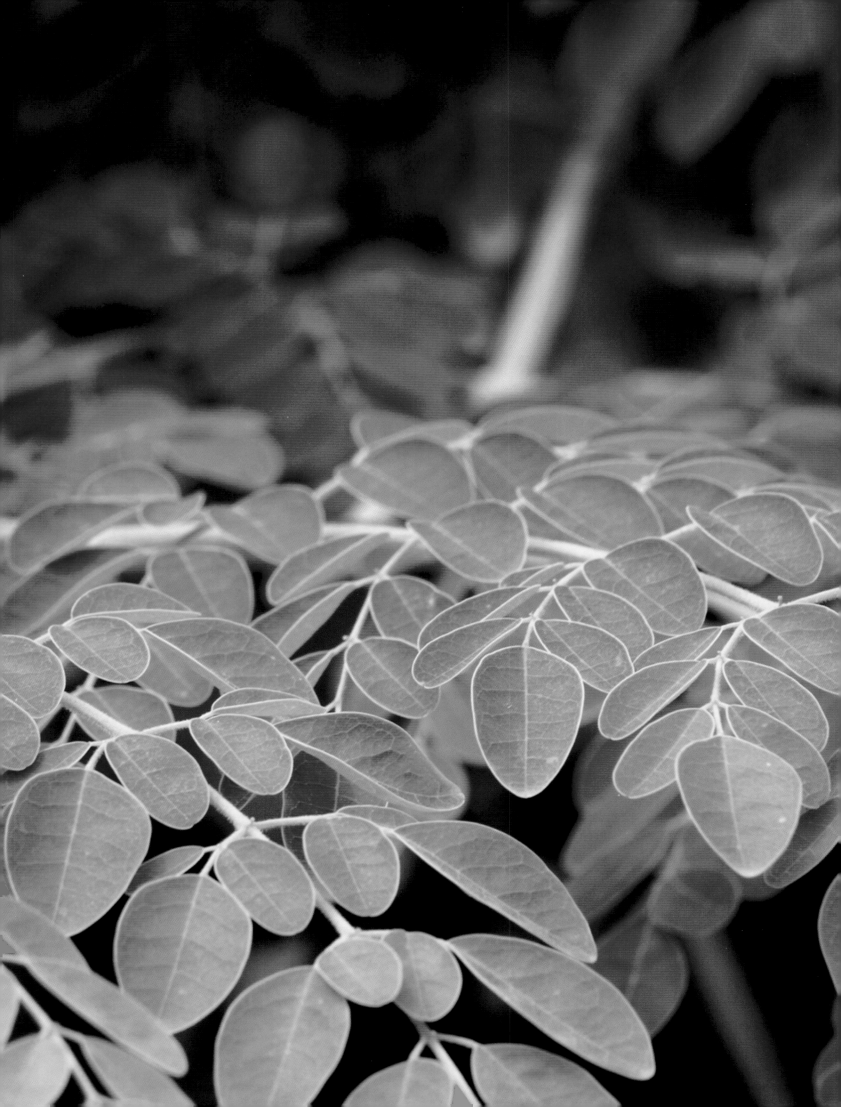

THE BALINESE SUPERFOOD

Most people in the United States have never heard of it, but in many places it's known as the "Miracle" tree or sometimes the "Giving" tree.

In Bali, they call it "Daun Kelor." It's the moringa tree.

Moringa is very important in the Balinese culture. Westi tells me the tree has a "magical spirit." In Balinese traditional lore, practitioners would fight black magic with moringa tree stems, using them to direct bad energy away from the body.

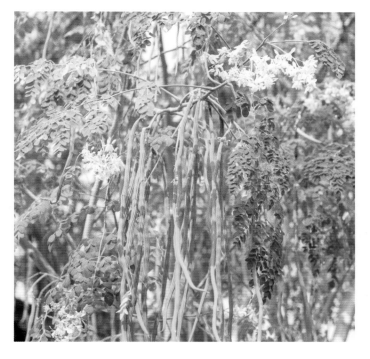

The leaves of the moringa tree contain micronutrients, vitamins and every essential amino acid, which is rare for a plant.

"A REMARKABLY COMPLETE SET OF NUTRIENTS."

In practical use, moringa is what I think of as a real superfood. That's because we're not talking about one fruit or leaf with an abundance of only a few vitamins.

Almost the entire moringa tree is edible. That includes the pods, leaves, seeds and roots.

The leaves have a remarkably complete set of micronutrients, vitamins and every essential amino acid. That's rare for a plant.

Look how moringa is head and shoulders above these common foods for nutrient content:

Moringa Nutritional Values vs Various Foods

Nutrient	100 g Dry Moringa Leaves	Other Foods
Vitamin A	18 mg	Carrot: 1.8 mg
Calcium	2000 mg	Milk: 120 mg
Iron	28.2 mg	Spinach: 1.14 mg
Potassium	1324 mg	Banana: 88 mg
Protein	27.9 g	Yogurt: 3.1 g
Magnesium	368 mg	Broccoli: 19 mg
Fiber	19.2 g	Whole Wheat Bread: 6.8 g

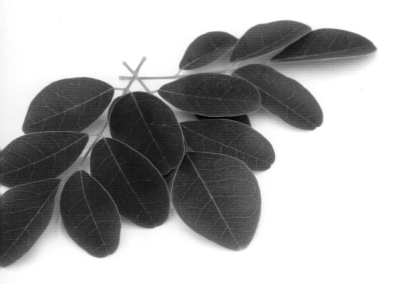

And nutrition is only one benefit of eating moringa. When researchers looked at extracts from the moringa leaf, they found that it was full of antioxidants, and is also very effective against diabetes.[1]

The leaf extract is also antibacterial and studies show that it kills human tumor cells.[2]

Westi told me that when he was a child it was more common to eat all parts of the moringa tree. Today, villagers use the leaves mostly as a "super vegetable."

In Bali and Africa, they use Moringa to filter water. You crush the seeds and run water that may be tainted through the powder, which filters out many impurities. It's a bit like the way we would use a charcoal filter in the West.

My friend in South Africa, Dr. Josiah Kizito, uses moringa extensively. He is a well-known researcher and expert in natural-healing methods, especially in the use of healing plants.

He has used moringa to revitalize many of his patients, who once suffered from extreme weight loss and were bedridden, plagued by all kinds of other illnesses.

Lelir told me that in Bali they use parts of the moringa tree in a poultice to ease childbirth. But they also use it as a nutritious superfood with many other traditional uses:

Life-Giving Horseradish Tree

(Moringa oleifera)

Balinese name: Daun Kelor

Nowadays, Balinese women often have their babies in a hospital. But not too long ago, that wasn't true. Even today, dukun bayi — our term for midwives — stay busy attending to home births in many villages.

Back in the 1960s, something strange started happening. More and more women were having convulsions while giving birth. Convulsions are a serious complication. I've read that half the women who have convulsions while giving birth die.

This problem spread with the use of a new kind of rice in Bali. The government in Jakarta introduced a faster-growing rice that allowed an extra planting every year.

But this fast-growing rice didn't have as much nutrition as our traditional rice. And the missing nutrients resulted in pregnant women having convulsions while giving birth.

But very few women died, because our dukun bayi knew about daun kelor — the horseradish tree.

The midwives kneaded the leaves of this tree together with red onion and some coconut oil. Then they massaged it into the woman's body. Very quickly, the convulsions would stop.

In many villages, the wood of the horseradish tree is a favorite fencing material. That's because most insects don't like it. If you build your garden fence with horseradish wood, you'll have a lot less trouble with bugs.

When I was a little girl, my mother made a savory soup using the leaves of the horseradish tree. The basic recipe was a favorite in Bali for many generations. And it's very healthy.

Mother would boil water and add chopped onion, garlic, chili, galangal, pepper, coconut oil and salt. Then she'd add chopped young leaves from the horseradish tree. We thought of it as a vegetable — sort of like the way you might think of spinach.

Horseradish leaves are high in protein, and contain several vitamins, minerals and several powerful antioxidants. So it makes a very nutritious soup. We think of these leaves as the Balinese superfood.

Horseradish tree also contains anti-inflammatory, antibacterial and antifungal compounds. It may help lower cholesterol and blood pressure. It may also help fight ulcers. It even promotes heart and circulatory health.

I make a scrub for rheumatism with the bark of the horseradish tree.

Horseradish leaf is a good source of quercetin and kaempferol — two very powerful antioxidants. Westi makes an antioxidant "juice" from the leaves.

— *Lelir*

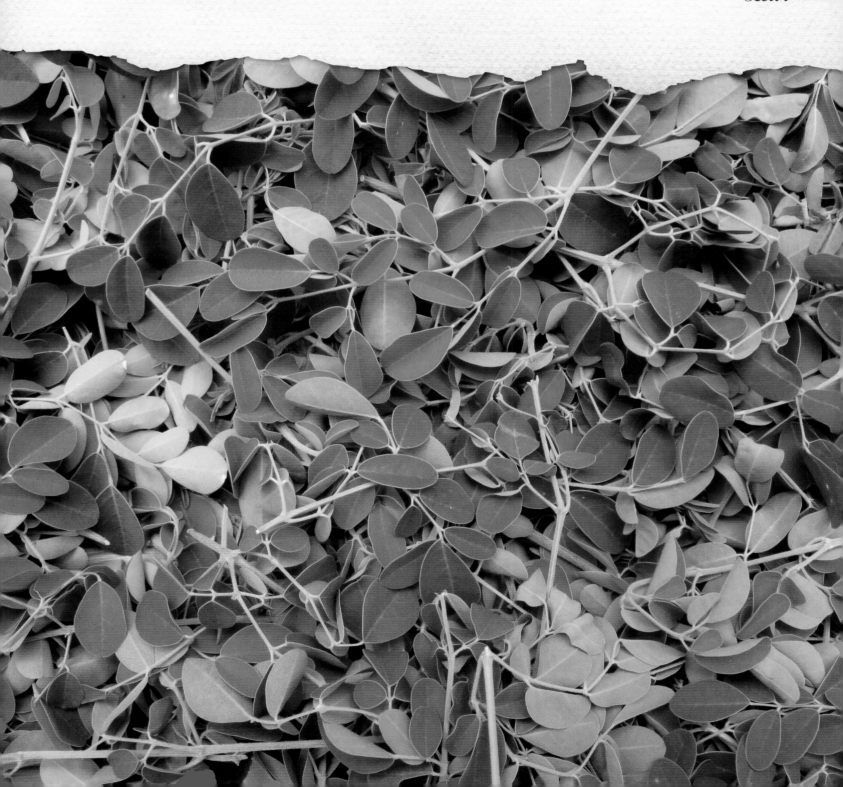

My Own Research and Discoveries

Plants that contain kaempferol, like horseradish, have been shown to reduce the risk of heart disease and cancer. Some components of kaempferol, called *glycosides,* have a wide range of medicinal and healing activities.

They include antioxidant, anti-inflammatory, anti-allergic, antidiabetic, anti-osteoporotic, antimicrobial, neuroprotective and cardioprotective benefits.[3]

There have been recent studies on horseradish and pancreatic cancer. Pancreatic cancer is one of the most dreaded cancers, especially since only 6% of those diagnosed with it live up to five years after the diagnosis.

From Pancreas to Prostate

The researchers tested pancreatic cells with horseradish extract alone and with a chemotherapy drug. They found the extract inhibited the growth of the pancreatic cancer cells and inhibited their pathway. The extract also increased the effectiveness of the chemotherapy drug against the cancer cells.[4]

Dr. Kizito told me he has had a lot of success using the moringa tree to combat prostate cancer.[5] What you do is rub the essential oil on the skin in the area of the prostate.

For other ailments, Dr. Kizito puts five drops of essential oil on the tongue.

Moringa also nourishes your skin. That's why Lelir uses it in her scrub. I recently came across an animal study that backs up the traditional Balinese use for horseradish tree. The extracts of the root and leaf relieve arthritis pain.[6]

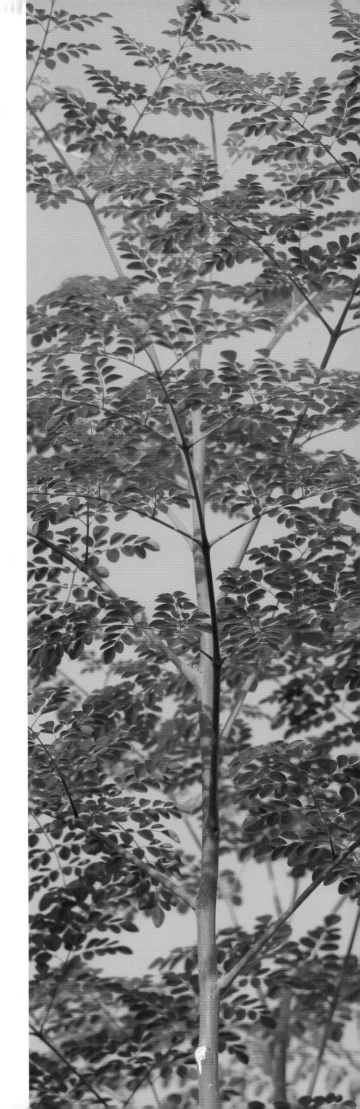

Westi's Balinese Moringa Soup

West told me: "For healing, the best quality of leaf to use is not the youngest or the oldest leaves, but those somewhere in the middle. They have the most nutrients and medicinal value."

So they use the young and old leaves as vegetables in their soup. And it's so simple to make.

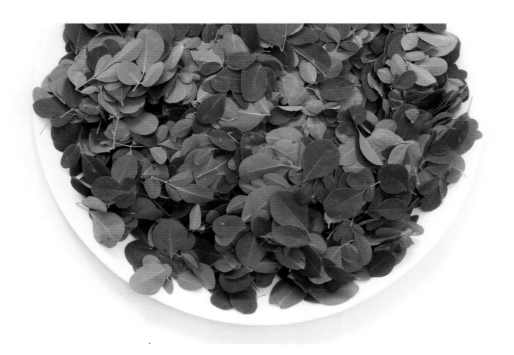

Take red onion, garlic, galangal, ginger, black pepper, pure coconut oil and salt in any combination you like.

Mix all of the ingredients together, add plain water and boil it all together.

Then, add the moringa leaves and even some fermented tempeh or tofu for a little bit of an Asian flavor.

Moringa

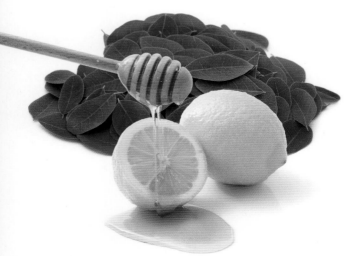

Westi's Antioxidant Juice

Put a small handful of fresh leaves in a blender with three glasses of water. Then add a little honey and lemon. Blend thoroughly. Drinking this juice gives your immune system a real boost.

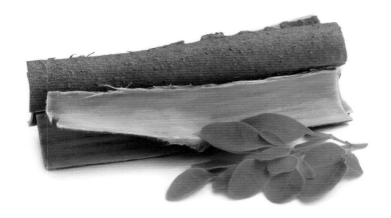

Lelir's Rheumatism Scrub

Using a mortar and pestle, grind together small amounts of each the following:

Bark of the horseradish tree	Clove leaves	Greater galangal root	Frangipani bark	Red rice

Mix the ground ingredients together thoroughly. Add enough water to make a paste. Massage into sore joints.

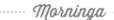
Moringa

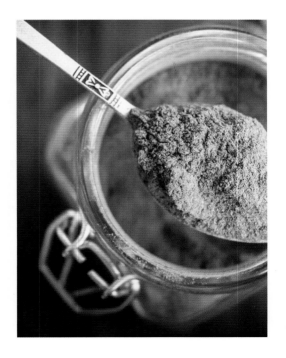

Hot & Cold Tea

Both hot and cold moringa tea are delicious. To make it cold, just add 1-2 tbsp of moringa leaf powder and a slice of fresh ginger root or some freshly squeezed lemon juice to 16 ounces of water. Stir thoroughly and allow it to sit for an hour to brew.

For hot moringa tea, use ½ to 1 teaspoon of moringa leaf powder in 8-12 ounces of hot water. Allow the tea to steep, covered for about 10 minutes.

When I tried it, I added a little bit of sweetener made from the African katemfe fruit, but a little honey will also do the trick.

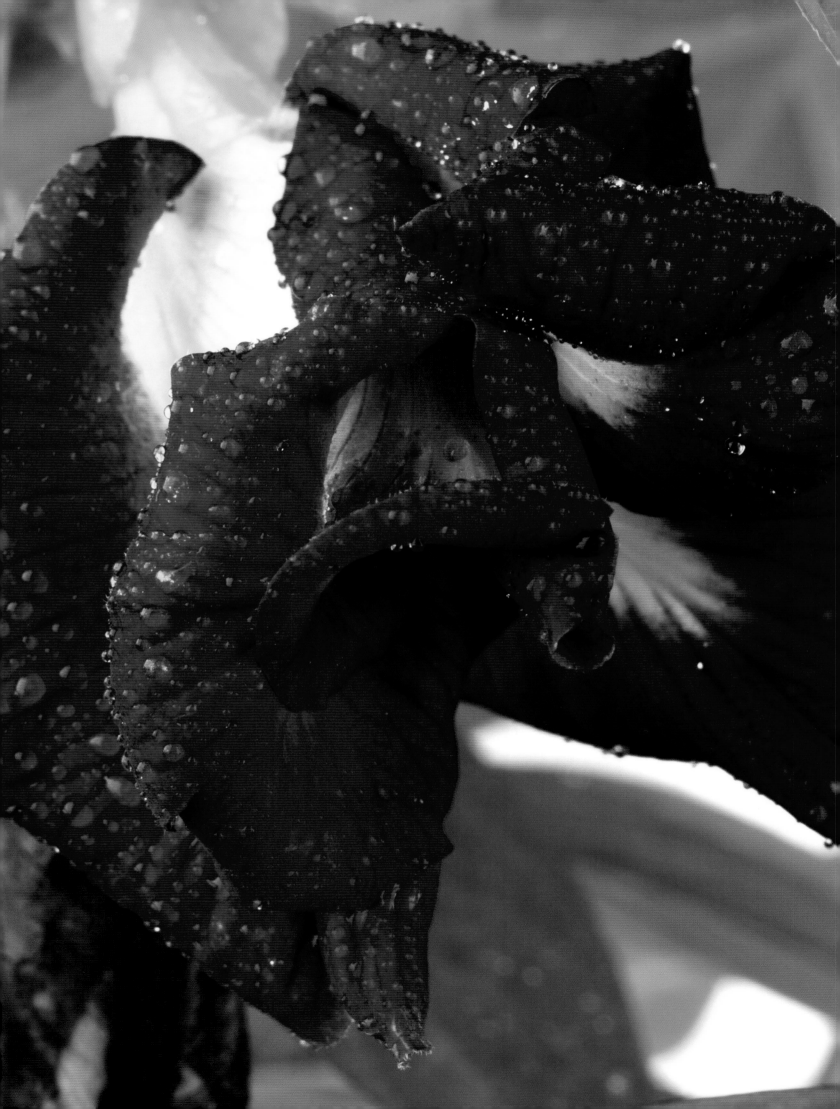

BRAIN POWER
IN A BEAUTIFUL BLUE PETAL

You can't get to Lelir and Westi's hometown of Ubud by plane. It's in the middle of the Balinese jungle.

You first land at the Bali Ngurah Rai Airport in Denpasar. Then you drive deep into the densest, greenest rainforest you've ever seen.

But first you have to land. What a ride! From the air it looked more like we were about to try to stop a marble going 300 miles per hour across the width of a desk.

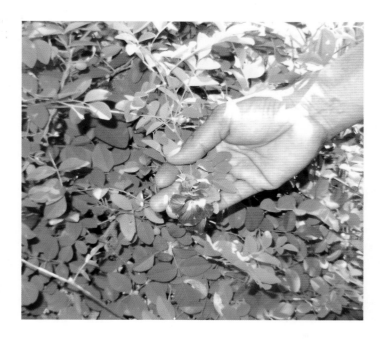

Westi showing me a butterfly pea from his garden.

> "I DON'T SCARE EASILY, BUT I WILL SAY I HAVE A BETTER APPRECIATION FOR OUR FIGHTER PILOTS WHO LAND PLANES ON AIRCRAFT CARRIERS."

I don't scare easily. But I will say that I have a better appreciation for our fighter pilots, who land planes on aircraft carriers.

Fortunately, the sliver of land on which the Denpasar airstrip is located also connects Bali to its tiny resort island of Kuta. It's a popular vacation hangout for vacationing Australians.

Have some fun and take a look at it on a map some time.

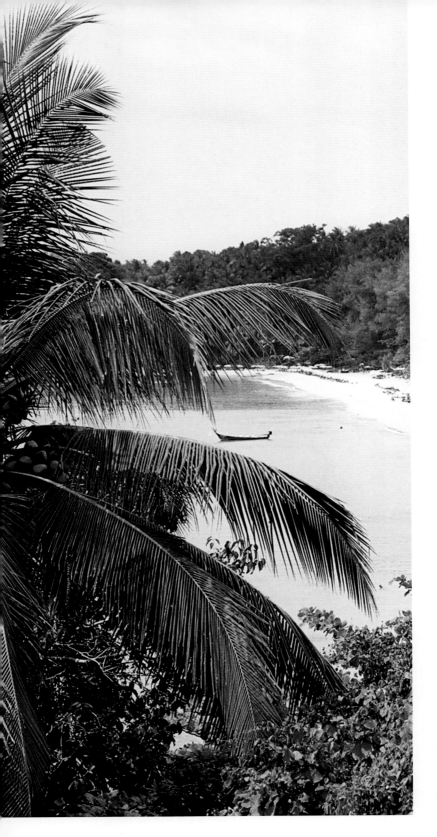

After relaxing on the beaches of the resort island of Kuta, I headed north through the jungle to Ubud.

After relaxing on the beach for a day of recovery, I headed north to Ubud. It was there in a quaint little village I got my last little bit of luxury before heading even farther into the jungles of Bali.

I've been in hotels all over the world and have had the privilege to stay at the very best. The Breakers in Palm Beach, the Ritz in Manhattan. In Los Angeles I've stayed where the Hollywood rich and famous stay.

But I have to admit, this Four Seasons was the most incredible hotel I've ever stayed in.

The hotel is a collection of buildings and cottages built into the cliffs that hang over the banks of the Ayung River.

Just getting to the lobby means crossing a very high bridge that hangs some 70 or 80 feet over the lush, dense greenery and the rushing water far below. At the end of it, there is a huge koi pond... which is on the roof of the lobby!

It was the most spectacular hotel I'd ever seen. It's built into the mountainside on various levels. Every level is open to the air — even the restaurant and rooms.

Everything is made from solid wood and looks handmade — all teak and mahogany, both of which grow wild on Bali. Teak is great for outdoors because it's very hard and water-resistant, which is why they use it on boats.

My room was a cottage at the bottom of the gorge, almost at river level. Every night, when I went to sleep in my open-air room, I fell asleep to the sound of the rushing river.

There were plants on top of plants and the mood is set by the sound of the river. I could have spent the entire time just relaxing there.

I was amazed by the sheer denseness of the green and the colors of the flowers.

My cottage was surrounded by star fruit, water apples, mangoes and gloriously tall coconut trees covered with green coconuts.

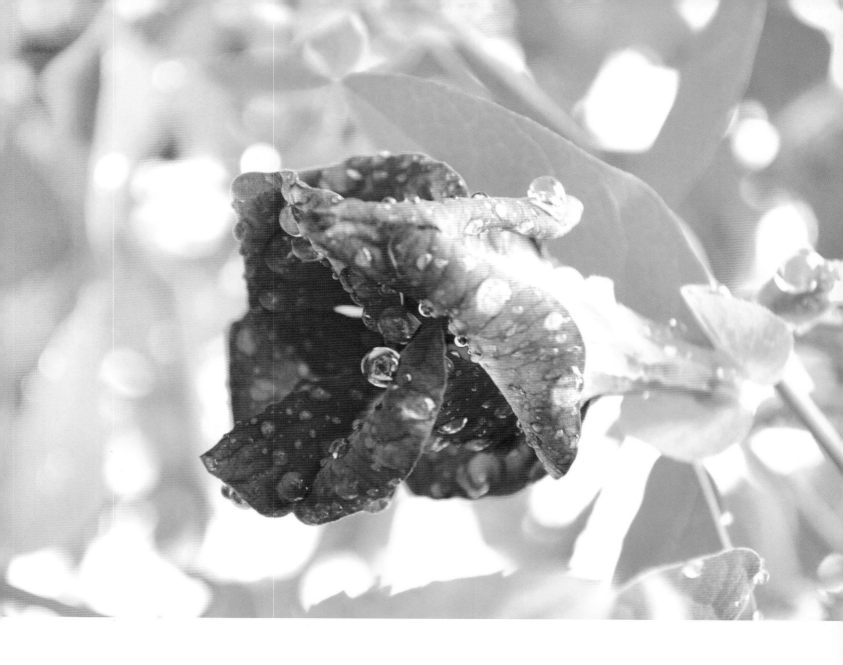

Flower Power of the Butterfly Pea

The most spectacular flower I saw was the butterfly pea, because of its deep purple color.

You can also see white, light purple and pink variations of this flower, which I discovered depends on the flavonoid concentration. Flavonoids are plant compounds that have a lot of health-enhancing and protective properties.

The butterfly pea is everywhere, because the vines grow wild and the Balinese use the flowers extensively. They use them to decorate the small cymbals for religious ceremonies, but the flowers are religious offerings themselves.

The Balian name for the flower, *Bunga telang,* comes from the Indonesian words for having clear vision. That's because besides being brain-boosting, among a host of other things, traditional herbalists on Bali use the roots to cure eye diseases and the flowers to cure eye infections like conjunctivitis.

Lelir explained the importance of the butterfly pea to Balinese tradition...

A Cultural and Medicinal Mainstay

(Clitoria ternatea)

Balinese name: Bunga telang

Bali is famous for its handicrafts — especially woodcarvings. If you walk into almost any shop near our beautiful beaches, you'll find hand-carved animals, masks and other figures.

But most of these carvings aren't made by artists. At least not by artists, as you might think of them. You see, in Bali most rice farmers also carve wood.

Our lovely island has always been Indonesia's breadbasket. We grow enough rice to feed our own families... the families of our neighbors... and many people beyond.

Growing rice — especially on terraced hillsides — is hard work. But it isn't work that pays the farmer well. So Balinese farmers have always had to find other ways to make ends meet between growing seasons.

When your island is covered with forests, carving wood is a natural choice. So our rice farmers carve many of the items they use around their homes. And many decorative objects to sell in the markets.

Other farmers create beautiful paintings. Their paintings reflect the vivid greens and blues of Bali... the jungle, the sea, and especially the sky. If you haven't seen the sky here, it's hard to describe. But it's an especially deep blue — almost like a jewel.

It isn't easy to find a color to match this shade of blue. But we have a secret that does it. The secret is a delicate flower we call "Bunga telang" — or butterfly pea.

Butterfly pea grows everywhere in Bali. It clings to shrubs and bushes growing around our rice fields. You'll also find it growing in or near temple gardens.

Its blooms are a deep blue and shaped a little like a butterfly. We make a dye from the flowers for painting and as a food coloring. We also use butterfly pea in religious ceremonies.

Dark blue and black are the colors of mourning in Bali. So the butterfly pea has become an important symbol at Balinese funerals. Offering butterfly peas in honor of a passed loved one is a sign of your respect and sadness.

Black is also the color we connect with the north and water. When the rainy season was late, our ancestors would offer butterfly pea flowers to Wisnu. They believed he brought the annual rains from the north, so they would present him with the deep blue blossoms to win back his good favor.

Our ancestors always preferred natural ways. Westi and I – along with many younger Balinese – understand the wisdom of this. We try to keep the natural traditions alive. Many of those traditions revolve around food.

The lovely blossoms of butterfly pea make a striking blue food coloring. Our ancestors used it to make a unique blue cake.

This may seem strange to you, since Western cakes are usually white (vanilla), yellow (richer, moister) or brown (chocolate). But Balinese cooks have always tried to make their food visually appealing... and one result is the blue cake we now serve on special occasions.

Of course, like so many other plants, the butterfly pea has medicinal uses. I learned how to use butterfly pea from my parents. It eases chronic itching and relieves conjunctivitis – or "pink eye."

To treat conjunctivitis, we pick the blossoms early in the morning. That's when it makes the strongest medicine. We take these fresh blossoms and steep them in a glass of clean water for about 20 minutes. Then we wash the eyes with the water.

This treatment usually clears up conjunctivitis within a few days.

I also use the same mild solution to ease itching. If your skin is itchy, just wash it with water used to steep butterfly pea blossoms. This will ease the itchiness quickly.

Because it's so soothing to the skin, I use butterfly pea to color some of my bath salt formulas, too.

In my studies at the university, I've discovered many Balinese herbal medicines are perfectly suited for traditional uses like these. Butterfly pea is a perfect example.

You might think that a flower used to make dyes is a strange choice to treat conjunctivitis. But research has shown that butterfly pea contains antimicrobial and anti-inflammatory compounds.

It also contains chemicals with anesthetic and anti-itching properties.

Best of all, butterfly pea is gentle and completely safe. It can't hurt the delicate tissues of your eyes. It doesn't even sting. It's my first choice for children who come down with pink eye.

— *Lelir*

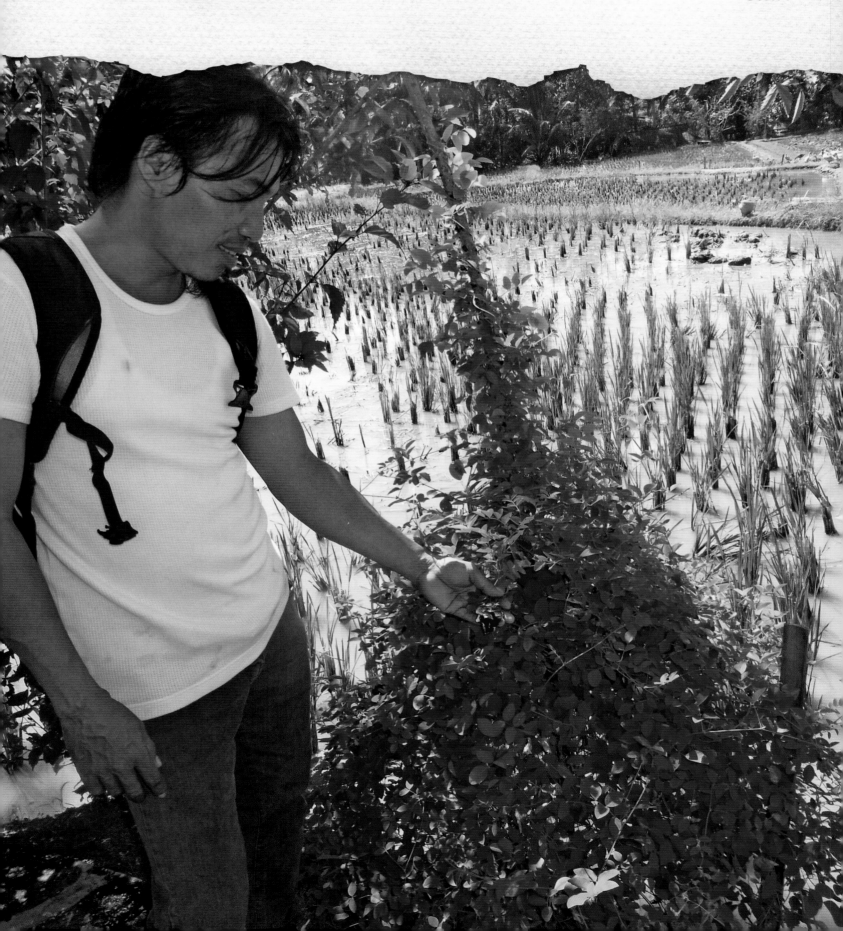

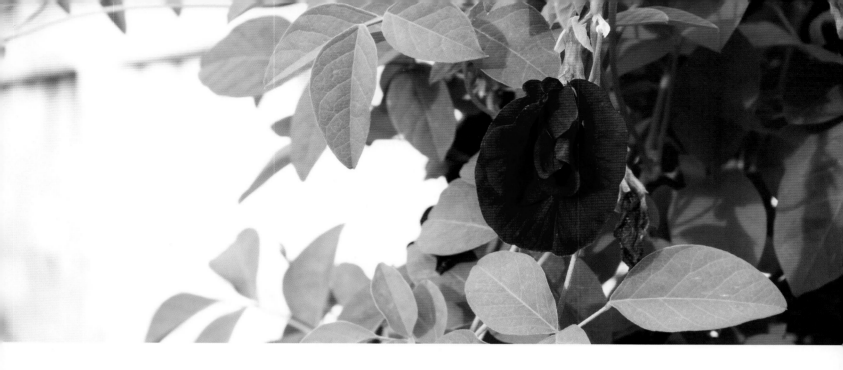

My Own Research and Discoveries

This is one plant that has so many healing properties, I could probably write a book about it alone.

Memory booster	Anti-inflammatory
Lowers blood pressure	Pain relieving
Antistress	Diuretic
Anti-anxiety	Anesthetic
Antidepressant	Lowers blood sugar
Antimicrobial	Insecticidal
Antipyretic	Anti-asthmatic

They use all parts of the plant on Bali. The roots, seeds, flowers and leaves have been used for centuries.

Butterfly pea is one of the few plants that has *cyclotides* in it. These are peptides that have antitumor properties and cause cancer cell death because they can penetrate the cancer cell membrane.

A recent study at the Chinese Academy of Medical Sciences in Beijing found butterfly pea to be very effective against certain lung cancer cell lines.[1]

Dry the leaves and grind them to a fine powder and, much like the famous extract of the periwinkle flower (vinpocetine), butterfly pea will enhance your memory and brain power and give you a calm, relaxed focus.[2]

Bali's Secret Salad Sensation

Natural medicines aren't studied in the U.S. as much as they are in the rest of the world, so I had to keep digging through the research to find out why butterfly pea is so powerful. Finally, I discovered that a team of researchers from India found that butterfly pea increases levels of the neurotransmitter, acetylcholine.[3]

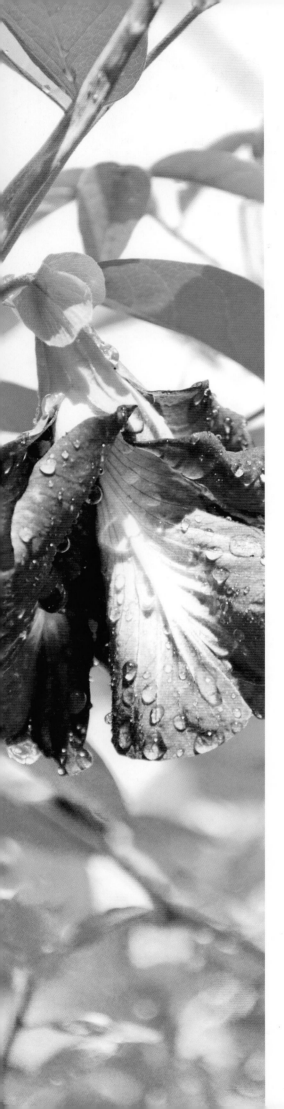

This is important for anti-aging, because acetylcholine is one of the brain chemicals that decreases the most with age. It's crucial for communication within the brain. A lack of it causes messages to travel slowly, to break down or stop traveling all together. That's why loss of memory and coordination as you age is a common consequence of low acetylcholine levels.

Butterfly pea reverses that. So it improves your thinking and balance naturally.

Traditional teas made from the leaves also improve eyesight and help relieve sore eyes.

And when you grind the leaves up with salt, it's a remedy for swelling.

The leaves, when you put them in a salad, will also improve digestion.

The butterfly pea has an unusual way of creating a seed. The flower dries itself on the vine, then turns into a bean pod. Seeds from these pods can be planted to grow a new vine.

You can use all the parts of the plant in salads or grind the leaves with a little water and use the liquid as natural food color.

To make your own Balinese purple dye from butterfly pea flowers, begin by placing a flower at the bottom of a small glass. Add a little bit of water, then push and grind at the flower with a spoon. The water will turn a bit blue. Then add a few drops of lemon or lime juice and the acid will make your dye turn purple.

When you add this to food, the result is a beautiful shade of light purple. The Balinese use it to color jams and even rice cakes.

I've also made a drink with butterfly pea flowers, added it in salads, and when I was in Bali, I ate the flowers picked fresh off the vine.

As I mentioned, the powder is very effective as well. Clitoria ternatea is one of four herbs traditionally used in an Ayurvedic brain-boosting mixture, called *Shanka Pushpi*.

Both the water and fat-soluble components appear to be bioactive and have been shown to enhance memory. So to get the full effect, eat butterfly pea components with a meal.

Balinese "Blue" Recipe

One of the most colorful desserts I had at a restaurant in Bali
was a serving of "blue" rice topped with coconut. I found out how they made it:

·· *Butterfly Pea* ··

Ingredients:

1 pound of rice	30 bunga telang flowers	5 ounces of coconut milk	½ tablespoon of salt
1 pound of grated coconut	8 ounces of palm sugar	8 ounces of powdered sugar	1 tablespoon of rice flour

Instructions:

1. First, you boil the butterfly pea flowers in water.

2. Cool the blue water and pour over the rice.

3. Soak the rice for an hour.

4. Strain and steam rice over high heat for half hour.

5. Pour the coconut milk and salt over the rice and mix well.

6. Cover the rice and steam for another 20 minutes. Let it cool and serve with banana leaves.

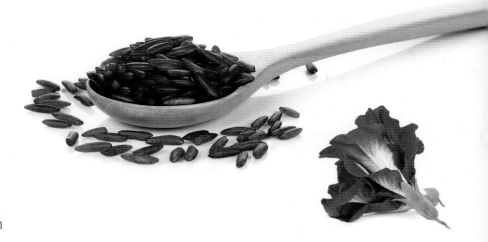

Now, melt the sugar in around 3 or so ounces of water.

Grate the coconut and add it in to the melted sugar.

Put the mixture over medium heat for 10 minutes or until it's sticky-looking.

Add the rice flour Blnd stir, then cool.

Roll the coconut/sugar/rice mixture into a ball and place it on top of the blue rice and serve.

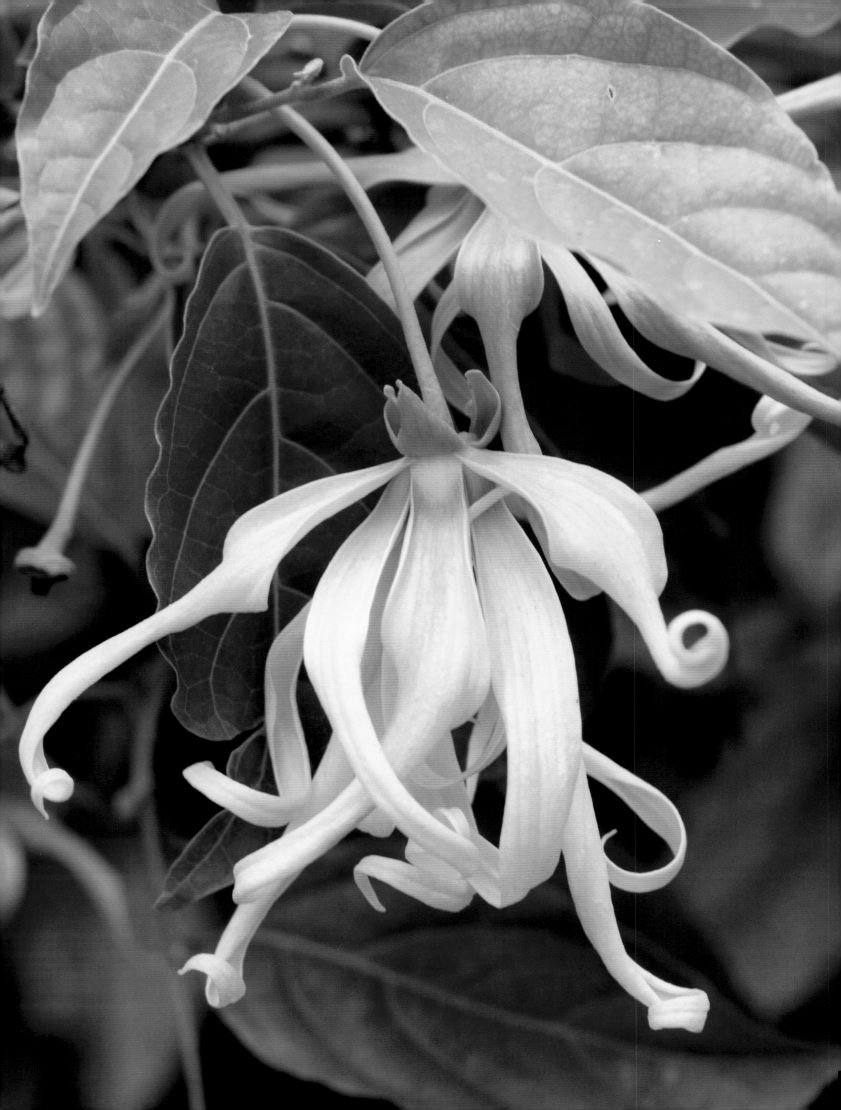

BALI'S JADE ORCHID: A HEALING PERFUME

While we were walking around Westi and Lelir's garden, a man ran up us. He was out of breath and sweat was pouring off of his forehead. His face glistened in the sun.

He said something in Indonesian and Lelir quickly ran into the house with him. The man ran out with a jar of tea and disappeared into the forest.

Westi turned to me. "That man's son has a fever. Lelir gave him a *champak* tea she made from the bark a few days ago. It helps reduce most fevers here on Bali." Westi showed me their champak tree. It wasn't in bloom, but it still had a wonderful smell.

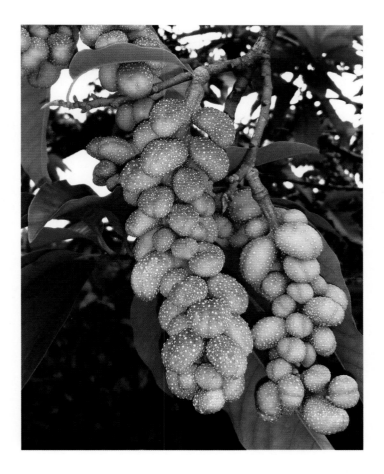

The champak tree, as well as its fruit and flowers, are truly beautiful, but they also contain a bundle of health benefits.

No Wonder it's Called the "Joy Perfume Tree..."

I learned about a similar tree called magnolia champaca, which has bigger flowers. But it's not as aromatic. They got the "joy perfume" name from the velvety leaves of the michelia flower, which is also known as the yellow jade orchid.

The champak tree has fruit, which looks like a cluster of big bumpy grapes. They ripen in late August and you can see them for sale in the markets on Bali throughout the fall.

Like most of the beautiful and fragrant flowers and plants on Bali, behind champak's lovely exterior is something even better: a bundle of health benefits.

Ease Fever and Promote Calm

(Michelia champaca)

Balinese name: Cempaka

We Balinese women are very lucky. Like most women, we like to smell good. But we don't have to buy our perfume from a department store. We have many perfumes growing right in our gardens.

One of my favorite scents is cempaka – or champak. In warm weather, champak trees come alive with deep yellow blooms and their scent fills the air.

It's quite a sight to see, because champak is no little bush. These evergreen trees can grow to 60 feet or more. So when a champak is in full bloom, there are hundreds of blossoms.

Champak is a close relative of the magnolia. The flowers are smaller, but the scent is just as strong. Champak is even used in some very expensive perfumes.

But in Bali – and in India, too – champak has a spiritual purpose. The essential oil made from the blossoms has a calming and balancing effect.

Priests often make a kind of scented water from champak blossoms. They sprinkle it on people as a blessing… or give them some to drink to bring peace and balance to their lives. This is why you'll see a champak tree growing just outside many temples in Bali.

I remember when I was growing up, champak was very important in our spiritual lives. My family would gather champak blossoms to make offerings at the temple. And if my parents wanted to show respect to someone special, they would put a champak flower in the person's hair. Because the champak blossom is holy, this is a sign of special honor.

Away from the cities, Bali is very peaceful at night. It isn't necessarily quiet, because the forest sounds are there… but it is peaceful. This is the best time to meditate, because there are so few distractions.

So sometimes my parents would go to the temple at night to meditate. And when they did, they usually brought champak flowers with them. As they sat quietly in the temple, the flowers' scent would fill the air.

The peacefulness of the temple and the flowers' perfume created a perfect atmosphere for meditation. My parents always came home from these experiences feeling calm, refreshed and renewed.

My mother and father also taught me other uses for champak.

The root is a purgative and good for clearing the bowels. My parents also used the flower to treat kidney disease. And you can make a tea from the bark to reduce fever. We've found champak works on most types of fever.

Champak is also excellent at healing and closing wounds and other sores. Cuts, scrapes and ulcers can all be healed. My mother taught me to grind the flowers, extract the juice and apply it on wounds or sores once daily. In a few days, the wound will be well on its way to closing and healing very cleanly.

— *Lelir*

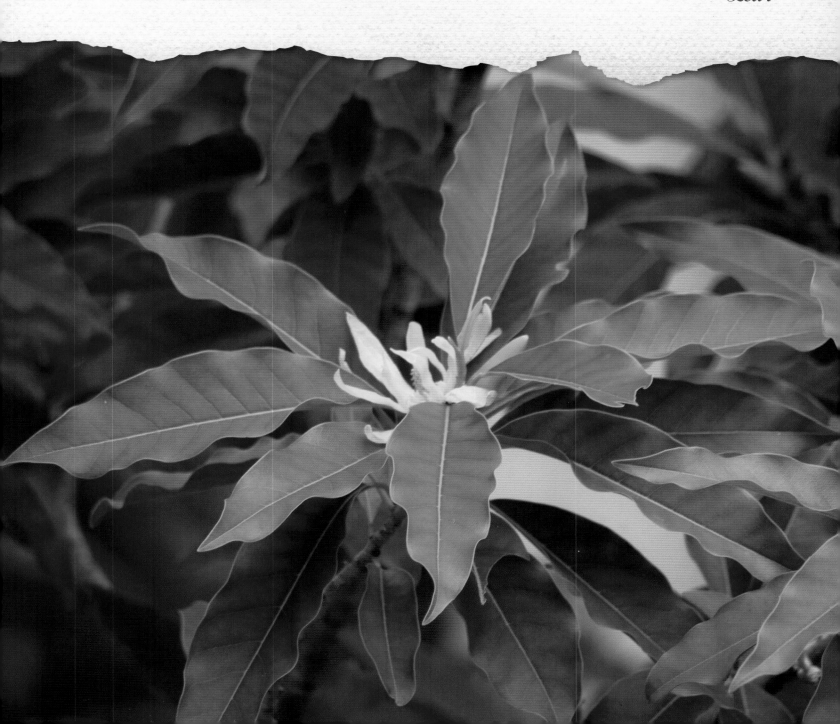

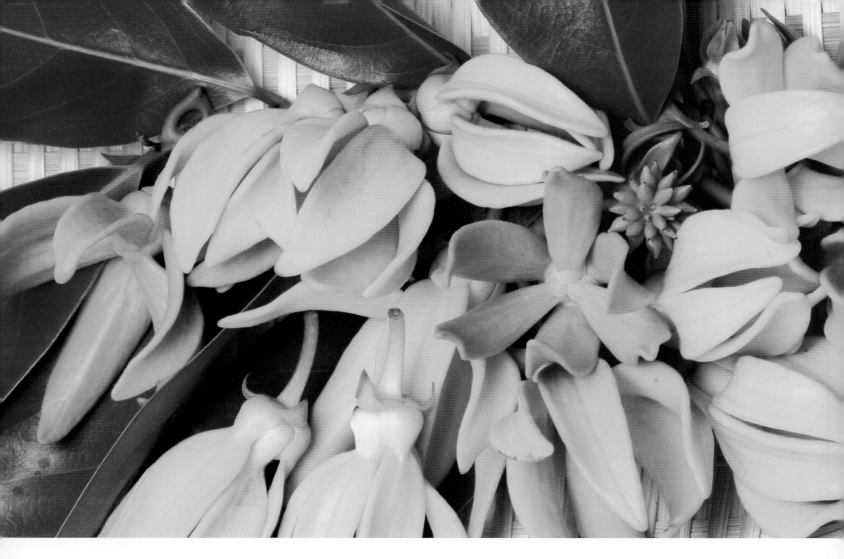

One of the world's most expensive perfumes, 'Joy,' uses this tree's blossoms in its formula.

My Own Research and Discoveries

Champak blossoms contain the powerful antioxidant, quercetin.[1] This is the same antioxidant in green tea. It has strong anti-inflammatory effects.

The flowers themselves are also powerfully anti-inflammatory.[2] They contain beta-sitosterol. Both quercetin and beta-sitosterol protect the prostate. These compounds have been shown to prevent prostate cancer and prostate enlargement (BPH).

Scientists in Papua New Guinea discovered that most parts of champak have antibacterial powers. The leaves, stems and root bark kill molds and fungi, too.[3]

In another study, researchers looked at the constituents of champak, and found that liriodenine is one of the more active compounds from the root and bark of the tree. Liriodenine is antibacterial and fights infection.

Quite a few studies show that champak is very effective for wound healing and cleansing.[4]

In India, champak is used to control blood sugar. University researchers recently put it to the test. They gave champak to two groups of rats. The first group had very high blood sugar. The second group had normal blood sugar.

After getting champak, the group with high blood sugar showed much lower blood-sugar levels. The animals with healthy blood sugar remained normal.[5]

Champak grows well in sunny areas and only requires a moderate amount of water. And it does well in temperatures down to the low 30s. If you live in a warm climate — like South Florida or Southern California — you might be able to grow it in your yard.

Champak makes an attractive addition to any garden. And when it's in bloom, the scent will promote feelings of peace and calm.

One of the world's most expensive perfumes, Joy, uses this tree's blossoms in its formula.

It's ironic that its beautiful scent, which women use to attract men, is used by women in India as a form of birth control.

An animal study found that champak has steroid-like compounds and high estrogenic activity, which make fetus implantation nearly impossible.[6]

In 2011, a study looked at many of the active components in the champak tree and found some of them showed high activity against breast and lung cancer cells.[7] It will be interesting to see the results of that research in the future.

This tree can be massive, and as Lelir said, many Hindus and Buddhists plant these trees near their temples. If you could make a bonsai tree out of it and stick it in your home, you'd have a delightful smell all year around.

Plus you could make tea that cures fever from the tree bark.

All you have to do is boil the bark powder for a few minutes,
then strain into a container and drink twice per day.

Champak

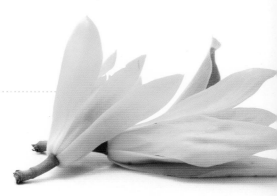

To make tea from flowers for indigestion:

Boil the flowers for 10 minutes and then let it steep for 10 more.

Cool and drink once a day for 3 days.

Or you can put the flowers in water overnight, then it's ready to drink.

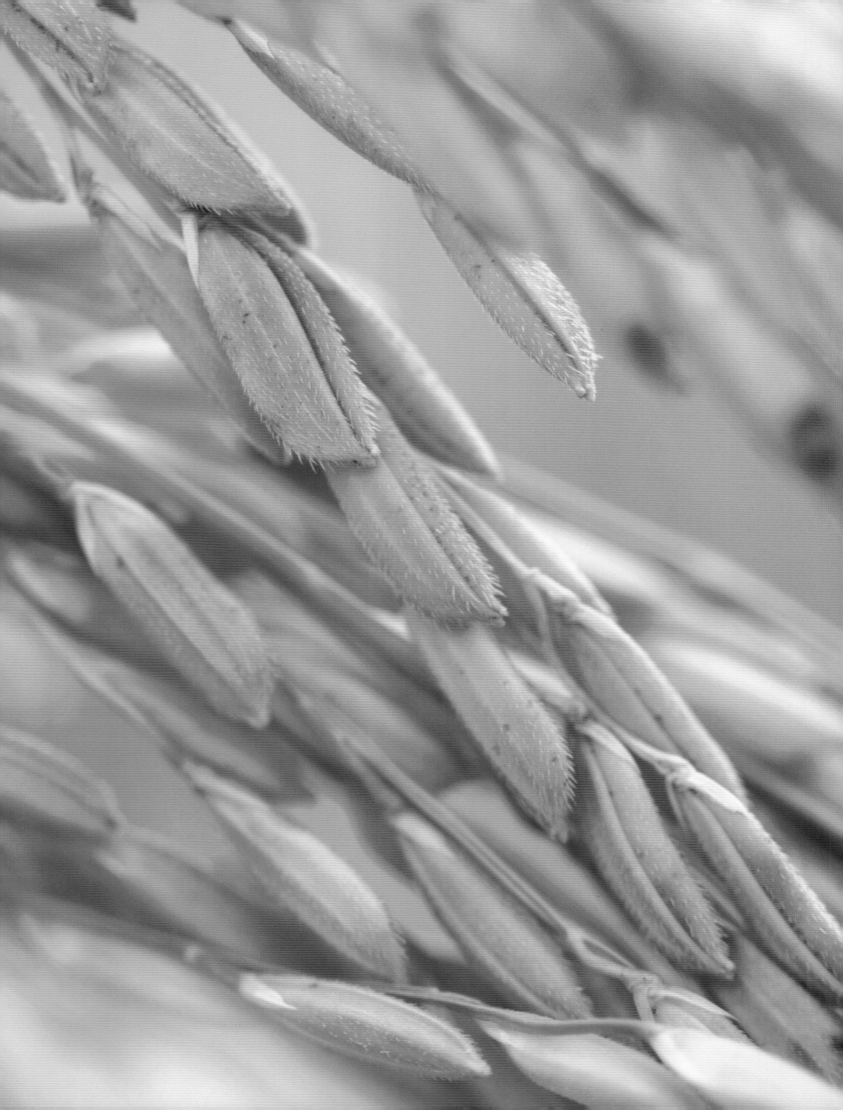

ANCIENT BALINESE GRAIN HAS HUGE HEART BENEFITS

Westi comes from a family of farmers. He's concerned about the use of fertilizers and the commercialization of the rural tradition of farming.

Farming has been their sustenance, and their main crop is rice, which they grow in terraced paddies. They also grow fruit trees and vegetables in little sections of those terraced paddies. The plots of land are pretty self-sufficient. They'll have chickens and a pig, and they barter with their neighbors. It's been that way for thousands of years.

"INCLUDING RICE INSTEAD OF OTHER GRAINS CAN JUST ABOUT CHOP YOUR RISK FOR HEART–RELATED ILLNESS IN HALF."

It Worked Very Well... Until Tourism Started

Developers started pushing the farmers out to use the land for the tourism industry. The remaining farmers started to use fertilizer on the land that was left to try to get more out of it. But Westi told me that when you use fertilizer, you get increased production for only a couple of years and then the land stops producing.

The reason is that it's a very fragile system. The water comes from rain — it's basically a tropical rainforest. The water falls in the mountains and flows downhill from there, and they use it to irrigate the rice fields.

They have canals that flood the paddies, which they open and close as needed for rice planting. They only flood the paddies when the rice has already grown and when they're composting.

And the traditional rice farmers use "organic pesticide." You and I call them ducks.

Instead of spraying chemicals on their rice, a staple of Balinese diet, they have done the same thing for thousands of years. They flood the fields and let the ducks in, and the ducks eat the insects. They eat anything that might be a pest and, in the process, their manure provides nitrogen and fertilization for the soil.

Then the farmers drain the fields, dry them and replant. And the whole process is started over.

One of the really amazing things I found on Bali is that there is always water. It comes down from the mountains and there are ancient stones that divert tiny slivers of the streams to water different plants and crops.

There used to be fights and feuds over water usage, but now they have a national system that maintains and regulates the flow of the water to get it to where it's needed. So now everybody gets an equal share.

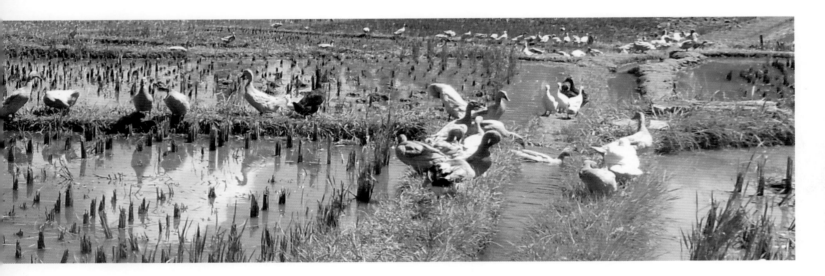

Rice farmers on Bali use ducks as an "organic pesticide," instead of spraying the kind toxic chemicals we have in the West.

You Can Hear Running Water Everywhere

The streams run for miles, and every so often they break off a little tributary to water a different field. Communal associations all share the water.

In this way, they use the existing irrigation system, which they never have to change, to go through the cycles they need to grow their rice crop.

The rice has to be wet at certain times and the fields have to be dry at other times. So they block and release the water as they need it. Sometimes they even grow other things in the dry fields between rice harvests.

It's an ingenious system that has worked well for millennia... and Westi tells me it gives them a very healthy and nutritious brand of rice.

Rice — More than Just a Grain

(Oryza sativa)

Balinese name: Padi

When you visit Bali, you'll find almost everything is different. Even time.

The traditional Balinese calendar — called Pakuwan — has 30 seven-day weeks. Once every 210 days — or once a year by the traditional calendar — we celebrate an important holiday.

Galungan celebrates the triumph of dharma (order) over disorder. The legends say that the god, Indra, came to Earth at this time to defeat an evil king, who had banished religion and brought great suffering to Bali.

Galungan lasts for 10 days. During this time, all the Balinese people honor their ancestors and the Hindu gods. It's a time of celebration and we decorate our homes and temples.

Walking down the streets in Bali, you'll see arches made of bamboo poles along the roads. People hang offerings from the poles and erect shrines at their bases.

During this celebration, many people believe the spirits of their ancestors visit their old homes. So we hold big family gatherings, pray at the village temples and visit with friends who have shown the family kindness.

Many young men also enjoy drinking brem during the Galungan holiday. Brem is a sort of wine fermented from rice.

To make brem, we take black Balinese rice and mix it with a little lime (pulverized limestone, not the fruit). Then we wrap this mixture in banana leaves and let it ferment for at least five days.

After five days, we unwrap the rice, making sure to save the liquid. The rice itself is delicious, with a sort of sweet and sour flavor. The liquid is the brem.

Sometimes, people mix brem with alcohol made from coconut palms. This makes a very powerful liquor we call "arak attack." It's 60% – 70% alcohol, so you can't drink very much.

We use rice for much more than making wine, of course. It's also the grain that feeds half the world's people.

Rice is extremely digestible. It is very gentle on the stomach. Plain rice is also a gluten-free grain, so people with celiac disease can eat it safely.

Rice flour – made by grinding rice – is the basis for most Balinese sweets. This makes them a little healthier than most of the wheat-based sweets in the West.

The rice plant – not just the grain – is also medicinal. To get rid of head lice, burn rice straw till it's black and then grind it to powder. Use this powder as a shampoo. It's remarkably effective.

You can chew young rice shoots to clear up indigestion.

We brew a tea from rice and galangal for young children who don't feel well. We crush the rice and galangal with a mortar and pestle and steep the tea till it's cool enough to drink. Then just strain off the solids.

You can also brew a tea from the roots of the rice plant. This tea is very effective for bringing down fevers. As my mother has gotten older, we use this remedy whenever she feels feverish. It's very gentle and has no side effects.

— *Westi*

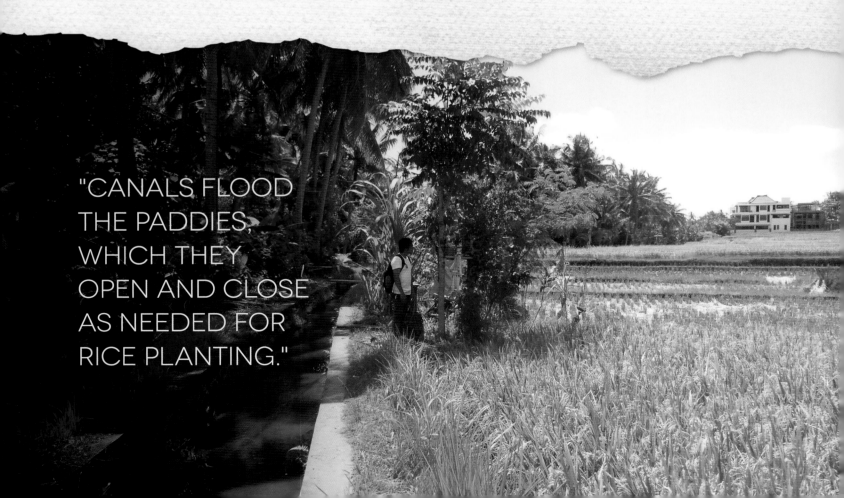

"CANALS FLOOD
THE PADDIES,
WHICH THEY
OPEN AND CLOSE
AS NEEDED FOR
RICE PLANTING."

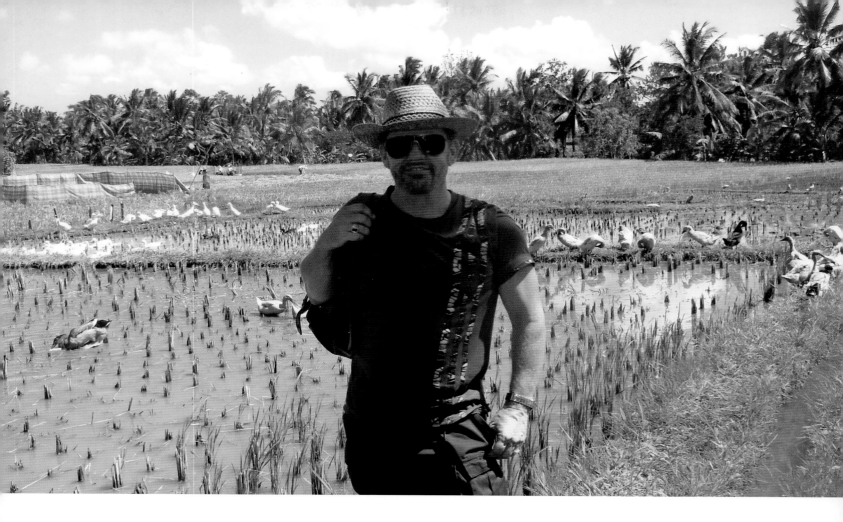

Westi took me on a tour of the rice paddies near Ubud. Rice has been the main staple on Bali since ancient times.

My Own Research and Discoveries

Westi has taken it upon himself to return to the native, natural systems that worked beautifully on Bali for thousands of years.

He's very educated and he's a treasure trove of knowledge about herbs.

He's got a college degree in agriculture and he gives tours to teach people farming the traditional way.

He shows visitors how the water system works, and how to rotate crops. And he reveals how, even in the 21st century, it's still possible to be completely self-sufficient in a relatively small space.

Westi wants to build a resort on the land he's inherited from his father and grandfather.

He wants it to be a healing center, a house where people can come for treatments, massage and herbal therapy. It will be focused on wellness and teaching sustainability, but the tourists will also get to take home fresh herbs from his private garden, which he took me to see.

They have two gardeners there to protect the plants and to pick what Lelir and Westi need to make their products.

Some of the herbs they grow are not well-known in the U.S. But even though rice is widely available in the states, it contains health benefits you may not know about.

For example, did you know that rice seeds can be anti-inflammatory?

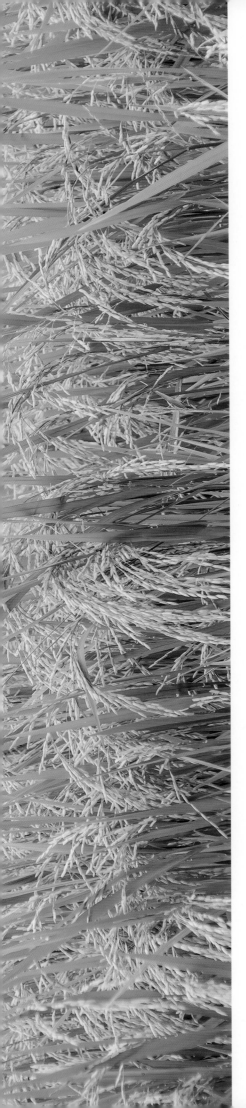

One recent study on mice shows that rice seeds suppress TNF-alpha, an inflammatory compound that is associated with arthritis and Crohn's disease.[1]

It also seems to help lower triglycerides, the blood fats that can lead to inflammatory and chronic disease, by as much as 30%.[2]

The journal, *PLoS One,* published a joint study by Harvard University and the Chinese Center for Disease Control and Prevention. It shows that for just about any measure of heart health you can think of, including rice instead of other grains can just about chop your risk for heart-related illness in half.

The study looked at more than 15,000 people from China. Those who favored eating rice over soy, wheat or starchy grains and tubers were:[3]

- 50% less likely to be obese.
- 51.9% less likely to have metabolic syndrome.
- 37.9% less likely to have high blood pressure.
- 41.5% less likely to have blood sugar problems.
- 14.5% less likely to have high triglycerides.
- 39.8% more likely to have higher heart-protective HDL cholesterol.

Also, the rice plant can help naturally ferment other foods. When the Japanese make natto, their natural soy food, they lay the cooked soybeans on cooked rice straw and tie the package shut to let a little heat and oxygen ferment it naturally.

I don't recommend eating rice as the main part of any meal, though. The Balinese use it in their dishes, but not as the main component.

The trick is to eat wild rice, which has a much lower glycemic load than processed white rice. That way, you get the benefits of rice without the inflammation or blood-sugar spike. Wild rice isn't always brown, by the way, so make sure you know what you're getting.

Also, coconut flour and almond flour are excellent choices to replace flour from wheat, bran, buckwheat, millet and other grains if you want bread. But if you can't find them, rice flour makes a good alternative.

How to Make Perfect Bali Rice

Westi and Lelir prepare their rice the way the Balinese have for centuries.

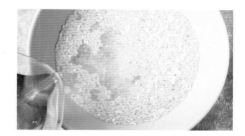

Rice

In the morning, Lelir washes the rice for a good 15 minutes. **To prepare it like she does,** you put the rice in a container or bowl, pour water in until the rice is just barely covered, and then get your hands right in there and knead it for a few minutes.

Let it rest for a few minutes and then repeat a couple of times.

Pour off the water and refill the bowl with fresh water, then let it stand for a good eight hours.

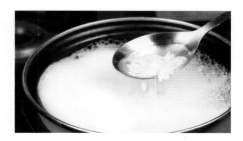

Pour the rice and water into a stock pan over medium heat and simmer until the water cooks off. You can add turmeric or ginger for a bit of flavoring.

Remove from heat and allow to cool and you have perfect rice.

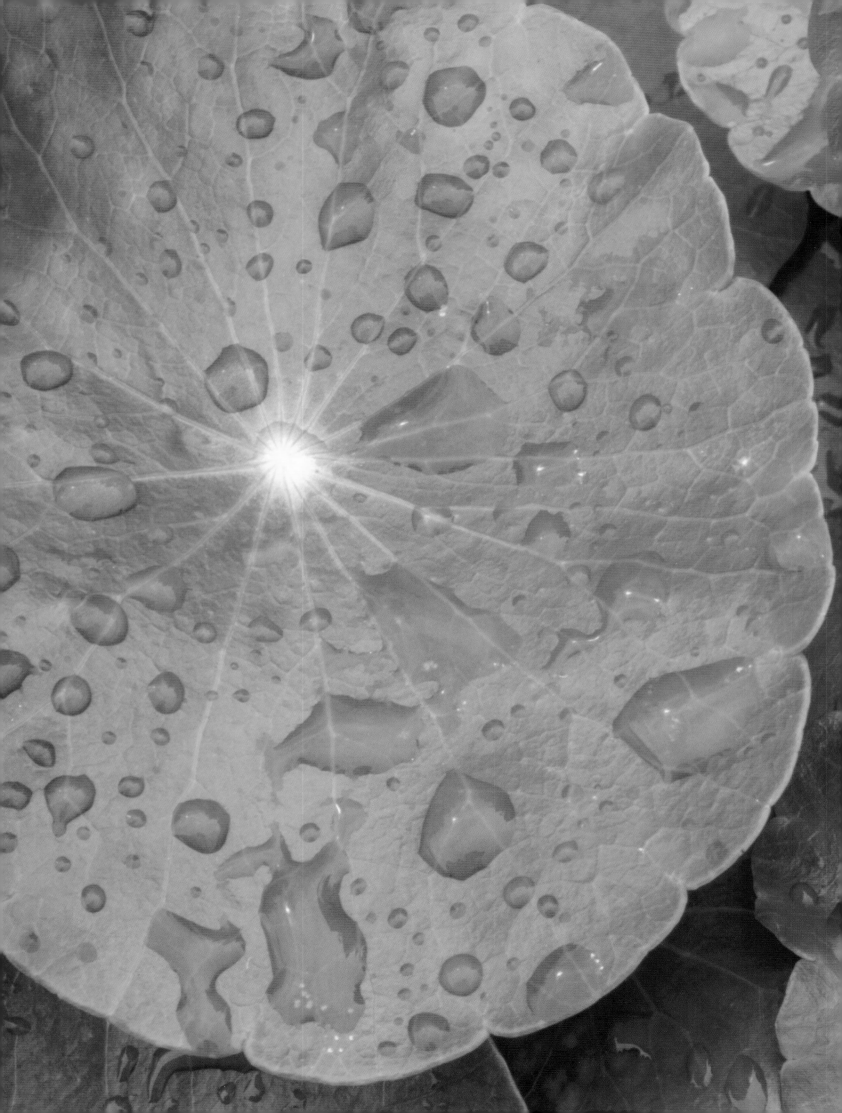

BALINESE SECRET FOR BETTER MOOD AND MEMORY

As I've mentioned, you can't fly into Ubud, Westi and Lelir's hometown. So I began my journey on Bali in Kuta, a popular hangout for Australian surfers.

From Kuta, I ventured deep into the lush rain forest. The mood was set by the incredible greenery and the sound of rivers rushing through deep gorges.

I could have stayed in Kuta and spent my entire trip just relaxing there. But it was time to trek higher to Ubud and from there, deeper into the jungle...

Medical Myth Shattered in Sacred Monkey Forest

One of the first places I wanted to see was the Sacred Monkey Forest of Padangtegal. It's an ancient Hindu religious site, but it's also the home of a species of monkey that helped us discover something very important for your brain.

The Forest of Padangtegal is really only 27 acres, but it has a hundred species of trees, a Hindu temple and the long-tailed macaque monkey. There are 605 of them there and they live in "troops."

They're fascinating, because some will come out and have a little interaction with the visitors, while others never have any contact with people.

I wanted to see them because of a study I read by Princeton biologists Elizabeth Gould and Charles Gross.

You see, for years, science believed that the adult human brain could not grow new brain cells. They thought we were born with all the brain cells we'll ever have — and that when the cells are gone, they're gone for good.

The study, published in the *Journal of Science,* detailed a new discovery by the biologists — the daily growth of new brain cells in the adult macaque monkey.

Because of this discovery, we now know your brain can grow new cells.

This is very important, because our brains shrink as we age.

Over the course of your life, your brain will lose five to 10% of its weight. The shrinkage starts around your 20th birthday.

Today, we can help prevent this consequence of aging by renewing the growth factors that decline with age. This is the best way to slow down brain shrinkage.

And we can do it with an herb that's native to Bali and Southeast Asia, just as macaque monkeys do.

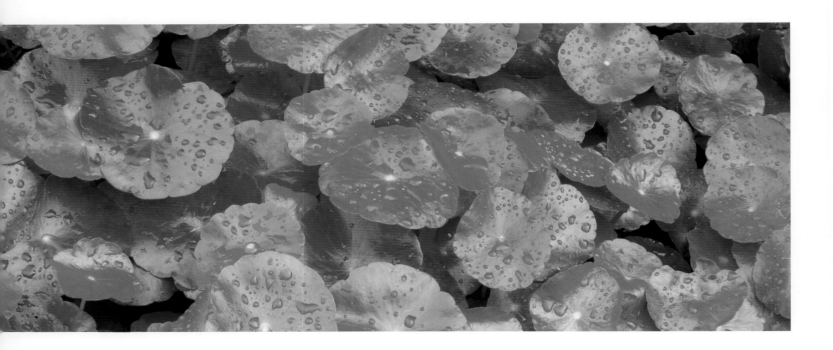

Ayurvedic Herb Grows New Brain Cells

It's an herb called *gotu kola.*

When I traveled to India, I found gotu kola there, too. It's one of the most important herbs in the oldest system of medicine in the world, Ayurveda medicine.

As I've said before, I always have faith that something works when I see the same tradition of use spring up in totally unrelated places around the world.

Ayurveda also uses goto kola to reduce anxiety, reduce fever and treat skin conditions. It also improves circulation and has an ancient link to longevity... Westi tells me that his ancestors believed elephants who ate gotu kola leaves lived longer than those that didn't.

However, it's the brain-boosting activity of gotu kola that makes it most interesting for me.

I know losing memory and brain power are two of my patients' top concerns.

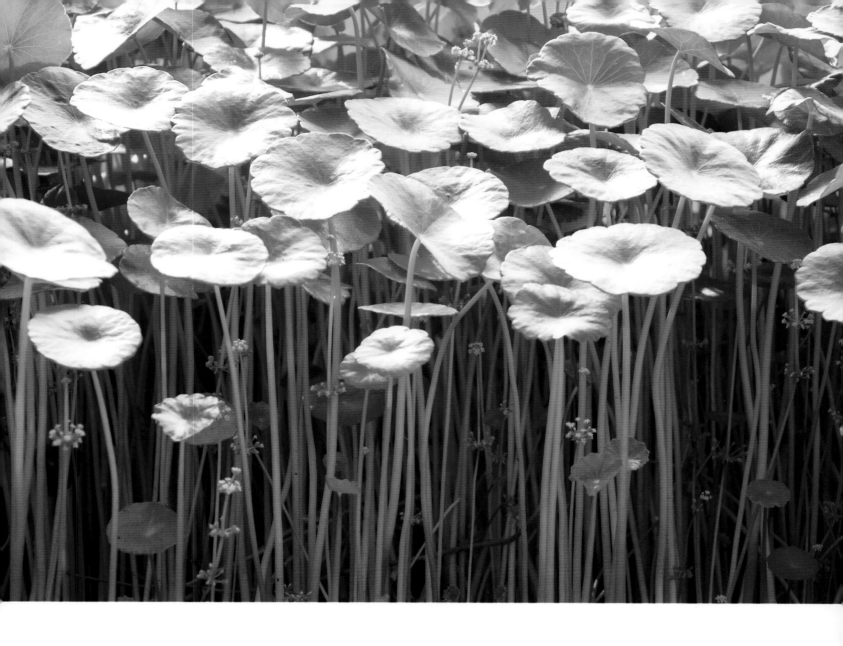

So I was pleased to find clinical trials that show gotu kola can help spur growth in brain cells.

In a recent study, gotu kola extract helped increase neurite growth in mouse brain cells, proving that the extract was responsible for this growth.[1,2]

In a new study on human brain cells, researchers treated the cells with different concentrations of an extract of gotu kola (centella asiatica).[3]

However, there is also another healing benefit of gotu kola. Contained in the gotu kola plant is asiatic acid, which has been known to fight and induce cell death in tumors. In a recent study, asiatic acid was also found to inhibit the growth of non-small lung cancer cells.[4]

Gotu Kola is used by the locals as something of a "first-aid kit" with many traditional uses. Westi gave me the inside story on some of them...

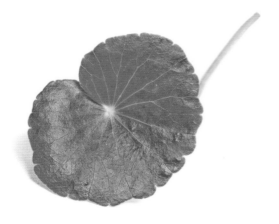

Herbal First-Aid Kit

(Daun piduh)

Balinese name: Gotu Kola

Most visitors to Bali spend much of their time along our beautiful southern coast. This is understandable. The main airport is just outside Denpasar in the south. Our southern beaches are truly a paradise. And there are many modern hotels nearby.

Far fewer visitors make it here to Ubud in Bali's interior. But even fewer get all the way to the northern side of the island. That's a shame, because Bali's northern coast is unique.

In the north, there are lovely black sand beaches. There is little surf here, so it's a wonderful place to swim. In the mornings, you can catch a boat that will take you out to see the dolphins. Along the coast here, you can also dive or snorkel on the colorful coral reefs teaming with sea life.

There are also lovely spots to stop along the roadway from Denpasar to Singaraja on the northern coast. One is located about halfway between the mountain resort of Bedugul and Singaraja. It is called Gitgit Waterfalls.

When the Dutch ruled our island, many years ago, this area was a resort just for the rich landowners. The cool, refreshing waters seemed like a perfect spa for Europeans not used to Bali's heat and humidity.

Now these beautiful falls are for everyone. And they are a very special place to visit.

Today, there is a sign along the road and a parking area. You can drive to within about a 20-minute walk from the falls.

Don't be fooled by what you see along the first half of your walk, though. The government built a long concrete walkway – consisting of hundreds of steps – to make the walk easier for visitors. And one side of this walkway is lined with little stalls selling handmade crafts and soft drinks.

But as you get closer to the falls, you'll see the old Bali. Bushes and trees grow on both sides of the pathway here. You may notice the scents of nearby clove and vanilla plantations. The air gets cooler as you descend to the falls... they act like a natural air conditioner.

Gitgit is actually two falls. But you have to take a much harder hike to the upper falls.

Most visitors are satisfied viewing the lower falls. They tumble down about 115 feet into a small rocky basin.

The basin is surrounded by trees. Sometimes you can spot troops of wild monkeys who've come to drink the cool water. And here in the basin, the sound of rushing water is everywhere.

You may be tempted to take a swim... and swimming is allowed. But you should know about a local legend. According to the story, any couple who swim together at the falls will not stay together for long. This legend gives a whole new meaning to the saying, "Swim at your own risk."

On your climb back up to the parking area, watch along the pathway for a low, ground-hugging vine. It has bright green kidney-shaped leaves growing from a reddish stem. In season, it blooms with small white flowers.

This is daun piduh, or gotu kola.

Gotu kola grows wild across much of Bali. People here also cultivate it in their gardens. In Ayurvedic medicine, gotu kola is one of the most important herbs for rejuvenation.

It's also a handy first-aid treatment for bug bites and small cuts. We just crush a few leaves in our hands and rub them on the wound to cleanse and speed healing.

In Bali, gotu kola is sometimes called "the student herb," because it sharpens the mind. We also use it to combat senility. The leaves make a delicious, though slightly bitter, tea. You can prepare it just as you would any tea — either from fresh or dried leaves.

In our traditional medicine, gotu kola is used to cleanse the kidneys and purify the blood. It may also boost immune function.

We love to chop the fresh leaves very finely and sprinkle them on our salads. And we always keep dried leaves on hand for making tea.

— *Westi*

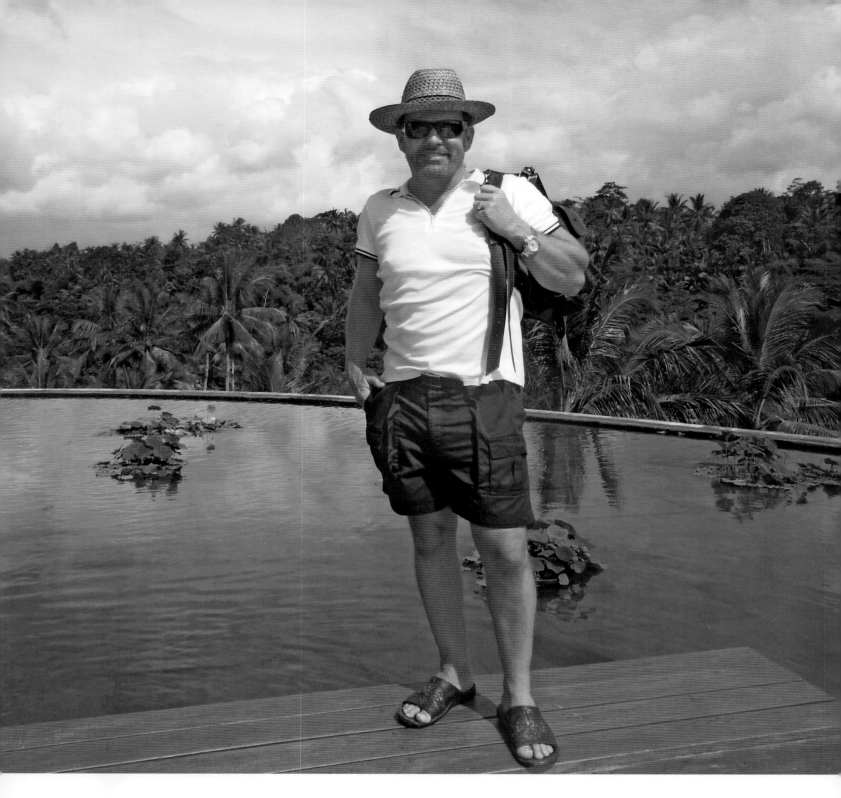

I'm surrounded by gotu kola — and I was pleased to find clinical trials that show gotu kola can help spur growth in brain cells.

My Own Research and Discoveries

Gotu kola comes in very handy to treat many skin conditions. Chemicals in the leaves — called "triterpenoids" — increase antioxidants and the blood supply to wounds. In a pinch, you can even use gotu kola on minor burns.

The leaves and stems are edible raw and they're quite pungent and aromatic, a lot like parsley.

Although some people like to eat the leaves on their own, I mix them with other green leaves.

COMMON WAYS TO TAKE GOTU KOLA

Gotu Kola

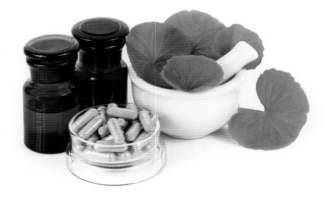

1. **As an extract.**
   Take 10 drops or from 10-20 ml per day.

2. **As a dried herb.**
   You can make a tea of the dried leaf,
   three times daily. Use up to 6 grams of dried leaf.

3. **As a powdered herb (available in capsules).**
   Take 400-600 mg, three times a day.

Gotu Tea

The fresh or dried leaves can be made into a caffeine-free tea (gotu kola is not a stimulant).

To prepare leaves for tea, dry them in indirect sunlight and store them in an airtight jar.

When you're ready to make your tea, crush a few leaves into a cup, then cover with boiling water. Steep for a few minutes, strain out the leaves and enjoy the hot, full-bodied tea.

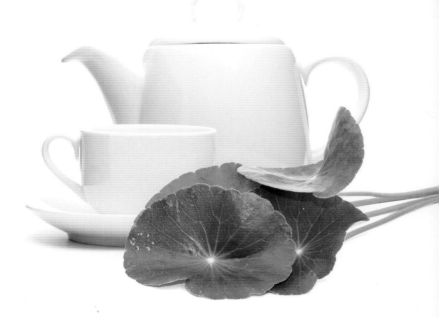

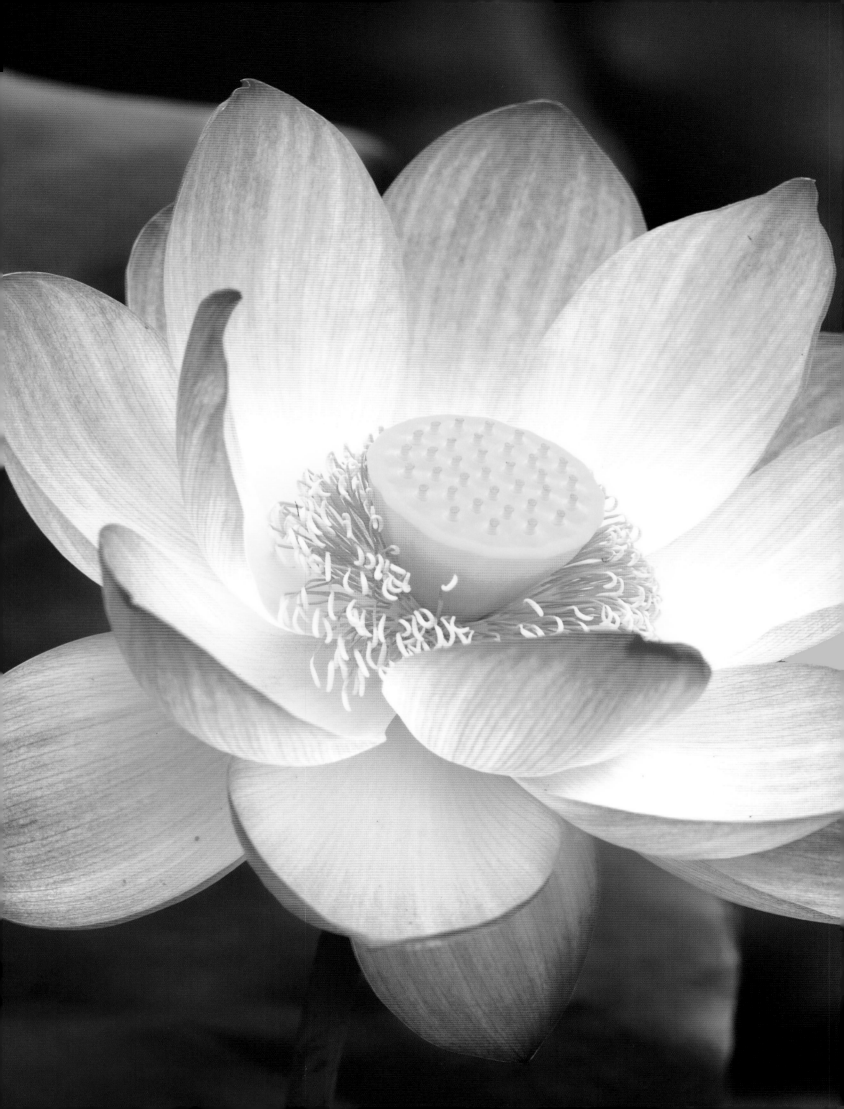

SACRED SLIMMING SECRET IS BALI'S MOST DELICIOUS HEALING FLOWER

One of the first things I noticed about the people of Bali was their friendly, broad smiles. They were the kindest, most compassionate people I've ever met. You can walk up to a total stranger in Bali and he'll treat you like you're a member of his own family.

I also couldn't help but notice how thin they all seemed to be... both women and men. There just didn't seem to be any fat people.

Naturally, I expected the women to eat like birds.

But I was amazed to find them eating rich, creamy and sweet foods.

Westi and Lelir helped me understand why.

Turns out, the women of Bali have a "slimming secret" that is virtually unknown to the outside world.

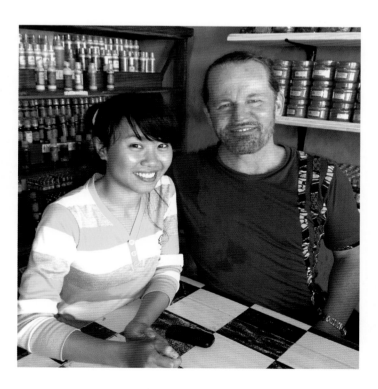

This young Balinese woman who worked in Westi and Lelir's shop is typical of the Balinese... very slim. I just didn't see many overweight people at all while I was in Bali.

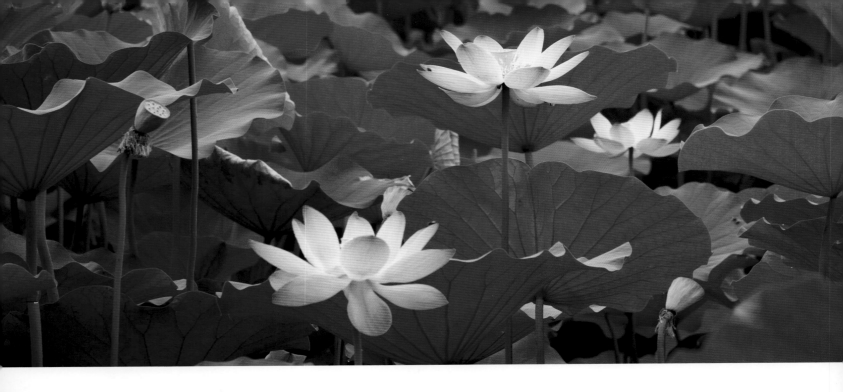

Drain the Fat From Your Cells

The most impressive fat-reduction herb in Bali borrows from their Indian and Hindu roots. It's called the "sacred lotus," and you may have seen it in Asian art, paintings and statues. And let me tell you, once you see it growing, you never forget it.

Even more than its appearance, I was a bit surprised to find that this might be the secret that keeps the Balinese so slim. The extract from its leaves can speed up the breakdown of fat... and over time, actually drain the fat right out of your fat cells.

In animal studies, the sacred lotus prevented an increase in body weight[1] and promoted the breakdown of fat.[2]

It worked even better when combined with workouts. The researchers found that it "significantly suppressed weight gain" when it was used together with workouts.

Because this effect is not very well known in the U.S., most of the research into the sacred lotus' power is being done in places where they actually use the flower.

For example, scientists at Inha University in South Korea tested a sacred lotus extract on human "pre-fat" cells. That is, cells that will turn into fat given the right conditions, like lack of exercise and poor diet.

Cells treated with lotus extract resisted turning into fat. The extract stopped all the processes that turn regular tissue into body fat.[3]

Who would have thought that the leaves of the iconic lotus flower could be such a powerful weight-reduction tool?

But it gets even better... because the Balinese have all kinds of health issues they treat with this alluring flower.

An Entire Pharmacy in One Plant

(Nelumbo nucifera)

Balinese name: Bunga Padma

"Wow! What is that?" the tall, pale man suddenly shouted. He was pointing at a large rosy blossom rising like a phoenix out of the water.

I was guiding a small group of Europeans on one of my herbal walks. As we walked along the edges of a flooded rice paddy, my friend had spotted the gorgeous bloom.

Almost every Westerner has heard of this flower, but very few have seen it growing. When they do, many have the same reaction as this man did. The sacred lotus is that dramatic... and that beautiful.

The lotus boasts rosy pink petals that fade to white at the base. Individual blossoms rise out of the water on sturdy, hairy stalks. They can reach a height of almost ten feet.

The crowning glory of the lotus is at the heart of each blossom, which is a rich golden hue. The effect is stunning.

The lotus isn't just one of the most beautiful flowers in the world. It's one of the most sacred, too.

Spiritual Elixir

According to tradition, the lotus is sacred to the Goddess Lakshmi, who brings spiritual and material abundance. Taken in any form, lotus is said to increase concentration, calm restless thoughts, dispel nightmares and open the heart center.

No wonder Padma – meaning "lotus" – is such a popular name amongst Hindus!

If you visit Bali, you'll find many Hindu temples here. In fact, there are so many temples, Bali is sometimes called "the Island of Temples."

In many of our temples, images of lotus blossoms are carved into the walls. And the gods and goddesses are often depicted sitting on lotus flowers. This is a symbol of their holisitc character, because the lotus is considered the most holistic of all flowers.

Heal Heart Trouble

Lotus has many uses – both as medicine and food. In Bali, we use every part of the plant – the stalks, the seeds, the leaves, the petals and the roots.

We cook the roots to combat diarrhea and heal hemorrhoids. The seeds work to heal heart trouble. We also use them to improve a sterile man's semen and heal impotence.

The flowers, filaments and the juice from the stalks are an effective heart tonic. According to tradition, the roots and seeds have anti-aging properties, too.

The roots and leaves promote weight loss. We also juice lotus roots to clear up acne and eczema. Porridge made from lotus roots eases nausea. And a poultice of the leaves helps lower fever and combat sunstroke.

Lotus is one of the most powerful healing plants I know. It's even a powerful aphrodisiac.

Meanwhile, back at the rice paddy, I smiled at the man's question. I'd heard it many times before.

"That," I said, "is a lotus blossom."

I stretched out, gently grasped the stalk, and drew it closer for my little group to inspect.

"Lotus is one of the most versatile plants in the world," I explained. "Let me tell you about the ways we use it in Bali..."

— *Westi*

"THE FLOWERS, FILAMENTS AND THE JUICE FROM THE STALKS ARE AN EFFECTIVE HEART TONIC."

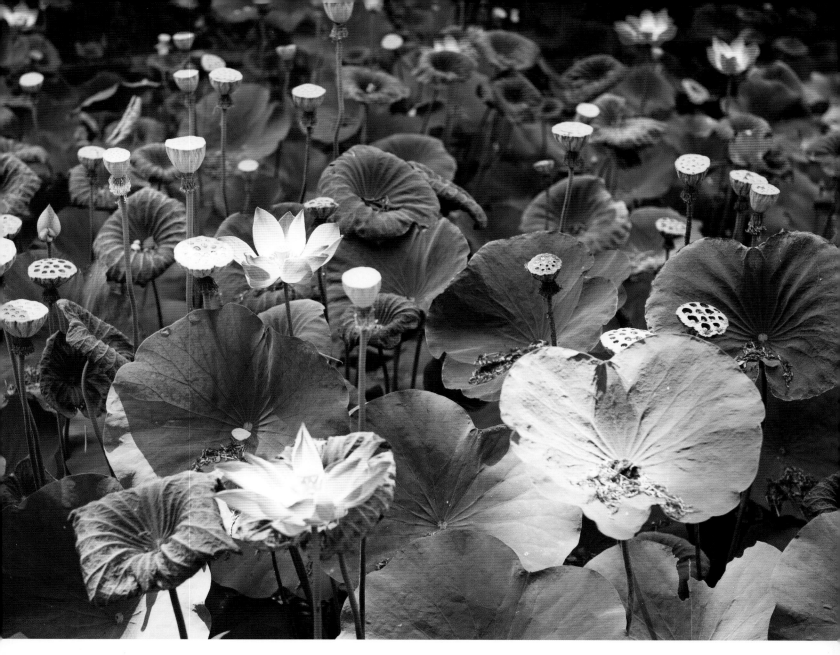

The sacred lotus is one of the most beautiful and versatile plants in the world, and can be used for numerous medicinal purposes — from weight loss to heart health. Essentially, it's a pharmacy in one plant.

My Own Research and Discoveries

I saw the large, pink petals of this sacred treasure of Bali blooming above the surface of freshwater ponds everywhere I went.

A few times I saw peddlers selling its unusual fruit, which grows right in the center of the flower and looks like the spout of a watering can. But most of the time I saw it carved into intricate stone statues outside of Hindu temples.

The sacred lotus keeps its pure and pristine look by the "lotus effect." Water simply rolls off, along with any dirt or dust particles, because the leaves have a complex nanostructure. It creates water resistance and minimizes adhesion.

Although it seemed to be everywhere I went on the island, very few outsiders know what this beautiful flower can really do.

A Tonic for Modern Diseases

Healers in Bali and India have used lotus as medicine for hundreds — probably thousands — of years. They didn't need scientific reassurance to know what was happening right in front of their eyes... people were healthier when they used the sacred lotus.

But now science is confirming these ancient uses and traditions, as well as the effects Balinese healers have always known, plus new effects against modern diseases.

For instance, the sacred lotus:

• Has anti-HIV potency.[4]

• Protects against diabetes damage (protects islet cells in the pancreas).[5]

• Has a strong antioxidant power.[6]

• Can reduce blood pressure.[7]

• Works against deadly melanoma.[8]

• Lowers triglycerides.[9]

A special compound they've isolated from the sacred lotus, called "neferine," kills lung cancer cells[10] and kills off the most common and deadly kind of liver cancer cells.[11]

The seeds and rhizomes also lower triglycerides.

But what is really interesting to me is that the lotus is a brain-power booster. One of the major components of the lotus is allantoin. When researchers tested this compound in animals, they found a number of remarkable transformations — like its ability to increase cognitive abilities.

Also, allantoin causes growth of new, healthy brain cells.[12]

That means the lotus may one day give us a natural cure for diseases like Alzheimer's, helping you regain your memory and cognitive abilities because of its ability to grow new brain cells.

As time goes on, I expect we'll see increasing proof that this beautiful flower is an entire pharmacy in one plant.

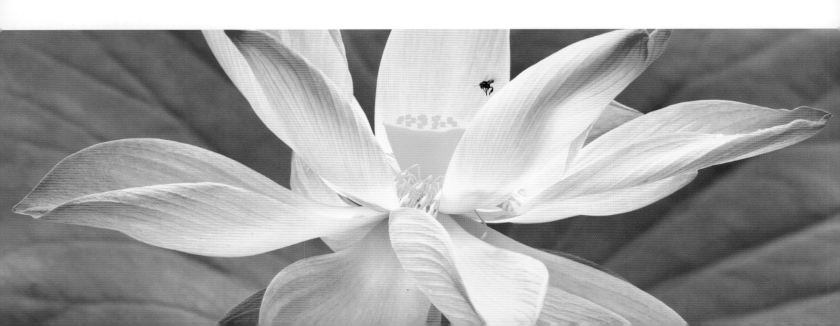

Delightful Delicacy

Did you know that the entire sacred lotus is edible? You can substitute coffee for a roasted and ground-up lotus seed. You can cook the root and eat it as a vegetable or pickle it in vinegar. You can also eat the leaves raw or cooked.

A popular recipe in Bali is to wrap the leaves around rice, mushrooms and different kinds of vegetables, and then bake it. Then you eat it like a sort of stuffed cabbage or a cooked lotus leaf wrap.

You can make this in a wok right at home, like I do.

1. First, heat up a wok on the highest temperature setting you have. Add just one tablespoon of oil and stir fry whatever vegetables you like for no more than a couple of minutes. Set those to the side for just a minute.

2. Add a bit more oil and stir fry the rice and set that aside.

3. Take your lotus leaf and lay it in a large bowl. Spread the stir-fried vegetables in the center of the leaf, and add the rice around it.

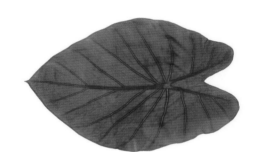

4. Now, fold the lotus leaves around the rice and vegetables. Press down until it's flattened.

5. Steam the entire thing for around four minutes. Then take the bowl out of the steamer or off the steam, and turn upside down on a plate.

Sacred Lotus

Another delicacy in Bali and India, too, is the matured stem of the lotus flower. They are very nutritious and taste delicious, so the Balinese eat them often.

Lotus contains a lot of iron, calcium and are an excellent source of dietary fiber. Because of this, Balinese women who are pregnant and need extra nutrients eat them.

The stems should be crisp and fresh. Make sure to wash them thoroughly to remove any dirt, because this part of the flower grows in the ground.

Then, peel off the thin outer sheath and slice it for a salad or chop it into fine pieces to use in a stir fry, like I do.

You can get the extract as a powder and make a tea with it, or boil it down to make a decoction. Look for powder that's made from the flower and the leaves. You can also use the whole fresh flowers as a garnish for your soups and main dishes.

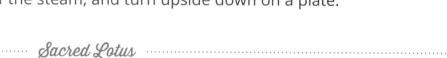

I like using the stamens to flavor my lotus tea.

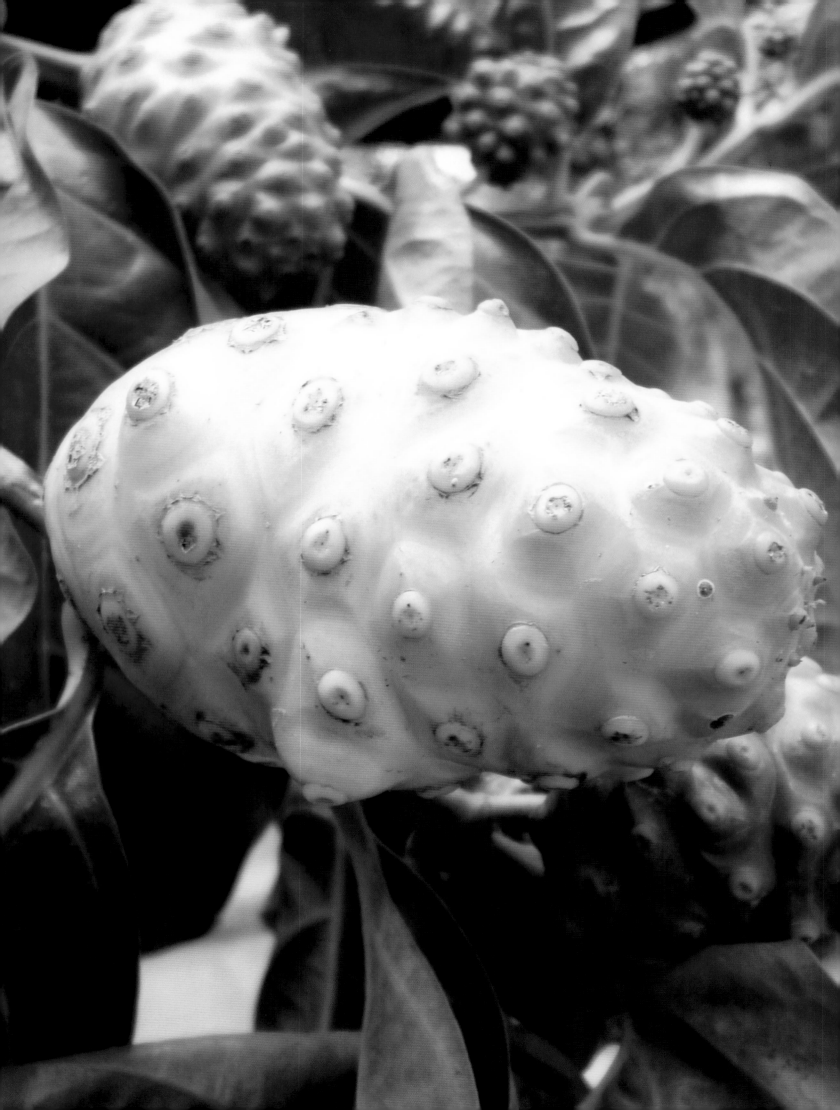

MAKE YOUR BRAIN YEARS YOUNGER WITH THIS TINY SUPERFRUIT

Mulberry trees became famous, largely because they have huge, green leaves that silkworms love to get fat on.

They became so important during the time of silk trading from Asia that the trees were imported all over the world to help feed silkworms.

Fast forward to today and these trees are hot all over the world for another reason: anti-aging.

Their fruit can keep your brain young.

The journal, *Annals of Neurology,* recently published a study that was one of the first to show that a compound inside the Indian Mulberry fruit can delay brain aging.

Other studies have shown that its berries can also boost brain performance. But that's not what I'm talking about here.

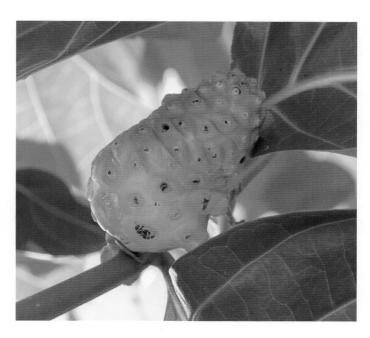

On Bali, herbal healers like Lelir use the Indian mulberry for anti-aging, to boost immunity and as a delicious refreshing drink.

In this study, those who ate more foods with anthocyanidins — the sugar-free plant flavonoids that give intensely colored fruits

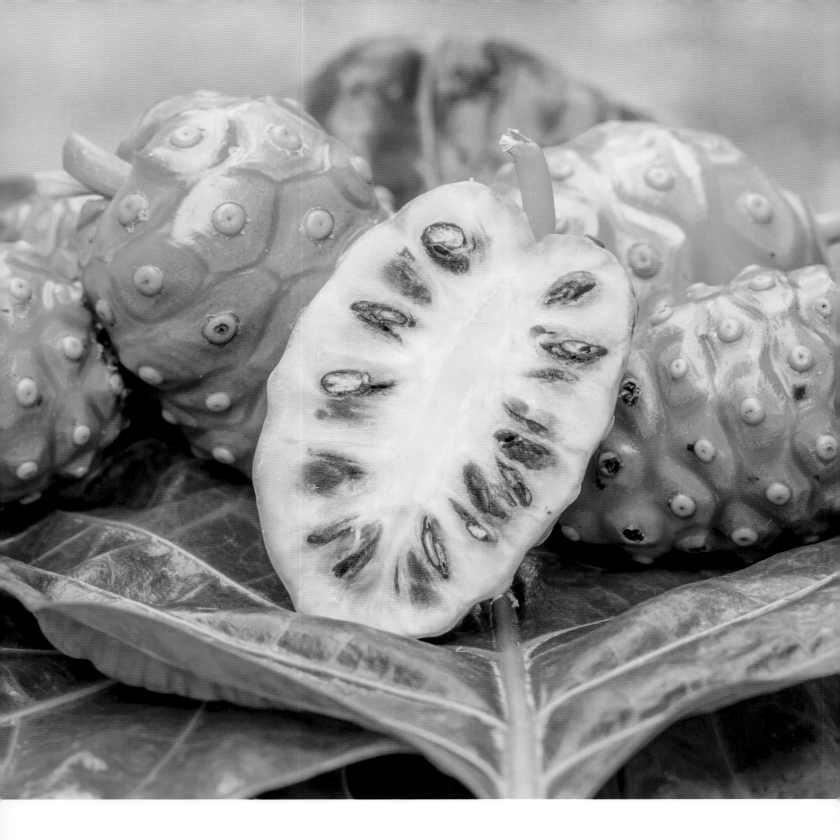

and vegetables their coloring — showed a delay in brain aging of up to 2.5 *years*.[1]

Researchers looked at evidence from the famous Nurse's Health Study, a study that's continually followed 121,700 female nurses between ages 35 and 50 for more than 30 years now. They have been surveyed periodically on the food they eat, and 16,010

of them who were at least 70 years old were tested for cognitive function.

Those who took in more anthocyanidins kept their brains younger.

It was the first time a published study put together the data on how anthocyanidins promote anti-aging.

Inflammation Fighter

In other studies, anthocyanidins were found to have protective effects on other parts of your central nervous system, not just your brain. For example, they appear to prevent inflammatory processes that lead to nerve injury.[2]

Preventing inflammation, and how doing so can help in anti-aging, is the biggest topic at the biggest anti-aging conferences in the world. When I speak at these gatherings and talk to other doctors, the huge problem of inflammation is something we see in people who visit our practices all over the world.

Anthocyanidins are unique, because they stay intact in your body so they can really deliver their benefits, like working against inflammation and brain aging. Other plant nutrients break down faster and can lose their punch.

Plants with the most color usually have the most anthocyanidins. These include blueberries, red grapes, red cabbage and cranberries.

In Malaysia, their native mulberry is full of anthocyanidins.

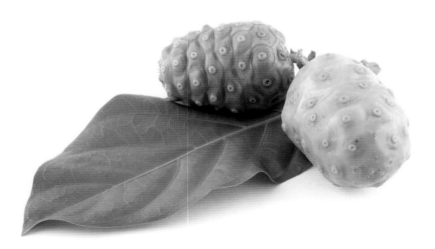

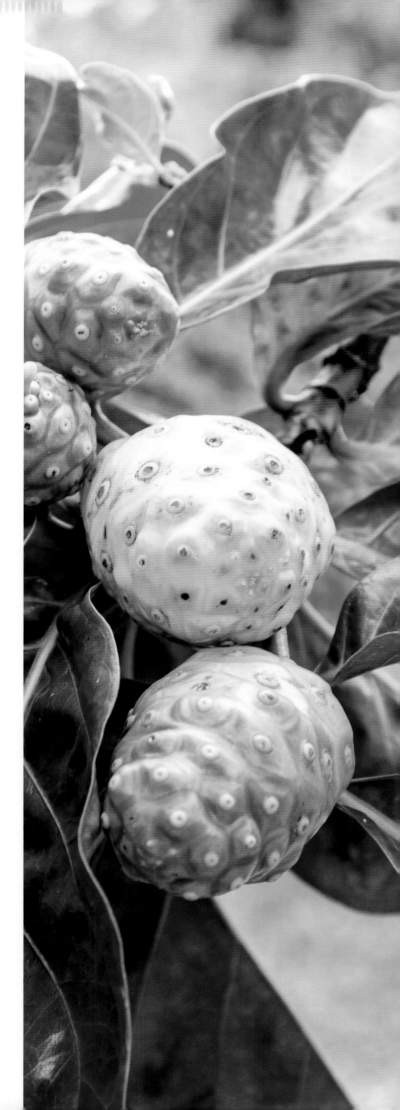

Indian Mulberry
Relief for Skin Problems and Nausea

(Morinda citrifolia)

Balinese name: Tibah

Indian mulberry is the ugliest fruit I've ever seen. It's pale yellow and almost looks like golf ball-sized clumps of frog eggs hanging from the tree. This fruit is actually a cluster of "cells," each containing a seed.

But the juice is popular in Bali and many homes have Indian mulberry growing in their back yard. And the fruit is very healthy.

Years ago, one of our neighbors brought home a piglet and kept it in his back garden. Right in the middle of the garden was an Indian mulberry. When the fruit ripened, it would fall from the tree. And each time a fruit would fall, the pig would run over and gobble it down.

The neighborhood children used to watch and laugh, because that pig really loved its mulberry fruit. But it also grew to be the healthiest pig any of us had ever seen.

Indian mulberry grows wild all over Asia and the Pacific islands. It's also a popular garden plant. We'll put five or six ripe fruit in a glass jar and cover it tight. Then we sit it out in the sun for a day or two to ferment.

After a couple of days, we pour off the juice and drink it. It's delicious, and we believe it strengthens the immune system.

We strain out the seeds from the "jelly" that's left in the jar. The jelly is very good for treating pimples, boils and other skin problems.

In Bali, we eat the grated fruit — it mixes in well with many foods. Or we'll mix the finely grated fruit with water and drink it. This is especially good for nausea and intestinal upsets.

— *Westi*

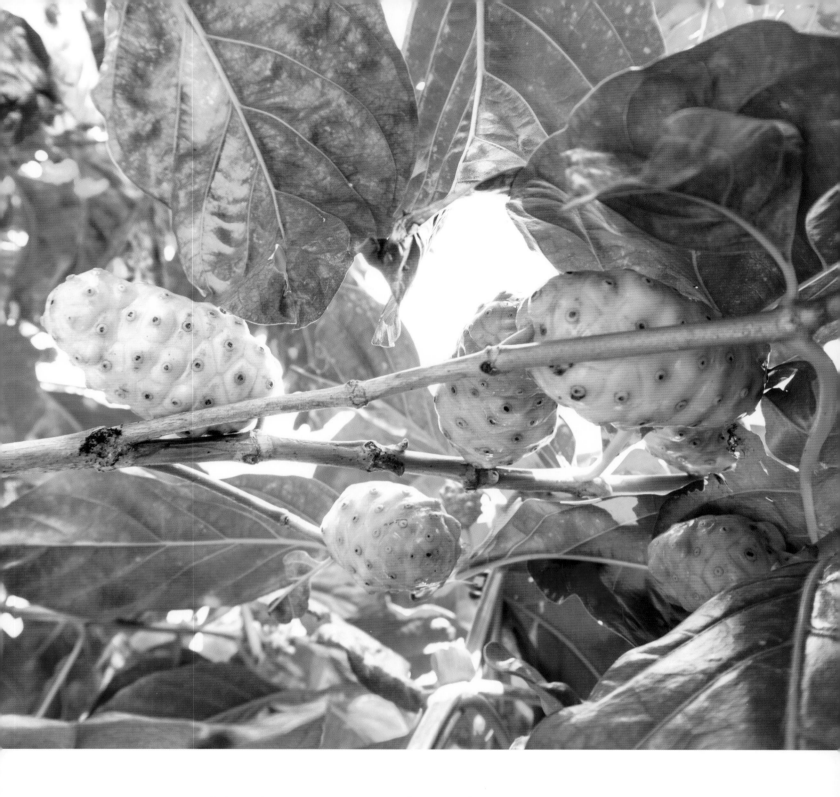

My Own Research and Discoveries

A few years ago, Indian mulberry became popular in Europe, and its popularity rose later in the U.S. Companies sold the juice under its Hawaiian name "noni."

What most consumers of the juice didn't know was that the "dry" part of the fruit holds most of the nutrition. But the juice still has some nutritional value.

Indian mulberry has been used in Polynesian folk medicine for more than 2,000 years. That's a long tradition of use, backing up the richness of this tree. It's no wonder, too. Indian mulberry has been found to survive and thrive in the most diverse places. From dry, humid and windy areas to wet, salty land, and even lava rock.

It's a resourceful tree that adapts well to new environments. It also self-propagates and has active regenerative properties that cause easy spreading. I've also read that in some places, it's seen as a persistent weed.

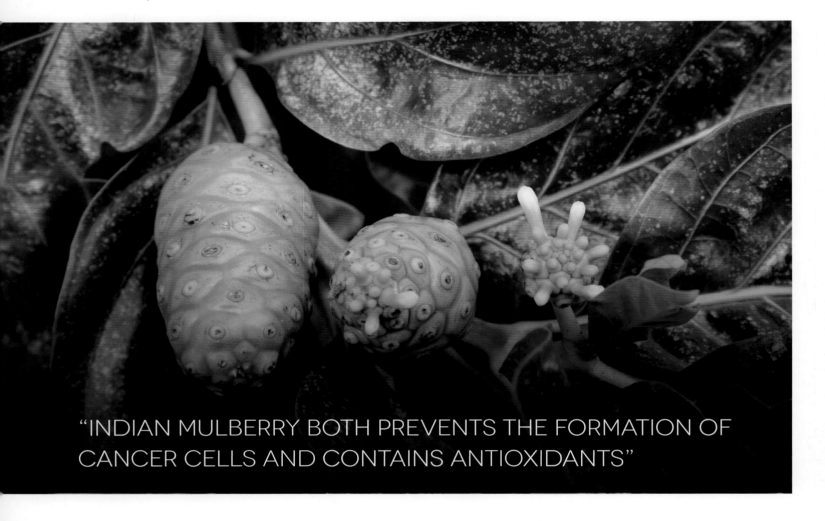

"INDIAN MULBERRY BOTH PREVENTS THE FORMATION OF CANCER CELLS AND CONTAINS ANTIOXIDANTS"

Potent Protection Against Cancer

But once again, as pesky as some people see it, Indian mulberry has potent cancer-fighting powers. Carcinogenesis is the formation of cancer cells. Indian mulberry prevents this formation, and also contains antioxidants.[3]

Indian mulberry is also a good source of linoleic acid, a known acne fighter.[4] This explains why the jelly left over in the jar is used by Westi and Lelir to treat pimples, boils and skin problems.

Thai doctors gave Indian mulberry extract (made from whole fruit) to a group of patients just before surgery. They gave a second group an inactive pill. After surgery, far fewer in the mulberry group experienced post-operative nausea.[5]

This backs up the traditional use of Indian mulberry for nausea.

And in animal studies, Indian mulberry reduces reflux and helps reduce acid damage.[6]

In Westi's garden, his Indian mulberry was tall, probably 15 feet. Westi told me that the fruit and flowers grow continuously year round. I've been thinking about planting one in my back yard. It should grow easily here.

Eating the Fruit

Here are some quick, traditional ways to eat the fruit:

1. Consume the fruit raw.
2. Cook unripe fruit in curry.
3. Cook fruit and consume with coconut.
4. Use fruit in teas.

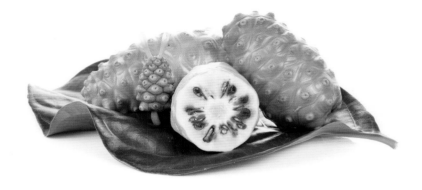

Eating the Leaves

Here are some quick, traditional ways to eat the leaves:

1. Cook as a veggie and eat with rice.
2. Wrap around fish before cooking and then eat along with the cooked fish.
3. Use leaves to make teas.

Indian Mulberry

Indian Mulberry Juice

As I mentioned earlier, Indian Mulberry juice doesn't contain most of the nutrients found in the fruit. And the fresh fruit is hard to find outside of Asia and the Pacific Islands. But you may be able to find the powdered fruit at health food stores or online.

You may be lucky to have a local farmer who grows and sells fresh noni. A silkwood farm may have them. But the berries are very tender and spoil more quickly than some other fruits. That's why you normally see Indian mulberries sold frozen or dried at local health-food stores.

Pick a fully ripened fruit. Place in glass jar with a small amount of water. Seal jar tightly, and let it sit for one week to ferment. Strain the juice through something like cheesecloth. Store in the refrigerator.

Even though Westi and Lelir are used to the taste and enjoy it, the juice might not taste that great at first. Mixing with other juices may make consumption more pleasant.

Noni Extract

You can also buy extracts in capsule form, which will usually have part berry and part leaf extract. The most powerful ones contain 25% or more anthocyanidins. They are available online and in many Asian specialty stores.

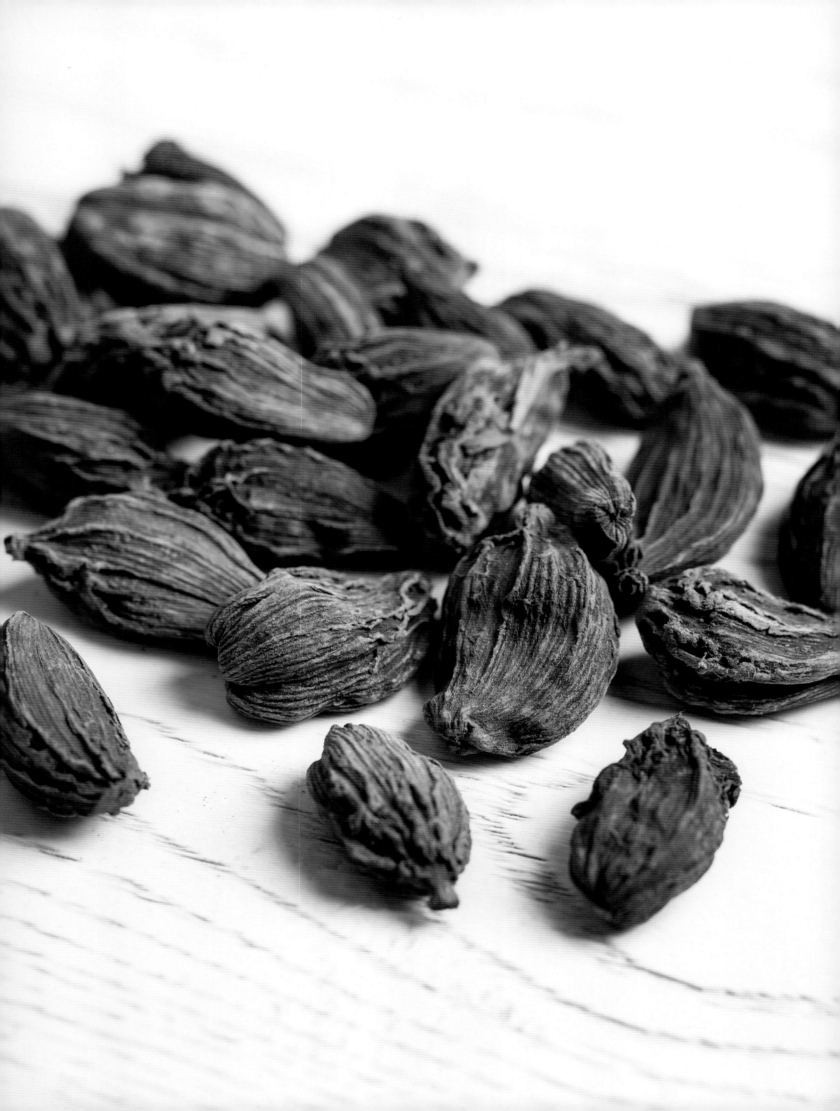

ANCIENT QUEEN OF HERBS CURES COUGHS, ASTHMA

(AND KILLS CANCER CELLS, TOO)

I can't complain, but sometimes I still do.

For instance, it's great to travel. I have a lot of stamina, and plenty of enthusiasm... but it's a very long trip to the opposite side of the world!

And it gets even longer when you have to wait eight hours, plus another year.

You see, I had a little difficulty getting to Bali the first time I was scheduled to go...

Oops, My Mistake

"This passport won't get you into Malaysia."

"What does that mean? My passport's not expired... is it?"

The ticketing agent wouldn't let me on my flight, so I was hoping there was just a misunderstanding.

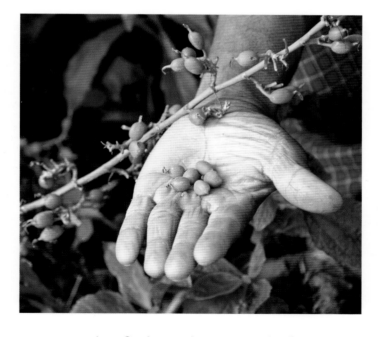

Java Cardamom is one example of why I wanted to visit Bali

"No, it doesn't expire until next month. But you can't enter Malaysia unless your passport is good for three months after you arrive."

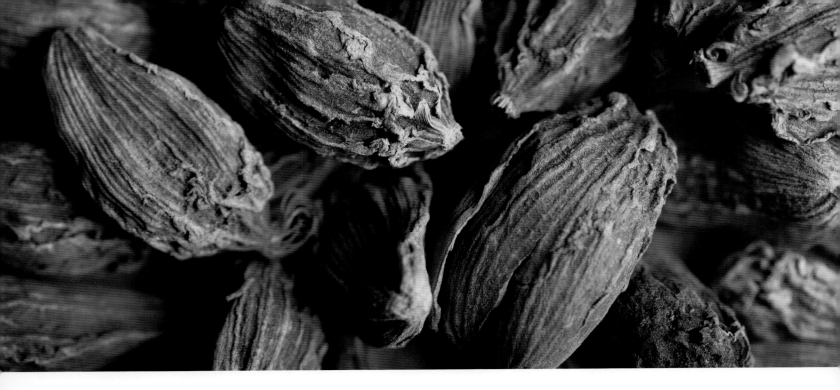

Cardamom seed pods are just one of the hundreds of useful plants I encountered on my trip.

I have to admit, I didn't know that.

I turned to my assistant S.D. "That doesn't sound like what the Malaysian government told us..."

"THE OIL EXTRACTED FROM CARDAMOM IS A POTENT ANTISEPTIC THAT KILLS BACTERIA, ESPECIALLY IN THE MOUTH WHERE THEY CAN CAUSE BAD BREATH AND INFECTIONS."

"The organizers of the anti-aging conference connected me to an official who told me, 'As long as your passport is good at the time, you're OK. There shouldn't be any problem,'" S.D. said.

Turns out, the official S.D. spoke with was wrong. So she got on her phone right away to see what we could do.

She got in touch with an expediting service that tried its best to get it fixed that day, so I

could make it to Malaysia on time. But you know how the U.S. government works sometimes.

After waiting in the terminal for almost three more hours, S.D. got one last call.

"They can get the extension, but they can't get it processed and delivered to you until tomorrow."

So I spent the whole day at the Fort Lauderdale airport only to be sent home.

The officials at the airport didn't seem very understanding when they said, "Well, don't you know you have to do those things in advance?"

I missed my flight and my speaking engagement in Kuala Lumpur... and my first trip to Bali.

But it's on me. I should have checked my passport and made sure. Luckily, the anti-aging conference's organizers were very gracious and arranged for me to speak there the following year.

So, one year later, I made my way to Bali for my first visit.

Queen of Herbs
Cures a Cough

I spent a day in Kuta, the Australian surfer hangout.

But I left the next day and made my way into the jungles of Bali and up the mountains into Ubud...

I was exhausted after flying for more than 24 hours, giving speeches for two days, and being on the go for four straight days.

By the time I got to Westi and Lelir's housed, I had a bit of a tired cough.

Lelir went right out into their little garden, gathered a few ingredients and made me a tea that took my cough right away.

The leaves she used were something she called "kapulaga." Turns out it's the Indonesian form of a very old and powerful herb, cardamom.

The Balinese cardamom is called "Java cardamom" *(Amomum compactum)*.

Cardamom also has a pod that produces seeds. The oil extracted from cardamom seeds contains cineole as its major active component. It's a potent antiseptic that kills bacteria, especially in the mouth where they can cause bad breath and infections.

Cardamom also helps guard against the ulcers you can get from drinking alcohol and the stomach bleeding that comes from aspirin.

I had encountered this ancient herb in India, where they call it "queen of herbs." There they sometimes chew the leaves for fresh breath and make formulas that treat asthma and coughs, just like in Bali, as Westi soon explained.

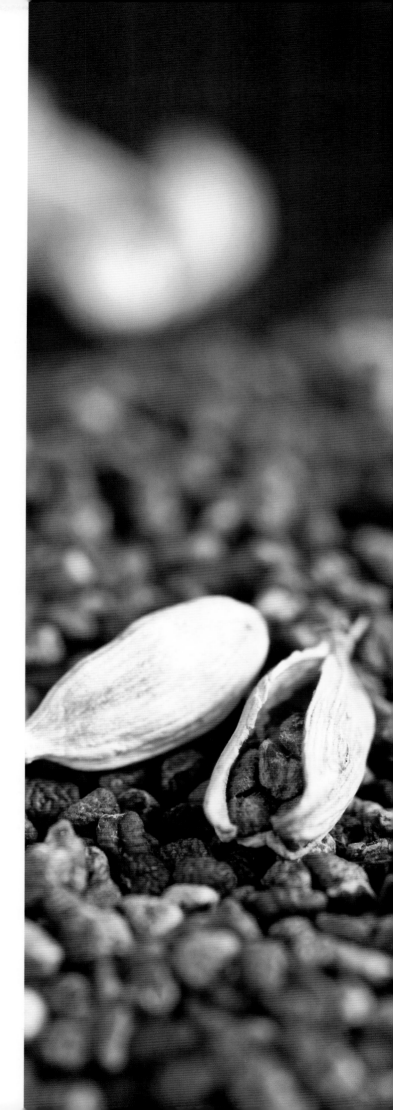

Flavorful Tea Eases Asthma

(Amomum compactum)

Balinese name: Kapulaga

When Lelir and I started out, we had a little shop and a garden. Over the years, the little shop grew and moved into a larger building. Our herb garden took over my family's rice fields. And we hired a few workers.

Hiring workers was a big decision, but we just couldn't handle all the work ourselves any more. It felt like a lot of responsibility. But it soon turned into something else. We hired people who shared our interest in herbs... and they soon became friends.

Before long, we were all sharing a cup of herbal tea before we started work in the morning. We use this time to plan our workday and to share news of friends and family.

Early on, Lelir noticed that one of the women would come in wheezing or out of breath some mornings. She had asthma. So we changed her morning tea.

We started giving her a cup of tea made from red ginger, long grass and an herb we call "kapulaga." Soon, she was having less trouble breathing. After a couple of months, she was feeling almost normal.

Now she keeps a supply of this tea at home, too.

Cures Symptoms of Head Colds

Kapulaga is better known in the West as "Java cardamom." In Indonesia, you'll find it almost everywhere.

Here in Ubud, cardamom grows in many gardens. But it also grows wild along nearby roads and trails. It's also common along riverbanks. And, of course, you can buy it in any market.

The plant grows about chest high and bears pods that hold fragrant seeds. We use the seeds most often — both for cooking and medicine — but the root is also useful.

Cardamom is a mild decongestant and also calms coughs. It aids digestion and acts as an antispasmodic. It has stimulant activity, too. The plant's roots reduce fever and act as an expectorant.

One of the easiest ways to use cardamom is to just chew a few seeds. This is a quick way to treat a sore throat or ease asthma.

I think cardamom is more enjoyable as a tea. So if I have time, I crush a teaspoonful of seeds and steep them in a cup of hot water. This tea not only soothes a sore throat, it also helps settle an upset stomach.

I never have to worry about running out of this handy remedy. Every kitchen in Bali is stocked with cardamom. We use it in curries and to flavor all sorts of food, from coffee to sweetbreads.

— *Westi*

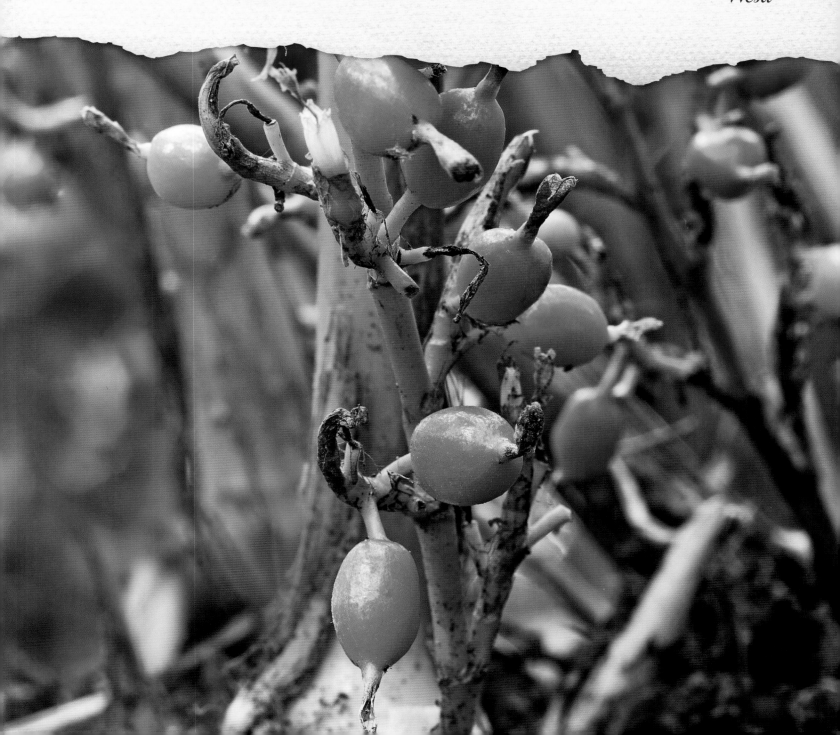

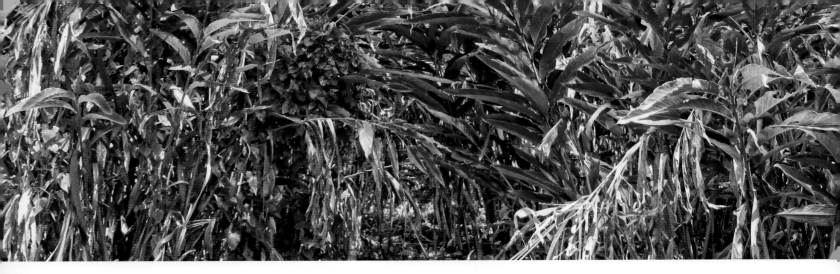

The jungles of Bali are a treasure trove of useful plants, like cardamom.

My Own Research and Discoveries

Cardamom is very good at killing microbes like strep, staph and E. coli, which can cause serious illness.[1]

A recent study backs up the traditional Balinese use against asthma. It comes from the Korea Institute of Oriental Medicine.

Doctors discovered that cardamom extract lowered levels of several compounds that trigger restricted breathing in asthma.[2]

Cardamom also slashes levels of one of the most destructive free radicals in the body, ROS (reactive oxygen species), and lowers levels of several molecules called cytokines, which can inflame the lungs.

And, even better for asthmatics, a high dose of cardamom reduces immunoglobulin (Ig)E in the blood. This is important because (Ig)E binds to allergens and triggers inflammation.

Cardamom Component Kills Cancer Cells

But, as you've discovered throughout this book, many natural plant compounds are also anticancer, and the cineole extracted from cardamom seeds is one of them.

Different forms of cineole from different plants all have cancer-killing properties.

A cineole that relieves congestion, 1,8-cineole, comes from the eucalyptus tree. This cineole kills leukemia cells[3] and three different human tumor cell lines, especially colon cancer, a very deadly malignancy.[4]

Cineole is also what gives sage oil its anticancer properties. It protects against overexposure to ultraviolet radiation, as shown in clinical trials.

Another active ingredient is nootkatone, obtained from ground pods. Nootkatone is a citrus aromatic, usually taken from grapefruit and used in fragrances. In its plant form, nootkatone is very adept at reducing inflammation, especially in the skin.[5]

Preparations

Lelir and Westi's traditional recipe for easing coughs, congestion and sore throat with cardamom is delicious and slightly sweet all on its own. They call it simply "Healing Cough Tea" in Indonesian.

First, you combine 1 level teaspoon of each of the following:

Java cardamom	Lemon grass	Fennel seed	Ginger root	Cinnamon bark

Place all of the spices in the bottom of a 24-ounce bottle. Add 24 ounces of boiling water and cap the bottle. Steep for 15 minutes, strain and enjoy.

This tea is naturally sweet, so you won't have to add any sugar or honey. Plus, you don't have to wait for a sore throat to enjoy it. Drink it anytime for the delicious flavor. Cardamom has a strong, very spicy and exotically sweet taste.

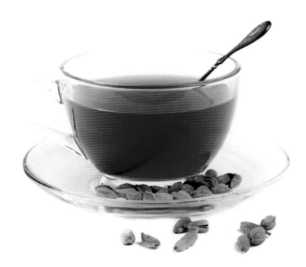

······················ *Java Cardamom* ······················

If you want to get some cardamom seeds yourself, you should know that there are three types: green cardamom, black cardamom and Madagascar cardamom. In Bali, they grow the black cardamom.

It's best to get the seeds while they're still in the pods, because after you remove them from the pods, they lose a lot of their flavor. Ground cardamom has even less flavor.

For example, you can store the pods and they'll keep their flavor for two years in an airtight container away from sunlight. The seeds will last maybe a year, but after you grind it, the powder will only last a few months.

It's very difficult to find the pods in grocery stores, but you can find them in Asian specialty stores and online.

Cardamom is also a bit more expensive than more common spices. The good news is, a little goes a long way, so if you grind it fresh yourself it will be well worth the price.

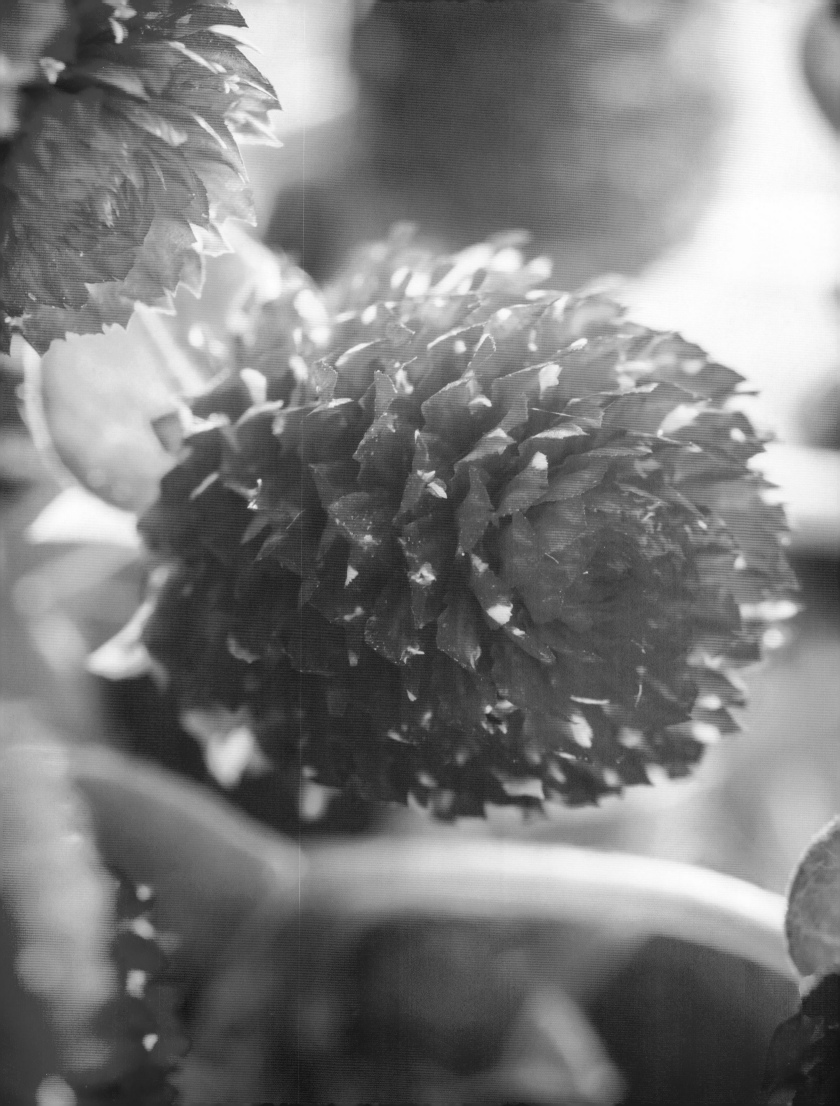

BALI'S BEAUTIFUL BLOOD PRESSURE CURE

I visit a lot of sites when I travel. I like to see as many people and as much of the local culture as I can, wherever I go. But Bali has a different speed to it that you don't experience anywhere else.

No matter how fast my friend Westi drove his truck or how many appointments I had, I never felt rushed. I never felt pressed for time.

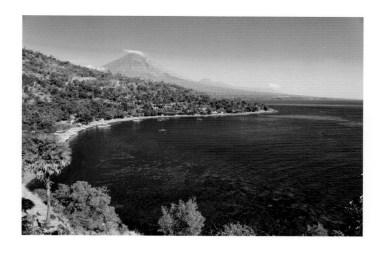

The coastline of Bali is very different than its dense interior.

"GLOBE AMARANTH CAN ALSO HELP YOU IF YOU HAVE CHRONIC INFLAMMATION."

In Bali, there's no urgency. Except maybe my stomach growling at me because I often forgot to eat. The time passes in such a relaxed rhythm you kind of forget about the regular, day-to-day things you're used to. No schedules. No reminders. Maybe Bali feels that way because it's an island.

Even the breeze is different in Bali. I remember standing at the edge of the Ngorongoro Crater in Africa thinking it was the wildest place on Earth. Bali is wild, too... but in a different way.

Africa is like a wild, untamed animal. But you get the sense that it's an animal about to be caged. Bali is wild in an unspoiled way, and seems like it will never change.

One of the things that sets Bali apart is the color. Westi and Lelir live in Ubud and to get there, you have to go through the middle of the densest, greenest rainforest I've ever seen. Like I said before, there were plants on top of plants. Green on top of green.

And everywhere I traveled, there were flowers. Not the occasional flower... but explosions of color on all sides.

Every pond, wall or doorway had flowers either growing on or draped over them. Flowers are very important in Balinese daily life. The Balinese use flowers both for religious offerings and decoration. But that's not all.

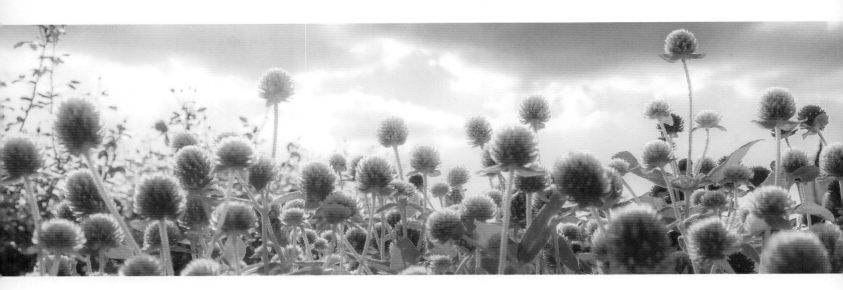

One Special Magenta Bloom Makes a Multitude of Medicines

Besides the beautiful sacred lotus, one of the amazing flowers you see everywhere is the globe amaranth.

The bulbs are a beautiful purplish red and they are like no flower you've ever seen. They just don't seem to wilt. The Balinese make garlands out of them and they last for weeks.

Its name is an English word for the Greek word "amarantos," which means "unfading." Because of this property, this little plant and its flower symbolize immortality.

Once you discover some of the powerful compounds contained within it, you'll understand why the ancient Greeks and Indians picked up on its anti-aging benefits.

Treatments at many of Bali's health spas often end with a floral bath that includes globe amaranth. The Balinese believe flowers are a link to the spiritual world. So after a spa treatment that cleanses you of real impurities, the flower bath cleanses your impurities symbolically.

Even better, globe amaranth can also help you if you have chronic inflammation. It fights diabetes[1] and can even lower your blood pressure. Maybe that's why everyone on Bali seems so relaxed!

Besides its other healing properties, which I'll tell you more about in a minute, Lelir explained that the globe amaranth also had a very useful place for her large family as she was growing up.

A Simple Cure for Pink Eye

(Gomphrena globosa)

Balinese name: Bunga Ratna

During celebrations, Balinese temples are a sight to see. We deck them with flowers of every color. Every temple becomes a unique rainbow of color.

One flower holds a special meaning for us. Its globe-shaped blossoms are a deep reddish purple. And they never appear to fade. Even weeks after they've been picked, they retain their shape and color.

Our ancestors believed this "everlasting" flower — which we call Bunga Ratna — could bring us closer to the gods and goddesses. So we Balinese often use it to decorate our temples and offerings. But my parents taught me another use for this beautiful flower.

As I'm sure you know, children tend to pass around every cold, flu and other malady their friends bring to school. One child goes to school with the beginnings of a cold, and half his friends bring it home.

My brothers, sisters and I were no different. Every so often one of us would come home with a case of conjunctivitis — "pink eye."

When this happened, our parents would go out to the garden where they grew globe amaranth.

Mother would pick a few blooms and put some water on to boil. Then she'd add five of the flowers to a cup of boiling water. When the water turned blue, it was ready.

Mother would strain the flowers out of the tea and let it cool a little. Then she'd have us wash our eyes with the tea. We'd do this every day for a week. The warm liquid felt wonderfully soothing. Even better, by the time the week had gone by, our pink eye was all cleared up.

Globe amaranth grows in gardens and sunny spots all over Bali. Westi and I always have some growing in our garden... just in case our son comes home from school with a "little problem."

— Lelir

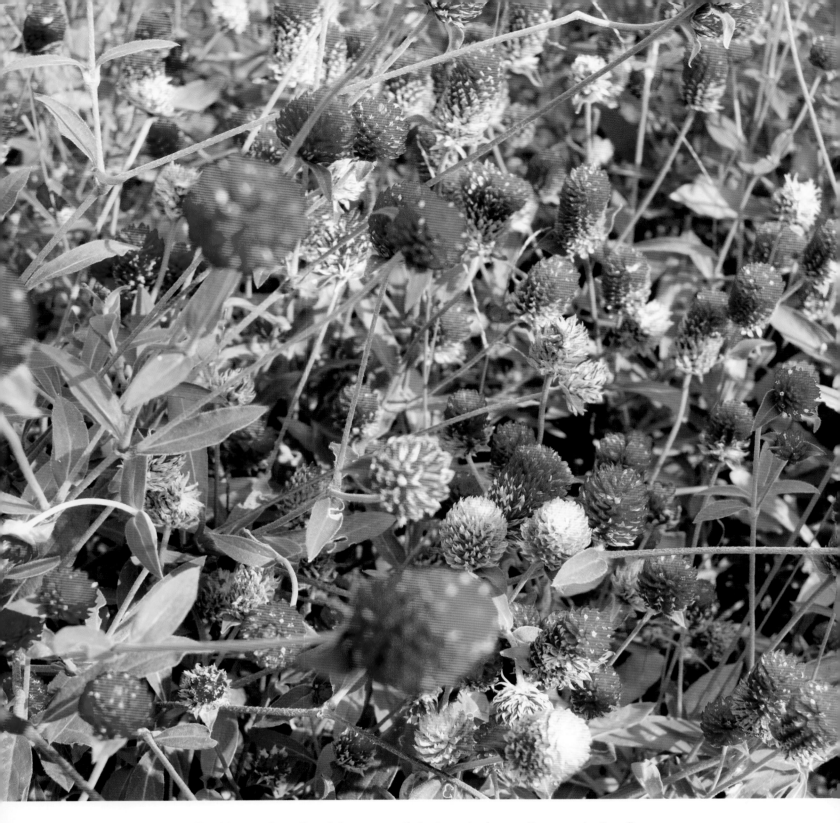

The blooms from the globe amaranth last weeks longer than most other flowers.

My Own Research and Discoveries

Science is only now slowly beginning to discover the many healing properties of plants that have been part of the oldest healing traditions in the world for centuries.

For example, have you ever heard of betacyanins? They are dark red plant pigments with powerful antioxidant health benefits. Globe amaranth has two unique betacyanins, isogomphrenin III and gomphrenin III.[2]

"THE FLOWERS, FILAMENTS AND JUICE FROM THE STALKS ARE AN EFFECTIVE HEART TONIC."

In China two scientists working with mice discovered that betacyanins have protective effects on the nervous system.[3]

These powerful antioxidants may be useful against cancer, too. When doctors in India exposed human leukemia cells to betacyanins, they began eliminating the cancer. The cancer cells began dying in a process called apoptosis, [4]

Globe amaranth is better known in places like Jamaica and the U.S. as bachelor button. It offers powerful medicine against prostate problems. In many countries they eat the sweet-tasting seeds from the dried flower pouches (the buttons) to aid prostate health. The unique healing antioxidant that helps in this is called gomphrenoside-1.

Bachelor button can help men who have a swollen prostate and have a hard time urinating — even if they've had the problem for years. But it's not only good for prostate health and cancer.

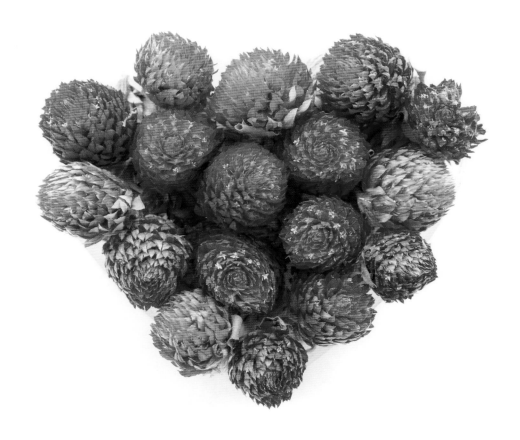

This Flower Also Packs Plant Power for Younger Cells and a Healthy Heart

Another of globe amaranth's powerful plant compounds is kaempferol. This antioxidant helps boost your skin's natural defenses against the environment because it fights superoxide free radicals, which age you faster. The free radicals damage the fatty layer of the cell, making it more prone to cellular attacks. Kaempferol stops that process. Kaempferol also helps defend your skin against ultraviolet radiation and blocks pain.[5]

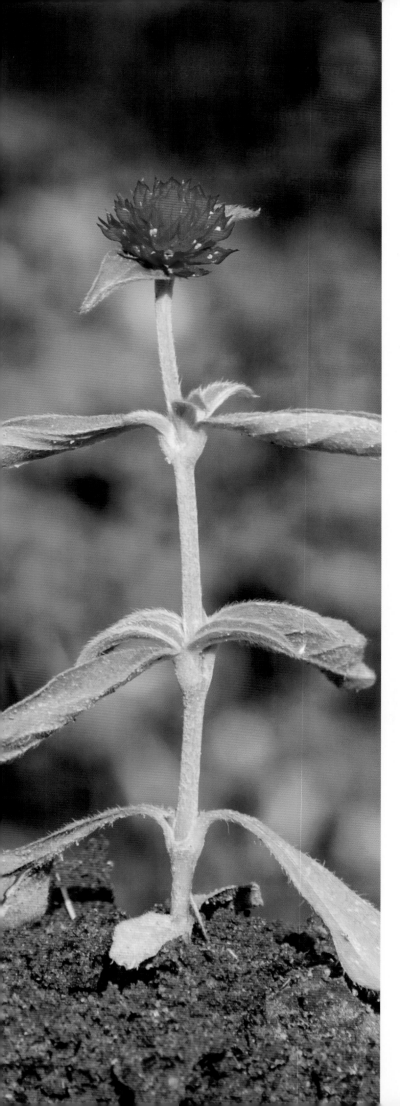

As I mentioned before, one of the best things about globe amaranth is that it lowers blood pressure. This has been a traditional use on Bali for centuries. But I found a little-known study that backs up how Bali's traditional healers, the Balians, have traditionally used this flower.

A team of Brazilian researchers from the Federal University of Piauí, Brazil, proved that globe amaranth significantly reduces arterial blood pressure without changing the heart rate.[6] This is very important because it means that nothing else in the body changes except blood pressure. Even a very small amount works very well.

Amaranth is easy to grow. You'll find these beautiful little purple-bulbed flowers growing in many places in the U.S., especially in Texas and the south. It's commonly used as borders for flowerbeds, and you can also use it for wedding pocket flowers (thus, the name bachelor button). It can grow up to two feet tall with a one-foot spread. It blooms in pink, purple and red. The flowers are often dried and sold as decorations.

They are known to grow in Hawaii like a weed and they grow easily around my home in South Florida. It likes warm climates and it survives well in hot summery days.

The little flower makes a nice food coloring as well. It livens up the look of your cakes, salads and teas.

Preparations

The globe amaranth flower is considered an anti-aging ingredient in Bali because it's so good for the skin. With so many marvelous benefits that make our skin and bodies healthier, kill cancer, reduce inflammation and protect our nerves, it's no wonder this plant is known as the immortal flower.

Globe Amaranth

To make an island tea with globe amaranth, simply steep the flower itself for 4-5 minutes. You can get the dried flower at many health food stores and online. You might see it in a Traditional Chinese Medicine section of a store, too. It's called Qian RiHong.

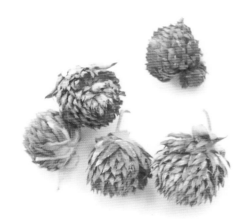

The thing about globe amaranth is that its long-lasting bulb is resistant to moisture. This means you need to stir it a bit while you're making the infusion.

Add the bulbs (along with the stems if the flowers are fresh) to the boiling water and let sit, agitating the mixture occasionally.

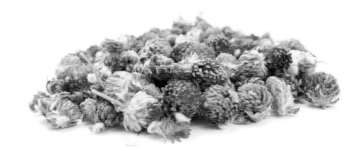

You'll get a purplish-red, caffeine-free tea that has a nice, sweet smell and a mildly sweet taste all on its own. But you can add a little honey to it if you like.

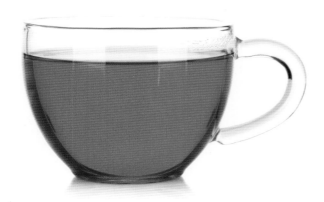

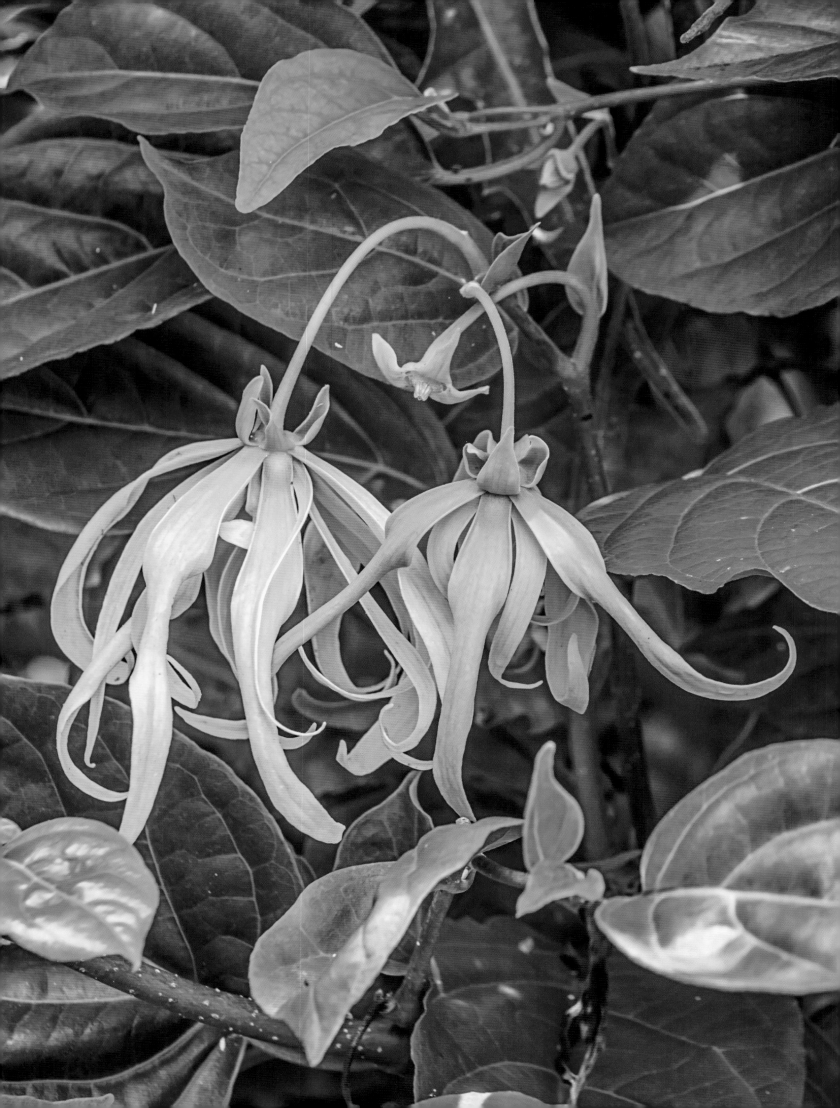

HEART CURE IN A NATURAL PERFUME

"We call this a cananga flower." Lelir picked one off of the small tree behind her shop.

"That looks like ylang-ylang," I said.

"Yes. It is smaller, but in the same tree family. Smell... it's very fragrant."

I took some of the yellowish-green petals. "That's beautiful. So it's a dwarf ylang-ylang tree?"

"Yes... it's small, so I can have it here by the shop. I use the flowers in my Jamu class, and for offerings. Most ylang-ylang trees are very tall."

Jamu, as I've already noted, is the name for the ancient group of natural cures and medicines they use in Bali.

"There are only a few flowers on this cananga tree. Where do you get the rest?" I asked.

"Down there we have a big ylang-ylang. You want to see it?" "Yes."

"Westi will show you."

And off I went around the corner and through the courtyard into their "backyard."

I ducked through the dense shrubs and came out in a clearing...

The shop is built on top of a steep hill. And in back, all over the hillside, grow trees and plants you can't even imagine.

There was a giant ylang-ylang tree with its soft, aromatic flowers that smell so good their oil is the base for the famous Chanel No. 5 perfume.

I'm holding an "ylang-ylang" flower. It's one of the most beautiful fragrances you'll ever smell.

I looked around and was once again taken by the incredible beauty of this place.

There were cacao trees full of cocoa beans, jackfruit trees with their giant watermelon-sized fruit hanging on the trunk, and teakwood. Teak is expensive, used for some of the finest woodworking in the world, and here were dozens of the trees just scattered everywhere.

Westi also has a durian tree, the tallest fruit tree I think I've ever seen. It's an unusual tree because the flowers bloom at night, so bats pollinate them. It was so huge I almost fell over backwards with my video camera trying to get it all in the shot.

Solitary Beauty

(Cananga odorata)

Balinese name: cananga, ylang-ylang

Cananga is a holy flower. It's very important to us for offerings in Bali, and we often choose to use it as a ceremonial flower.

The cananga flower is also a symbol that represents Balinese women. We believe that women should be able to live like a cananga flower. As you age you get more beautiful, more fragrant and stronger.

We don't usually do this with other flowers, but cananga is so special that there is a traditional Balinese ceremony where we put cananga in a woman's hair to attract a man for her to marry. The fragrance is so sweet and pure it is believed to be an aphrodisiac.

— *Westi*

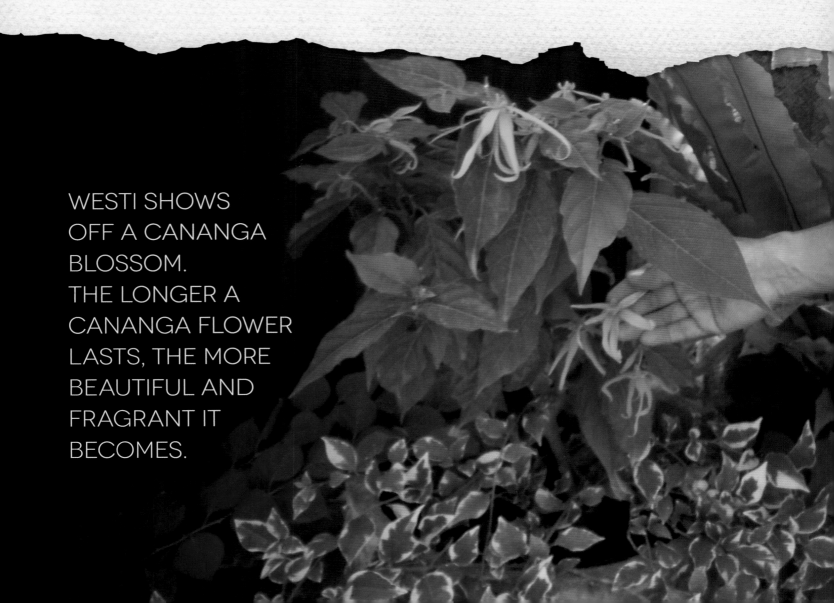

WESTI SHOWS
OFF A CANANGA
BLOSSOM.
THE LONGER A
CANANGA FLOWER
LASTS, THE MORE
BEAUTIFUL AND
FRAGRANT IT
BECOMES.

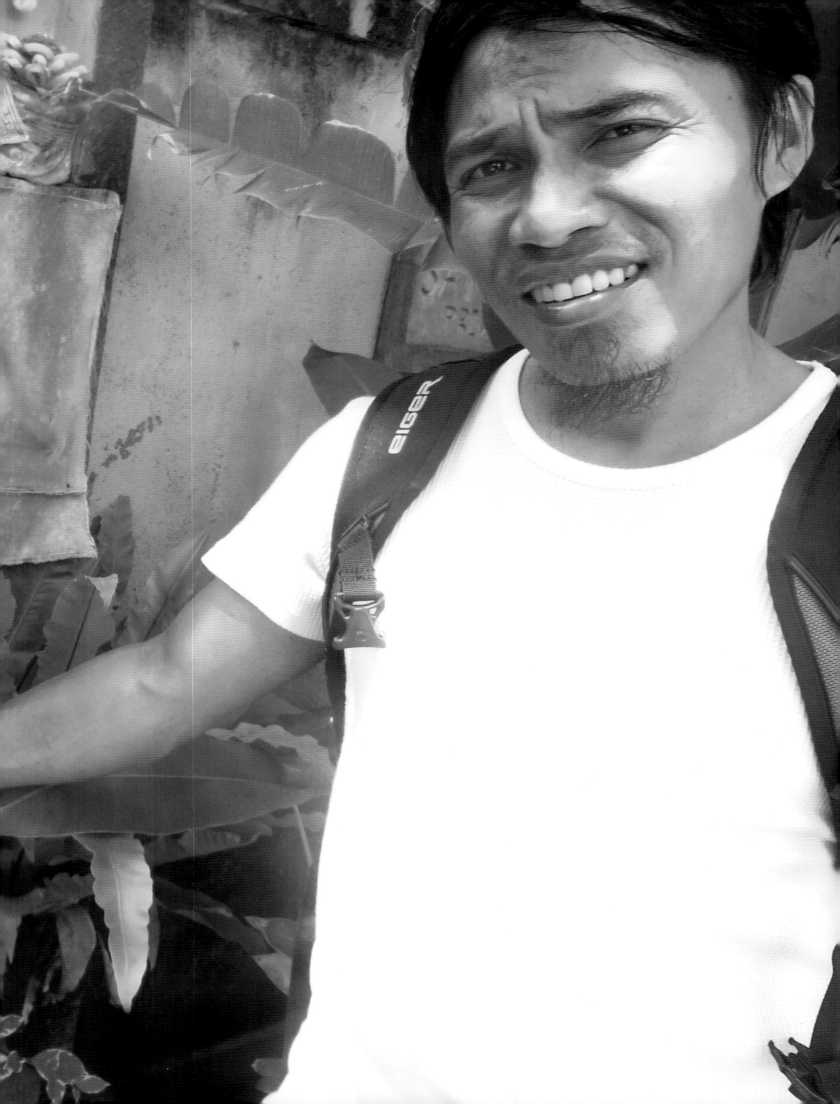

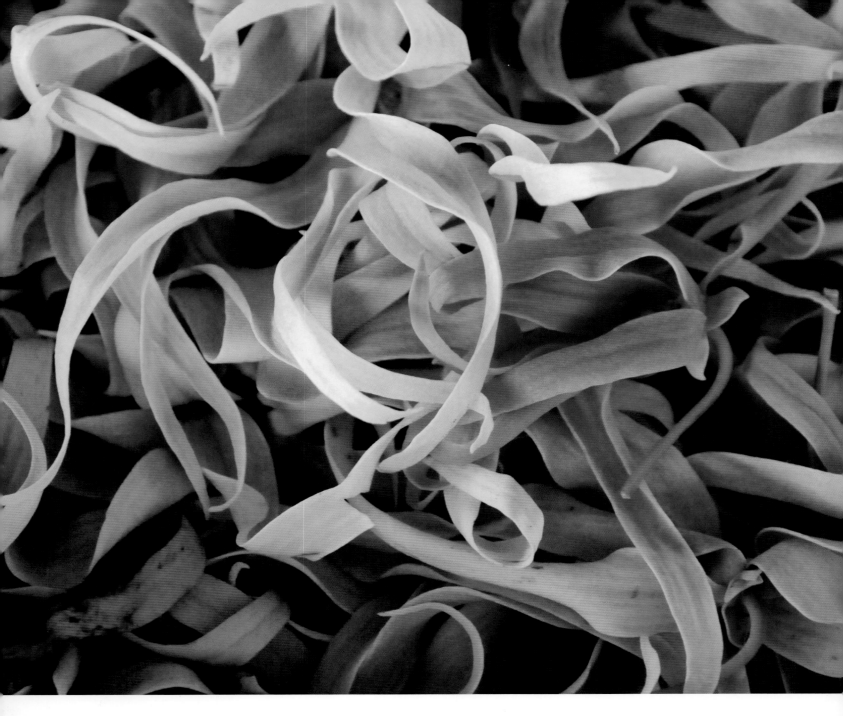

I have ylang-ylang growing at my house in South Florida.

My Own Research and Discoveries

Westi is very knowledgeable about the trees on Bali, their leaves and about the herbs he grows.

He's also very motivated to use his modern knowledge, together with traditional teachings. He's taken it upon himself to show people the traditional, sustainable ways of farming the small amount of land they have in Bali.

Westi talks about this a lot. It's the main thing he wants to accomplish with his education and the land he inherited from his father.

At his dream healing resort, he also wants to create a place visitors can get Jamu, which includes herbal massages and formulas.

The Balinese don't like pharmaceuticals and don't really trust Western-type medicine. So they come to Lelir and Westi's shop to get herbal cures instead.

When Lelir gives people ylang-ylang, it's usually in the form of the essential oil. However...

The ENTIRE Cananga Tree Carries Incredible Healing Properties

For example, inflammatory diseases like high blood pressure are rare on Bali, and cananga might be a reason why.

One of the most important traditional uses for cananga is that it lowers blood pressure.[1]

It also slows rapid heartbeat and controls heart palpitations caused by anger, anxiety and stress.

On Bali, birds love to eat the clusters of black fruit that grow on the trees. The little fruits are quite edible and reminded me of a juniper berry. Very tart.

And as it turns out, the berries have a nice little health bonus: They're anticancer.

I had to dig around to find good information on this, but I finally found a little-known study from the Graduate Institute of Natural Products at Kaohsiung Medical University in Taiwan.

Not only did they discover three plant nutrients they had never seen before, but they found that cananga fruit were able to kill liver cancer cells.[2]

The flower buds of the ylang-ylang could become a cutting-edge treatment in diabetes as well.

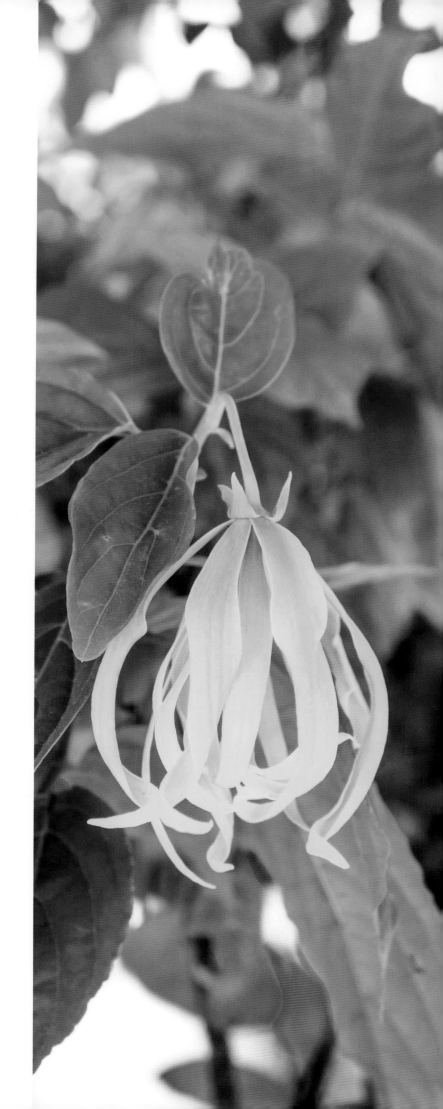

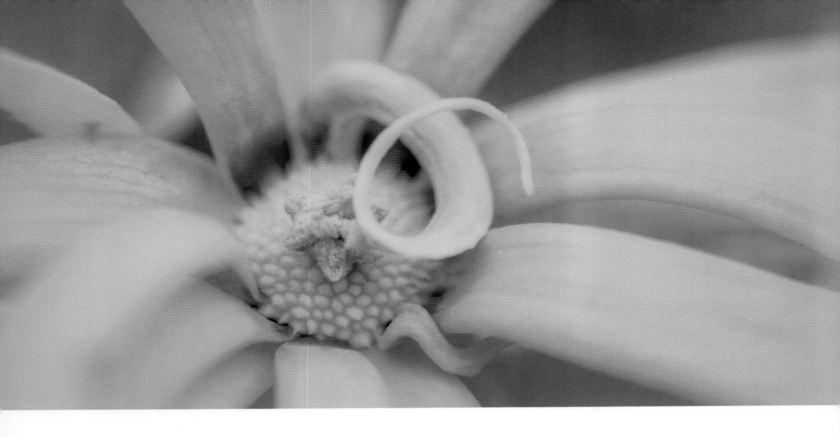

At Kyoto Pharmaceutical University in Japan, researchers have recently discovered that extracts from the buds stop the formation of aldose reductase.[3]

That's important because aldose reductase forms sugars in the body, which diabetics can't process well.

Even worse for diabetics, aldose reductase can cause a buildup of sugars in body parts that are not insulin sensitive, like the eyes and nerves. This can cause diabetic neuropathy, which can make people lose their eyesight and lose feeling in their extremities. Ylang-ylang flower buds stop aldose reductase from forming the sugars.

Scientists are studying the bark of the ylang-ylang tree because it's so strongly antibacterial that it can kill even gram-positive bacteria. Those are the worrisome bugs that antibiotics are now useless against.[4]

Ylang-ylang flowers have a chemical in them called geranyl acetate, which is antioxidant, anti-inflammatory and pain-relieving.[5] This may be why a traditional use for it in Bali is as a skin treatment.

Ylang-Ylang can reduce inflammation, skin irritation, redness and even eczema. It does this by normalizing skin moisture and secretions, and soothing and healing the epidermal cells that are irritated, infected or inflamed.

Ylang-ylang oil further helps by being antibacterial. That means it inhibits microbial growth and disinfects skin, skin rashes, cuts, wounds and scrapes.

The essential oil is also a sedative and antidepressant. Just smelling the beautiful fragrance will put you in a relaxed, happy mood. It calms nervousness, anxiety, stress and even feelings of anger and frustration, all while inducing a relaxed feeling.

Preparations

The essential oil of ylang-ylang is available from many Asian specialty stores and online. You only need very small amounts for aromatherapy, so the bottles will usually be 10ml or so. Look for 100%-pure, therapeutic-grade oil.

You can use ylang-ylang orally. It will wash away fatigue and anxiety and strengthen your nervous system.

If you live in the south like I do, you can grow ylang-ylang. Young plants are sold on sites like toptropicals.com and rareflora.com, or you can do what I do and visit gardenweb.com or davesgarden.com.

Cananga Flower

Lelir taught me a simple way to make a lovely cananga tea.

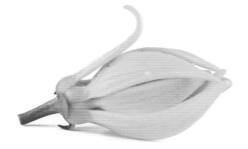

All you need are 10-15 grams of ylang-ylang flowers that have not bloomed yet (they will still be slightly green).

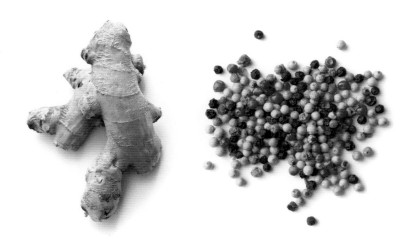

Add a bit of ginger and pepper, and crush it together. Then boil some water and strain it through the ylang-ylang mixture.

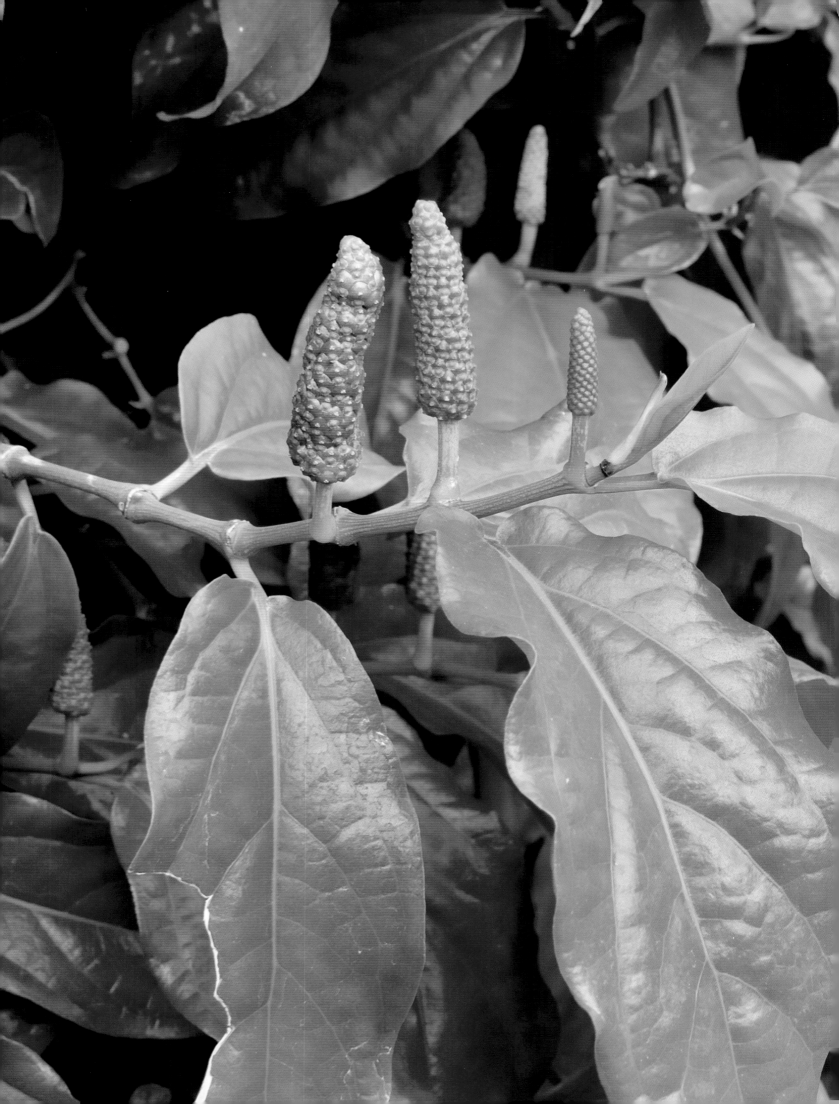

SPICE UP YOUR HEALTH…
AND YOUR LOVE LIFE

Most people think that hot, spicy food is bad for your health.

Yet the exact opposite is true. Hot peppers can make your eyes water and your tongue burn, but they also have healing power.

Peppers can help your body fend off ailments such as heart disease, cancers, cataracts, Alzheimer's disease and others.

Several widely separated cultures have used peppers for medicinal purposes for centuries.

Now, modern scientific research validates much of the traditional usage. Peppers can ward off the common cold and flu. They take away arthritic pain and help asthma sufferers. And they can stop itching and both internal and external bleeding.

But, one of the most ancient uses for Bali's long pepper is as an aphrodisiac. A sort of "love potion."

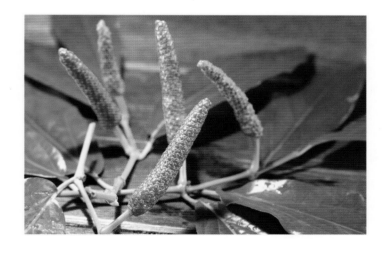

The Indian Long Pepper is'nt just hot, it has amazing healing powers and can ward off diseases like Alzheimer's, heart disease and cancer.

In fact, the ancient Hindu text the *Kama Sutra* directs men to mix long pepper with other spices and honey and, when applied to your body, it will "utterly devastate your lady." In a good way.

On Bali, another traditional use is as a powerful pain reliever…

Hot Relief for Pain... and Congestion, Too

(Piper retrofractum vahl)

Balinese name: Tabia Bon

Bali has so many beautiful and unique features. I've lived here all my life and still have so much to see. I imagine visitors can only scratch the surface.

But even if you get no further than our beaches, you should visit the famous black sand beach at Lovina. There you'll be close to another natural wonder you shouldn't miss. The hot springs at Banjar.

The natural hot springs are about a half-hour's drive from Lovina. They're set back from the road, so you'll have to walk a short way past a row of little shops. But it's worth the walk.

Long ago, the spring was divided into three tiered pools. Each tier still features a wall of dragonheads, "spitting" water into the pool below. Stone steps make access to each of the pools easier for bathers.

The springs are surrounded by forest and many flowering plants. It's a lovely spot, but Banjar is better known for something else.

The warm water is soothing enough, but it is also full of minerals – especially sulfur. Hot sulfur springs have been prized for their healing powers for centuries. Whenever the ancient Romans found one of these springs, they would build a bath there.

You see, the heat and sulfur are especially good for relieving the stiffness and pain of arthritis. So Banjar is not only beautiful, it's also a part of our island's healing traditions.

Indian long pepper is another Balinese tradition that eases pain. We call it "tabia bon," and my parents often found it useful – especially for toothache.

I can still remember my father taking dried long pepper, crushing it to a powder and making a poultice for neighbors with a toothache.

In short order, their tooth would stop throbbing and they could sleep comfortably. This made my father a very popular man.

Today we make a poultice from the mashed leaves to relieve rheumatism. It quickly warms and loosens the joints.

Of course, Indian long pepper is popular in recipes, too. Many Balinese families have it on hand. You'll often find it growing along garden walls and other quiet spots.

It's also an effective home remedy for congestion. It's one of those herbs that every Balinese grandmother has used.

When someone in the family is all stuffed up from a cold, you can make an infusion of the root in tea or milk. Then have the sufferer drink a little bit regularly throughout the day. It will soon clear up their congestion.

— *Lelir*

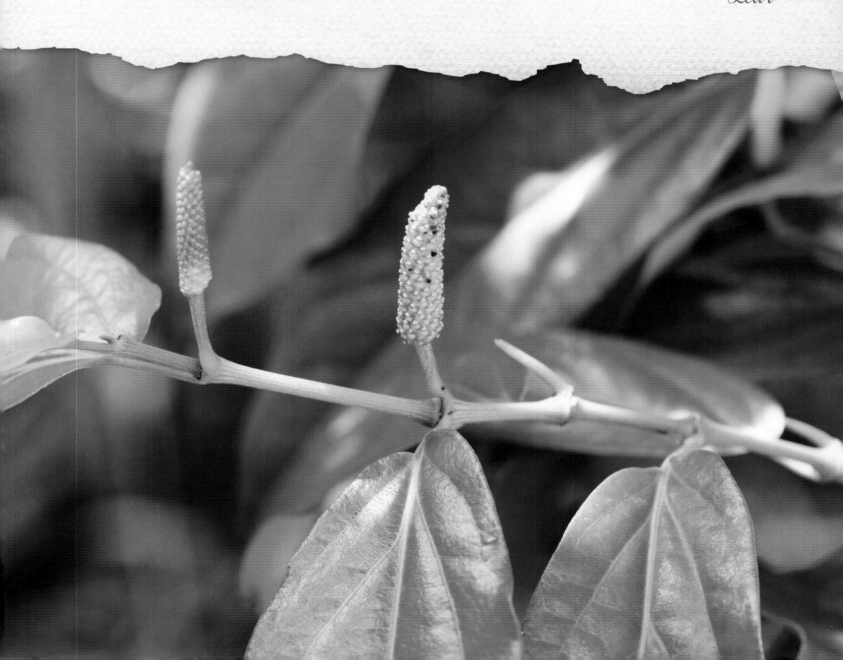

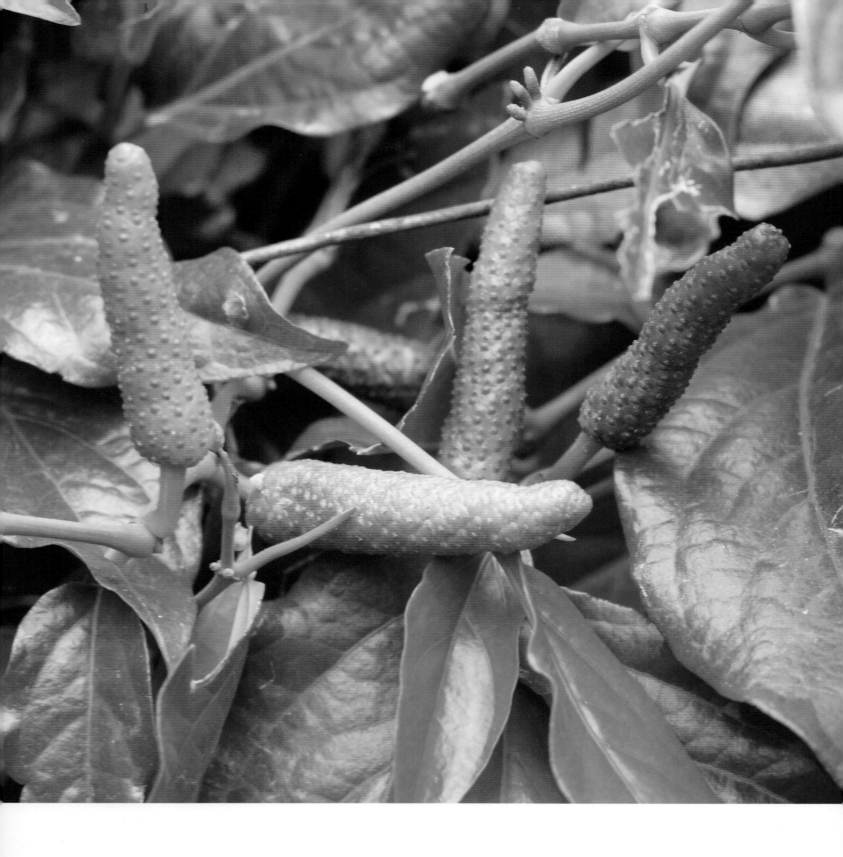

My Own Research and Discoveries

Long pepper contains a compound called piperine. One of the benefits of ingesting piperine is that it enhances the bioavailability of other nutrients, making them more easily absorbed.

Contrary to what many people think, the long pepper has no capsaicin.[1] However, even though you won't get the many benefits of that compound, the long pepper and its components like piperine, beta-sitosterol and other unique compounds, can:

Grow New Brain Cells. A new study shows that extracts from the fruit of the long pepper tree help enhance brain cell growth, even in very small amounts.[2]

Benefit Your Heart. Long peppers reduce triglyceride levels and platelet aggregation, while increasing the body's ability to dissolve elastin, a substance that thickens the aorta and increases heart disease. Cultures that use hot peppers like the long pepper liberally have a much lower rate of heart attack and stroke.

Fight Inflammation. Studies show that all of the components of the long pepper are more powerfully antioxidant than vitamin E, the standard against which all other antioxidants are measured.[3]

Lower Blood Pressure. When they give black pepper extracts to animals, the piperine lowers blood pressure across the board.[4] Even when they're fed a high-fat, high-carb diet, their blood pressure is still normal when they get piperine.[5]

Lower Blood Sugar. Long pepper lowers blood sugar levels and also prevents other complications associated with diabetes.

Improve Oxygen Uptake. Research tells us that the Indian long pepper may help improve the flow of oxygen into the body. Why is that important? Oxygen is your most powerful healing agent, detoxifier and cancer-fighter. More oxygen helps you prevent lung disorders, breathes new life into your bones and skin, and slows down aging.

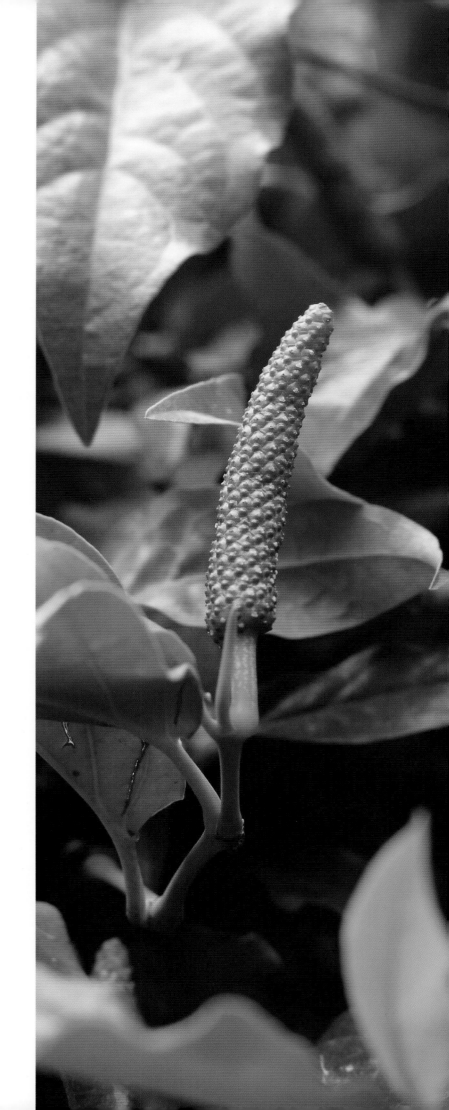

Drop A Few Extra Pounds. That heat you feel after eating hot peppers takes energy and calories to produce. After you eat them, they increase thermogenesis (heat production) and oxygen consumption in your fat tissue. Long pepper, in particular, seems to reduce both fat mass and the size of fat cells. In animal models, those fed a high-fat diet but also given long pepper didn't gain any weight at all. In fact, their fat mass went down, as did the size of their fat cells.[6]

Heal Your Prostate. In a review of several clinical trials, beta-sitosterol helped men with enlarged prostates improve urinary flow and volume *in every study*.[7] The native tribes living in Florida before European settlement recognized the benefit of plants containing beta-sitosterol, too. So it's been recognized for centuries by natural healers as a prostate protector.

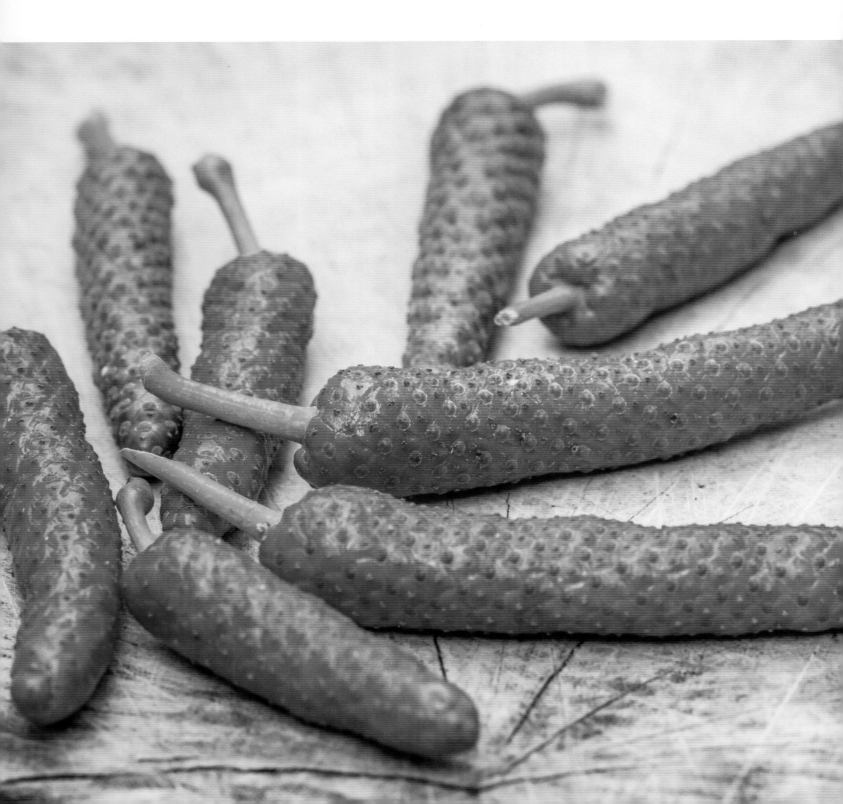

Preparations

If you like to eat peppers, don't listen to the "naysayers." Hot foods and those smoldering Indonesian dishes made with long pepper make excellent choices. They're full of vitamins, calcium and iron.

You'll be amazed at how easy it is to incorporate peppers into your cuisine.

.... *Indian Long Pepper* ....

I look for Indian long pepper when I shop and add it to my food in place of other peppers. They're quite good in salsa.

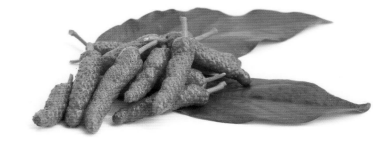

You can buy dried long peppers in bulk online and in many health food stores. You can also buy it ground.

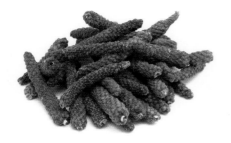

Long pepper is hotter than black pepper, and it has a kind of gingery hint to it. I like to put it on sautéed vegetables, like asparagus.

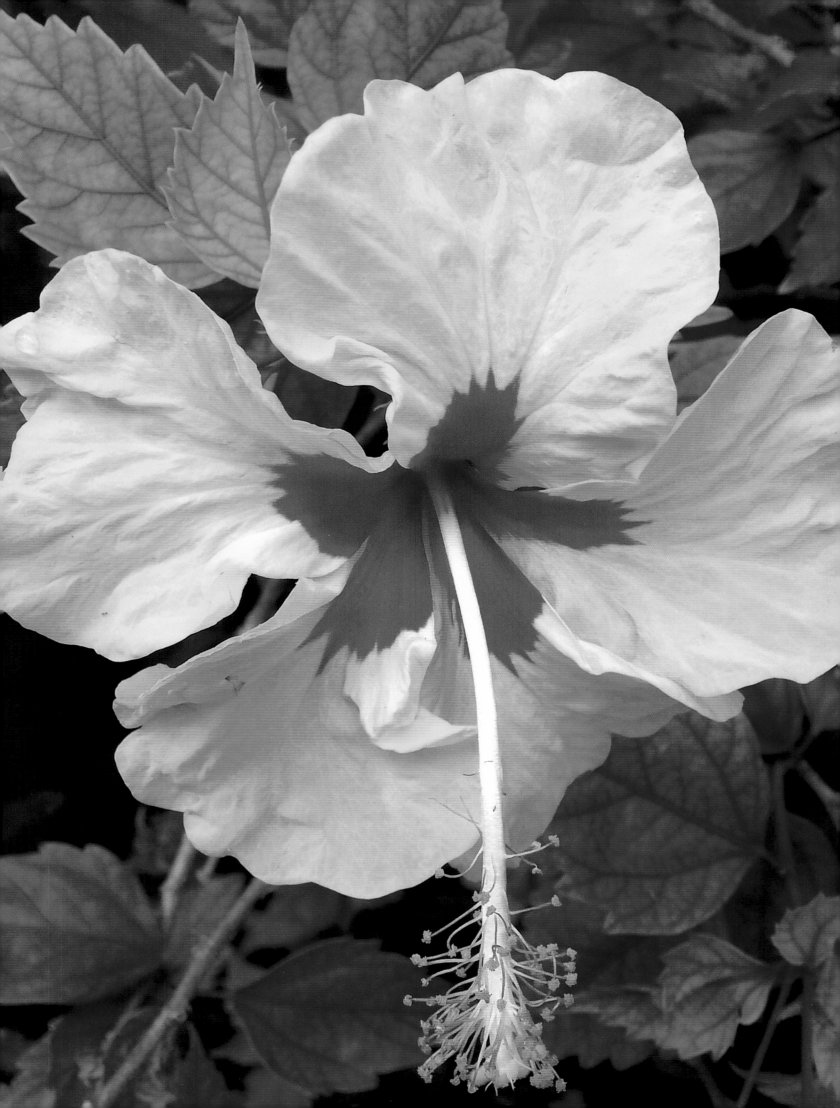

THE WORLD'S KINDEST BEAUTIFYING FLOWER

I've always been attracted to the healing practices of the ancients.

It's why I traveled to India... so I could track down the original source of the 5,000-year-old tradition of Ayurvedic medicine.

There I discovered many natural solutions for both health and beauty. Many of those traditions made their way into the Balinese Hindu tradition. This is how the use of hibiscus flowers came to Bali.

You may already be familiar with hibiscus. If you live in a tropical or sub-tropical area — like I do here in South Florida — you may even have one growing in your yard. But there's much more to this flower than just a pretty addition to your garden.

Hibiscus (also known as "rosemallow" and "Jamaican Sorrel") is often used in Ayurvedic natural beauty remedies.

This pretty flower has been a common treatment for hair growth in India and China for centuries — and there's modern evidence that it works.[1]

The leaves and petals of the hibiscus plant work to help improve the overall health of

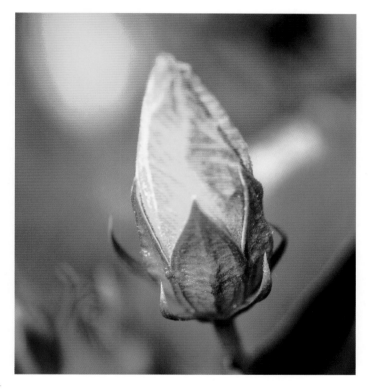

The leaves and petals of the hibiscus plant can prevent premature gray hair.

your scalp.[2] They can also leave your hair looking shiny and lustrous and help prevent premature graying.[3]

Traditionally, the hibiscus flower is used in hair rinses and shampoos. But when used topically, the hibiscus flower can darken your hair, so many women choose to take it internally instead.

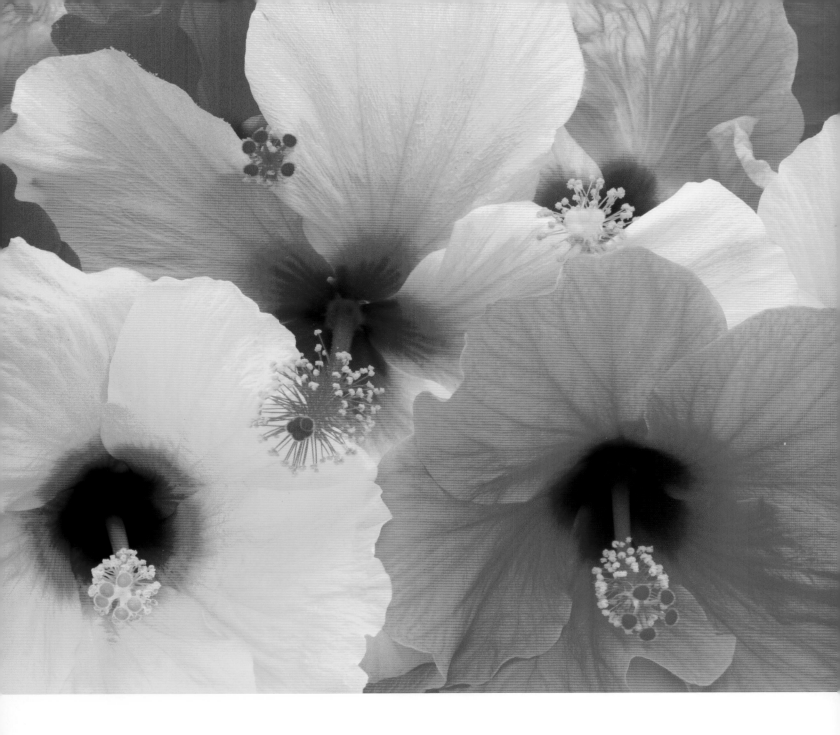

The Power of this Plant Goes Beyond Skin-Deep

It turns out hibiscus is also beneficial to your whole body. It guards against DNA damage. And anthocyanins extracted from varieties of hibiscus plants all over the world are being studied for their anticancer properties.

Powerful compounds in this plant can help tighten skin, reduce pores, improve elasticity and protect you from aging sun damage. All of that can leave your skin looking naturally firm, young and vibrant.

As I've said, I like it when cultures from all over the world use the same plant for the same remedies. It solidifies them as true healing agents. This is true for hibiscus as well.

I've seen it used in Jamaica, India and other remote places in the world. And as Lelir told me, it's used in Bali for some of the same reasons.

Yellow Hibiscus
Bali's Secret to Easing Childbirth

(Hibiscus tilaceus)

Balinese name: Daun Waru

Art and Balinese culture are linked together like blood and your heart. You can have a heart without blood... but it will be lifeless. Art has been a part of our culture for longer than anyone can remember.

Westi's father – like his grandfather, great-grandfather and great-great-grandfather – was a farmer. They were all also artists. For farmers, art has helped feed their families between growing seasons for countless generations.

I suppose this tradition started as so many others do... out of necessity. Long, long ago, farmers had to feed their families year-round. But the money they earned from their harvest didn't last a full year.

Balinese farmers have always carved useful items between harvest and planting times. Cups, bowls, spoons... anything their families needed. Wood was plentiful, and they had lots of time on their hands.

As their skills grew, these farmers found they could sell their carvings in local markets. People in towns and cities needed bowls and spoons, too. So farmers found a second source of income.

When tourists came to Bali, bowls and spoons evolved into decorative art. And as the reputation of Bali's artists grew, so did the market for hand-carved items.

Today, carvings made by Bali's farmers are sold around the world. Balinese art has become an important cultural export.

Here in Ubud, we have several small museums dedicated to art. And each looks at art in a slightly different way. Balinese farmers developed homegrown art. Bali inspired other artists who moved here from other countries.

Here in our city, these artistic traditions intersect.

Don Antonio Blanco was one of the most famous artists inspired by Bali. Don Antonio was trained as a doctor and traveled the world. But Bali seduced him. He settled here in 1952, married a Balinese dancer and painted in Bali until his death in 1999.

Today the Don Antonio Blanco Museum keeps this famous artist's legend alive.

The Neka Art Museum is a bridge between traditional Balinese art and art created by visitors enchanted by Bali. With such a mixture, this museum shows our island through the world's eyes.

There is also the Agung Rai Museum of Art – ARMA. This museum is dedicated to art done by Balinese painters and painters inspired by Bali. But ARMA celebrates Balinese art in an unusual way. It's also a small hotel – offering visitors to Ubud a chance to get close to Bali's art.

This growing appreciation for Balinese art gives us hope. Hope that people will also develop an appreciation of our herbal heritage as well.

Take, for example, the yellow hibiscus.

This large shrub grows practically everywhere in Bali. It loves our tropical soil. You can find it along roadsides, deep in our jungles and even cultivated in gardens. It's a lovely flower – worthy of cultivation for its beauty alone.

But yellow hibiscus has a special use here in Bali. We make a juice from the leaves to ease childbirth.

I've read that yellow hibiscus was also used this way in Hawaii. The leaves would be brewed into a slimy tea and given to pregnant women from their 7th month on. Regular use of this tea helps the baby come out easily.

Here in Bali, we soak the leaves for 3 or 4 days and make a tea from the juice. We give this tea to a pregnant woman from about the 7th month.

When I was a child, many people still had their babies at home. So my parents kept very busy brewing hibiscus tea. In those days, it was probably much easier to have a baby at home than in a hospital.

We also have another unique use for yellow hibiscus – and other types of hibiscus as well. It makes a wonderful hair treatment.

You take a handful of the young leaves and place them in a bucket or other receptacle and add some water. Then you crush the leaves in the water until the sap mixes well and it becomes an excellent hair conditioner.

— *Lelir*

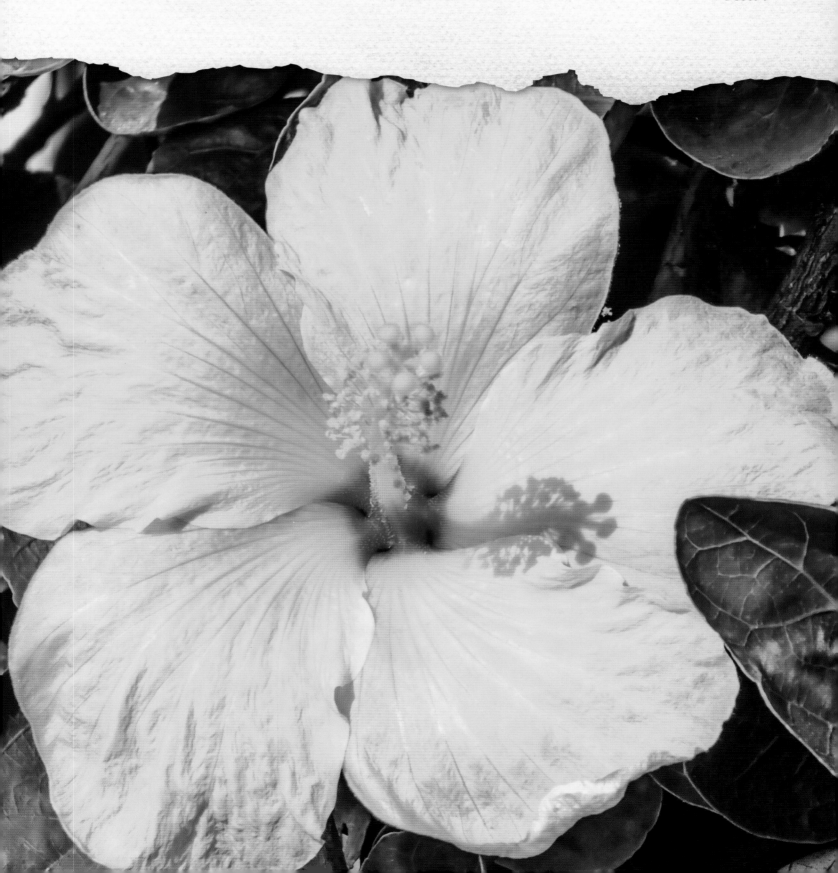

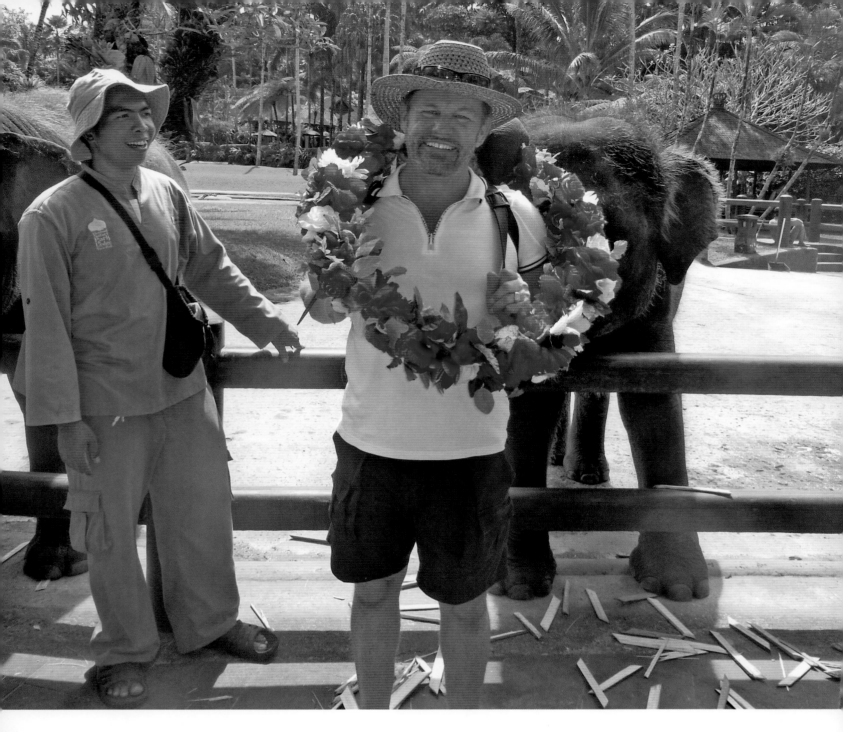

The Balinese are very fond of giving flowers as gifts. They gave me this wreath made of white and red hibiscus when I visited the Ubud Elephant Park Zoo.

My Own Research and Discoveries

One reason hibiscus is so kind to your body and skin is that it's loaded with healing antioxidants called "anthocyanins."

How powerful are they?

Potent enough to wipe out cancer cells.

At the Laboratory of Herbal Medicine and Molecular Oncology at the General Hospital in Taiwan, they discovered that anthocyanins from the root bark of the hibiscus killed almost 50% of lung cancer cells in one clinical trial.[4]

In Africa, I learned that traditional healers believe hibiscus gives liver protection.

Scientists at another prestigious Taiwanese research facility, the Institute of Biochemistry and Biotechnology, proved the herbalists right. Their study showed hibiscus anthocyanins induce liver cancer cell death and elevate liver-protecting gene expression.[5]

The prestigious journal *Molecular Carcinogenesis* reports that hibiscus anthocyanins are also effective against gastric cancer cells[6] and leukemia cells.

At the Birla Institute of Technology in India they found that anthocyanins from hibiscus also protect DNA from damage. They found a "significant correlation between antioxidant capacity" of hibiscus and that... "anthocyanins were the major contributors of antioxidant activity."[7]

In fact, I found over 750 studies on hibiscus and its health benefits.

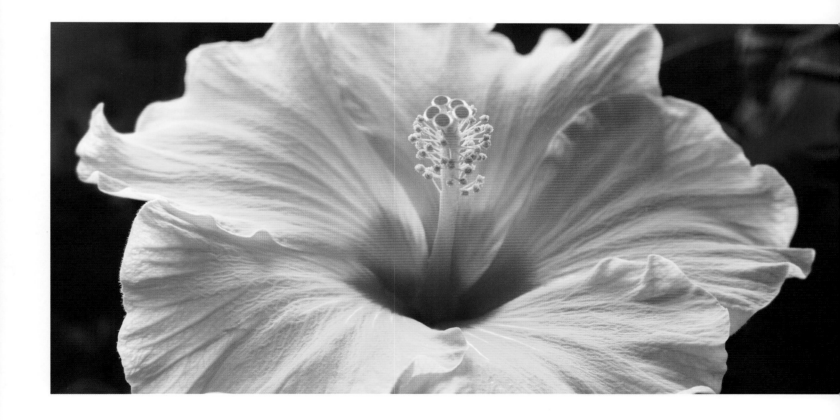

Younger, More Vibrant Skin

For your skin, these "super-antioxidant" anthocyanins protect skin cells from free radical damage, which can make you look tired and old. And they act as an astringent that tightens up pores and makes them appear smaller.

Although hibiscus is toning and tightening, it never strips your skin of its natural oils or dries it out. In fact, hibiscus has a high mucilage, or gel, content, which makes it a great moisturizer that can help improve your skin's elasticity and flexibility. That's exactly what you need, to give you that look of a flawless complexion.

Hibiscus also keeps your skin looking young because it's a natural sunscreen. Researchers in India have shown that hibiscus flower extract may protect against sun damage to skin by absorbing ultraviolet radiation.[8] Ultraviolet rays cause photo aging like discoloration and age spots that can add years to your face.

Yellow hibiscus does well in almost any tropical climate. It's rich in vitamin E and other antioxidants — especially plant sterols. These natural compounds are known to promote heart health.

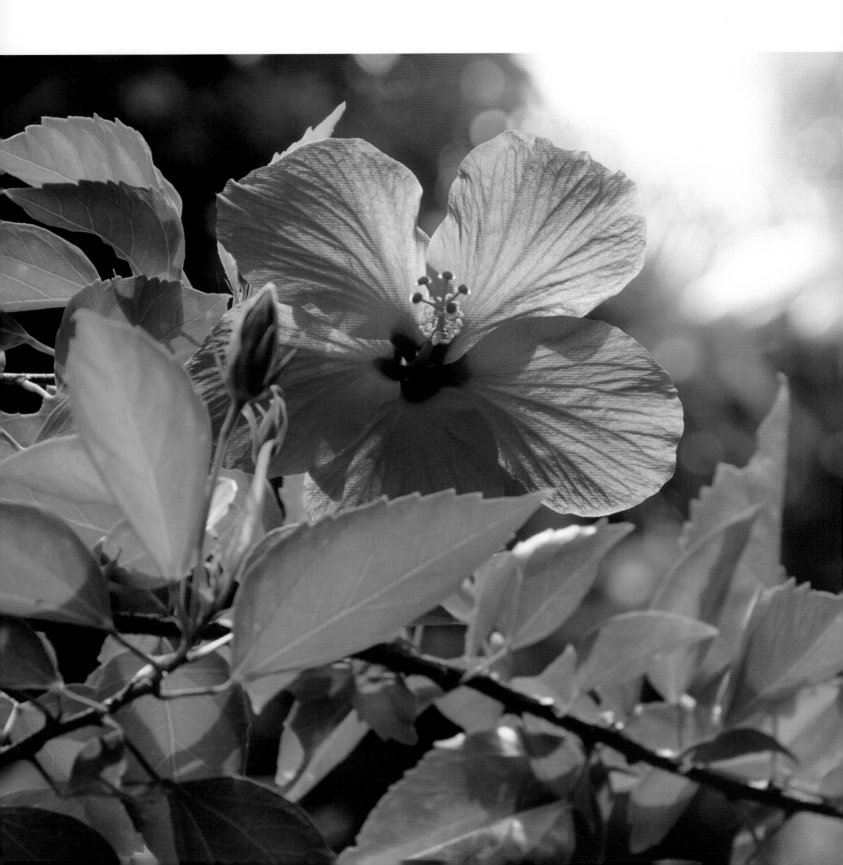

Here is What I Recommend

For antioxidant benefits, I recommend drinking two cups of hibiscus tea every day. You may also see it called sour tea, red tea or red sorrel.

Hibiscus

You can make your own hibiscus tea by steeping the petals of fresh or dried hibiscus flowers for 10-15 minutes.

The brewed tea will have a tart taste almost like cranberry.

You may want to sweeten it with honey or stevia.

Also, remember that hibiscus tea is very acidic, so it's best not to add milk because it could curdle.

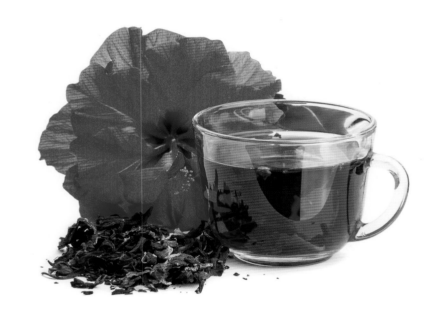

Celestial Seasonings makes a nice blend of hibiscus, rosehips, orange peel and lemongrass called "Red Zinger" that's widely available in supermarkets.

In beauty products, look for natural facial toners, serums and moisturizers containing hibiscus or an extract of hibiscus.

Also, luxury spas have recently started offering facials with light hibiscus acid peels.

And of course, you can find hibiscus in supplement form. 40 mg of natural hibiscus flower extract will restore that look of youthful beauty.

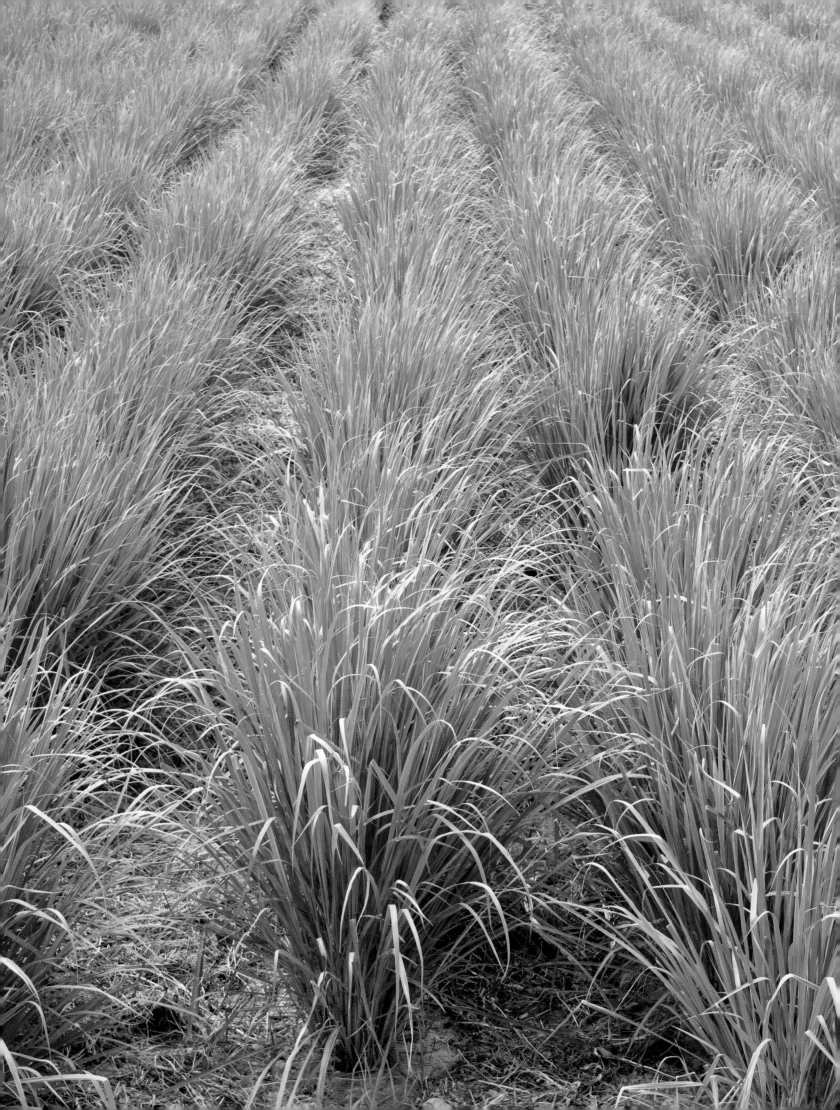

DRIVE AWAY PAIN

(AND MOSQUITOES)

They ward off mosquitoes in Bali with lemongrass. Specifically, citronella, a type of lemongrass.

Lelir and Westi showed me how they grow citronella *(Cymbopogon nardus)* in their huge herb garden. My own garden in Florida has just a fraction of what they have.

Mosquitoes don't like the smell of lemongrass, so they stay away. House flies don't like it either. In fact, researchers have found most bugs will avoid areas with the lemongrass oil.[1]

I'm sure you've heard of citronella candles for your backyard to keep the bugs away. But what if you're out walking around? Then you need to take lemongrass oil with you.

What I do is break open a couple of stalks and crush them in my hand. I enjoy the lemony aroma and then I dab it right on my skin instead of chemical bug spray.

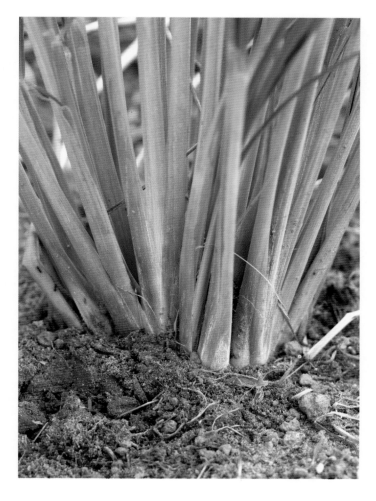

Lemongrass is a great natural mosquito repellent.

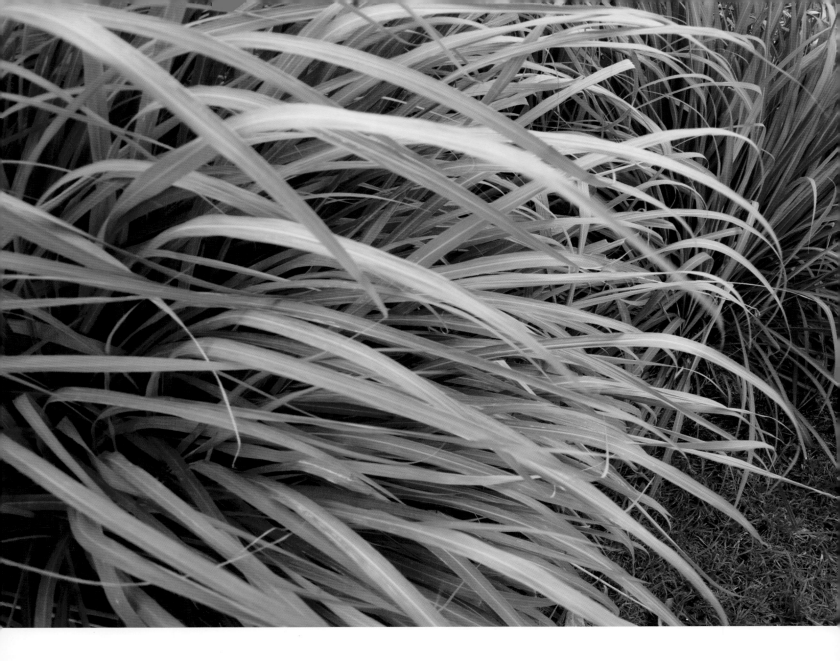

The Bugs Don't Like It, and Neither Does Fungus

It also makes a delicious tea ... because lemongrass isn't just for candles. It has a lot of health benefits.

That's why there are hundreds of lemongrass plants growing in Westi's garden.

Westi explained that his ancestors didn't exactly understand what fungal infections were, even though they experienced them quite often. But they have always used lemongrass for effectively curing these infections. Studies now back up this ancient use.

Researchers at the Indian Institute of Technology in New Delhi found lemongrass has incredible power against fungus. It destroyed 100% of the yeast C. albicans, which, when it overgrows, can cause infection and immune suppression.[2]

When doctors at the Federal University of Campina Grande in Brazil looked to lemongrass to treat a fungal infection that's common there, the essential oil from lemongrass *cured* 80% of the infections.[3]

Powerful Way to Purge Pain

Lemongrass is effective against chronic pain, especially connective tissue pain. The essential oil made from lemongrass is great at soothing ligaments, tendons and cartilage.

It's also good for relieving inflamed tissue from a sprain, tennis elbow or Achilles tendonitis. And it works for rheumatism and arthritis. In one study, animals given higher doses of lemongrass oil had 100% of their pain relieved.[4]

Traditionally, lemongrass is used in treating internal inflammation, not just acute inflammation and pain.

In one study lemongrass inhibited formation of cytokines, the inflammatory molecules that can cause dysfunction in the energy-producing centers of critical immune cells.[5] Many other studies on lemongrass have found similarly powerful, anti-inflammatory effects.[6]

Lemongrass protects the heart as well, by increasing antioxidants in heart tissue.[7]

And one powerful effect of lemongrass that most people don't know about is that it can raise HDL[8] and stop LDL cholesterol from oxidizing.[9]

Why is that so important?

When LDL oxidizes, it can form atherosclerotic plaque that can block arteries and cause heart attacks. Heart attacks are rare in Bali, and with powerfully protective plants like lemongrass in common use, it's not surprising.

Lemongrass oil is a powerful antifungal as well. One study showed that lemongrass oil vapor worked well against fungal growth. This means that using lemongrass as an aromatherapy would be highly effective against fungal growth.[10]

Lemongrass has a very important function in traditional Balinese cuisine and medicine. Westi told me lemongrass played a big part in one of his favorite parts of childhood.

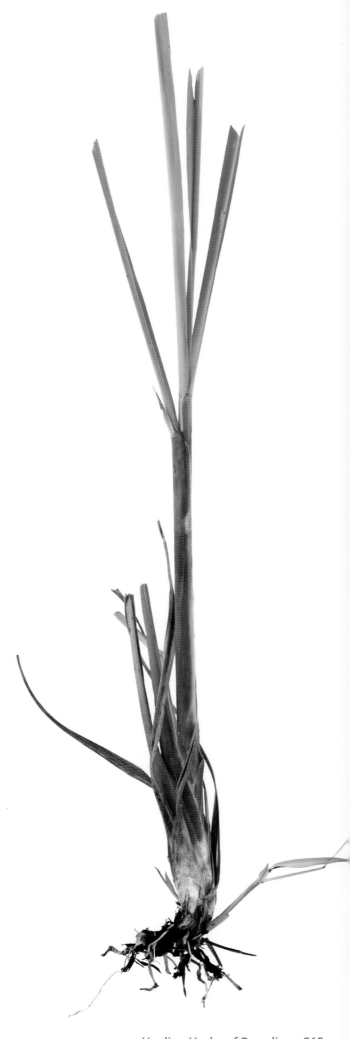

Delicious Lemongrass...

Always in the Kitchen

(Cymbopogon citratus)

Balinese name: Sereh

When I was growing up, the evening meal was an important time for my family. This was the one time of day when everyone was together, and our meals were lively events.

Mother always wanted to know what we'd learned in school that day and my father usually had something to share from his day in the rice fields... or stories of selling his carvings to local tourist shops.

Mother served up steaming bowls of rice and lots of fresh vegetables – whatever was in season. And, of course, we always had plenty of her homemade Bali hot sauce – called "sambal sereh" – on hand.

Even today, one taste of Mother's recipe can bring me back to my childhood in an instant. Almost everything tasted better when you added sambal sereh. It could turn even a bowl of plain rice into a feast.

One of the main ingredients in Mother's hot sauce was sereh – lemongrass. You'll find this herb growing in almost every kitchen garden in Bali. And not just because Bali hot sauce is so popular.

Lemongrass is one of the most versatile herbs. We use it to flavor foods... as an aromatherapy scent... to aid digestion... as an antispasmodic... even as an insect repellent.

This herb also eases diarrhea, kills many bacteria and fungi and calms fevers and flu. It's very effective against gastritis.

As you can imagine, rice farmers often suffer with athlete's foot. When the rice is young, the paddies are flooded and traditional farmers work barefoot or in sandals all day. In a hot, humid place like Bali, these are perfect conditions for fungi to grow.

For many generations, Balinese farm families have made essential oil from lemongrass and applied it to these fungal infections. The athlete's foot usually clears up within a week or two.

Lemongrass tea is delicious, with a warm, lemony flavor. We drink this tea on its own or mix the lemongrass with other herbs to make various herbal teas. But many Balinese also keep a spray bottle of lemongrass tea in the kitchen.

This may sound a little odd, but lemongrass contains citronellal, the same chemical found in citronella. Many people like to mist themselves with this tea before they go outside. It's an easy – and fairly effective – mosquito repellent.

Herbalists like Lelir and her parents also use lemongrass to relieve headaches.

But of all of the uses we have for lemongrass, my mother's sambal sereh will always be my favorite.

— Westi

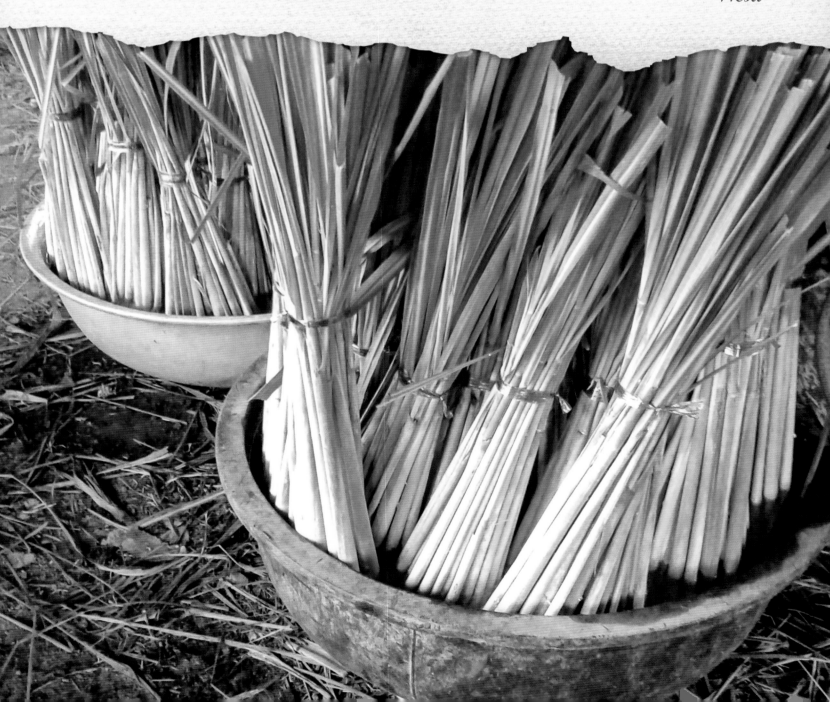

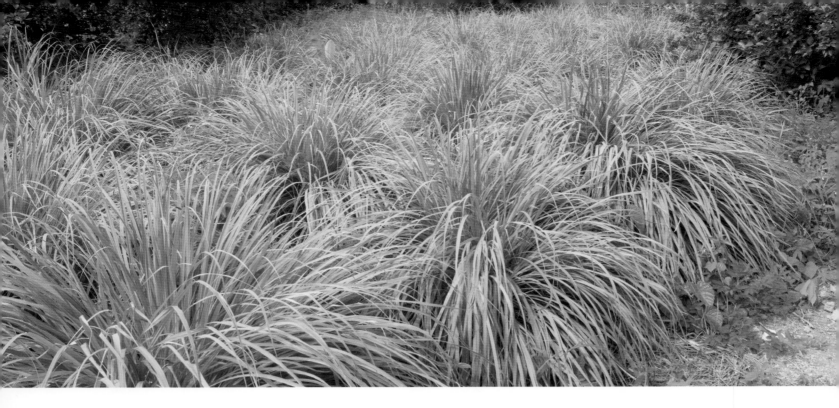

Lemongrass grows wild all over Bali and is used as a natural antibacterial and anti-anxiety agent.

My Own Research and Discoveries

Lemongrass has several benefits:

- Lemongrass is antibacterial, antidiarrheal and effective against worms.[11]

- In traditional Mexican medicine, lemongrass is used to reduce anxiety and calm people down. One study looked at lemongrass' calming effect. They tested it in mice and found that not only were the mice calmer and less anxious, they also seemed to stay calm no matter what. They were immune to annoying external stimuli like flashing lights.[12]

- Lemongrass can cure a stomach ache and even gastric ulcers. At Cariri Regional University in Crato, Brazil, scientists looking into lemongrass' effect on ulcers were shocked. They treated mice with lemongrass oil and then tried to give the mice ulcers... and they couldn't! Even using three different potent ulcer-inducers, the mice were protected.[13]

- Lemongrass also promotes the health of the friendly microflora in your gut that help you digest food and make B vitamins.[14]

- Many types of lemongrass relieve headaches, just as Westi described. Australian natives have used it as a headache cure for countless centuries.[15]

Researchers discovered that many kinds of lemongrass contain eugenol, an antiseptic oil that is a proven painkiller. Eugenol works by stimulating an enzyme called "UGT1A10" that converts chemicals and foreign substances to a water soluble fat that your body quickly flushes out, relieving aches and pains.[16,17]

That makes it ideal for treating headaches and inflammatory conditions. In fact, eugenol is almost as effective as aspirin.

Here is What I Recommend

Pain Relieving Tea

You can get lemongrass oil at your local health food store or on online. Look for pure Cymbopogon citratus on the label. It may also be labeled "Melissa oil" in Ayurvedic shops.

Tea made from the raw leaves relieves pain, too. I don't recommend the dried leaves for tea because they're fibrous and not very appealing floating in your tea.

I like to make the tea right from the plants in my yard. To make it, all you need are some fresh lemongrass stalks and a quart of water.

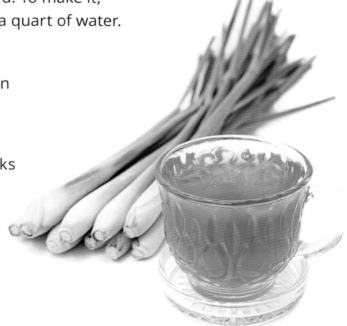

1. Boil the water, and in the meantime clean fresh stalks of lemongrass. Then cut and discard the green upper part of the stalks. The white part is what you make the tea with.

2. A trick I learned from Lelir is to tenderize the stalks by gently pounding them. This will release the oils into the tea.

3. Put the stalks inside a teapot and pour the boiling water over them.

4. Steep for 5 minutes and serve.

Bali-style Hot Sauce (Sambal Sereh)

Gather the following ingredients:

- Two lengths of fresh lemongrass
- Three medium red onions or shallots
- One chili pepper — choose one based on how hot you want your sauce
- Salt
- Salad oil

Remove the upper portion of the lemongrass — from where the "hairs" begin to grow on the stalks. (You can use these "hairy" parts to make tea.)

Finely dice the lemongrass, onions and chili. Mix thoroughly with a dash of salt and a few drops of salad oil.

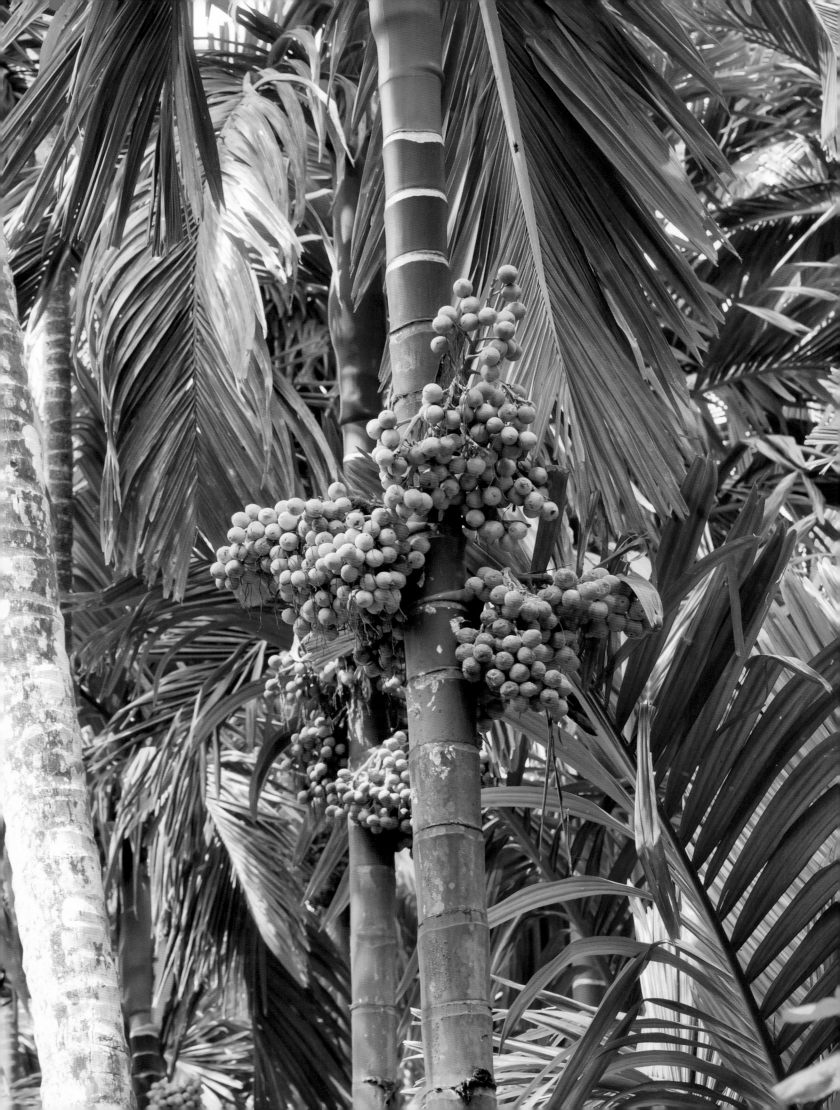

MORE OF BALI'S PAIN-RELIEVING SECRETS

As I mentioned earlier, I could have spent an entire trip in Bali just relaxing in the incredible atmosphere of the Four Seasons hotel... but it was time to trek into the jungle so I could meet with Ketut Liyer.

He's somewhere around 100 years old now and probably the most famous person on the island thanks to the book and movie *Eat, Pray, Love.* I love the line where the main character says to him, "You need to come to America," and Ketut tells her, "I don't have enough teeth to travel on an airplane."

Ketut was very interested in my coming to Bali. He said he had a dream I would come and he made a big deal of it. He told me that he's a ninth-generation healer and that he was happy I wanted to write about him and his ancient practices.

He gave me what he calls a reading. He analyzes you and tells you what your strengths are and what your future holds, and that kind of thing.

He said to me, "You very, very smart. You very strong. Smart and strong, very rare." Then he said, "You also very good. Smart, strong and good very, very rare!"

I don't know... maybe he says that to everybody. But I do admit he made me feel good about myself in a very short time.

I asked him how to do the most good with the time I have on this planet. He flashed a big grin. "You the smart one. You can figure it out."

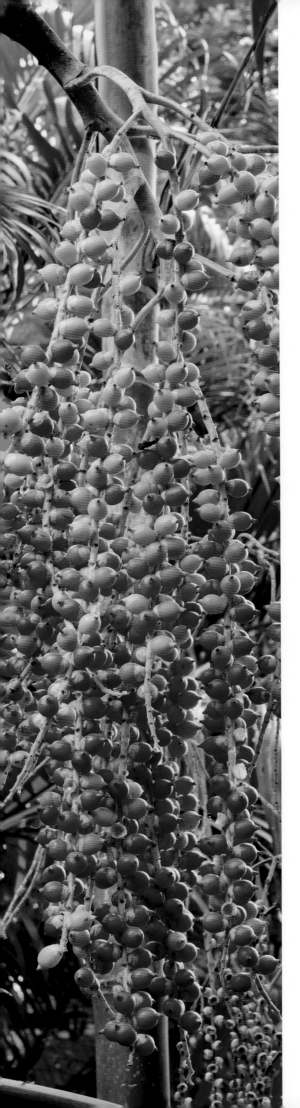

One of the Keepers of the Sacred Healing Texts of Bali

Ketut is a *Balian*. These are the traditional healers who have studied books inscribed on palm leaves called Lontars — the sacred healing texts of the Balinese. The Lontars have descriptions of illnesses, how to diagnose them and how to cure them.

Ketut is Hindu, like almost everyone in Bali. But the Balinese have their own version of Hinduism that has a bit of Buddhism mixed in. So it's very contemplative. Instead of being focused on festivals and rituals like most Hindus, they are more introspective.

For instance, they have three rules to live by they call the *"Tri Hita Karana."* The first is maintaining people-to-people relationships — making sure that everything you do affects others in a good way. In your work, your daily routine, every day you do things that help other people, maintain and strengthen relationships with other people.

The second is to maintain your relationship with nature. Your work and day-to-day activities have to support and strengthen your relationship with the world around you.

And the third is your spiritual relationship — your relationship with god.

It's a patient kind of approach and I like it because it's a very humble way of looking at things. Instead of saying, "Nature is wrong and we're going to fix it" like most Western doctors, Ketut's approach respects nature.

Balians have a sense of trust in your body's abilities. They tend to trust Mother Nature first.

That's why there is a long tradition of herbal medicine on Bali and why almost no one in Bali visits a Western-style doctor.

They're such a happy and sweet people and rarely upset or even hurt. But when they do have aches, pains, an upset stomach or just need a lift, there's a traditional remedy for that, too, which the Balinese have adopted.

Eases Pain and Aids Digestion

(Areca catechu)

Balinese name: Buah Jebog

In Bali, you will see many people with their lips stained red. Men, women and even older children. It's so common, we jokingly call it "Balinese lipstick."

But it's not from lipstick. These people with red lips aren't trying to color their lips at all. The red stain comes from chewing Buah Jebog – or "betel nut."

The first thing I should tell you about betel nut is that it isn't the nut of the betel pepper plant. It's from a palm called "areca" that grows all over Asia. But it's usually chewed wrapped in a leaf from the betel pepper plant, and that's how the name got mixed up.

Chewing betel nut is very popular throughout Asia. About 10% of the world's population chews it regularly. But it's hardly known to the outside world.

Here in Bali, families often welcome visitors to their homes by offering them a betel nut chew. It's almost the same as you offering your guests a cup of coffee. It's an important social tradition.

A basic betel chew is easy to make. You take peeled and cut nuts of the areca and mix them with a paste made from lime (the mineral, not the fruit) and water. These ingredients are wrapped in a betel leaf and popped in your mouth to chew.

In different parts of Asia, they add local flavorings. Some people put a little chewing tobacco in their chew. Others use spices. Here in Bali, adding tobacco is very popular.

When you chew betel nut, the first thing you'll notice is the very strong flavor... and that your mouth immediately fills with saliva. When you spit – you should never swallow – your saliva will be bright red. Your teeth and lips will also be stained red.

Fortunately, it takes the stain a while to become permanent. So you can get rid of the red if you just want to try betel once out of curiosity.

The chew is a mild stimulant. If you try it, you'll probably feel a little "tipsy" – almost like you've had a couple of drinks. Betel nut is known to create feelings of euphoria.

Just be aware it can be toxic in very large doses

The lime paste helps release the alkaloids in the nut. These chemicals cause the good feelings people get from chewing betel nut.

Chewing also helps you feel good in another way. It numbs your mouth. For many generations, we had no dental care here in Bali. Our elders chewed betel nut to relieve painful teeth and gums. Some still do today.

Chewing betel nut is a lot like smoking cigarettes in two ways. Most people don't enjoy it when they first try it. But if you stick with it for a week or so, it grows on you. And within a year, chewing betel becomes a hard habit to break.

The young shoots and flowers of the areca plant are often used safely as food. You can eat them boiled, fermented or even raw. But it is the nut that is most commonly used.

Scientists mostly ignored areca for centuries. They saw it as just another bad habit — almost like a narcotic. But here in Bali, we understand it has healing properties.

Besides easing pain in the teeth and gums, it aids digestion… and it's even known as an aphrodisiac.

But for now, betel is still used mostly for social purposes.

When you visit Bali — and you should — you will meet many warm and friendly people. Some will even invite you into their homes. If you notice a red stain on their lips and teeth, don't be surprised if they offer you a betel nut chew.

— Westi

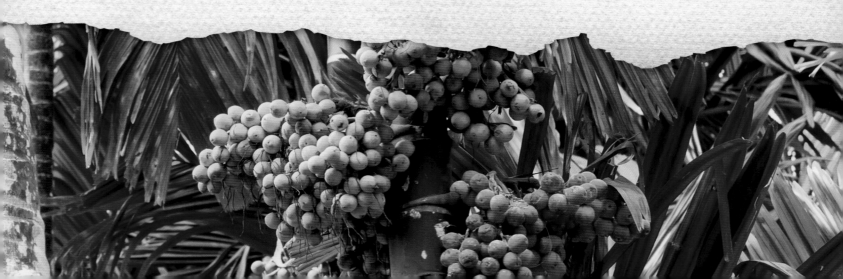

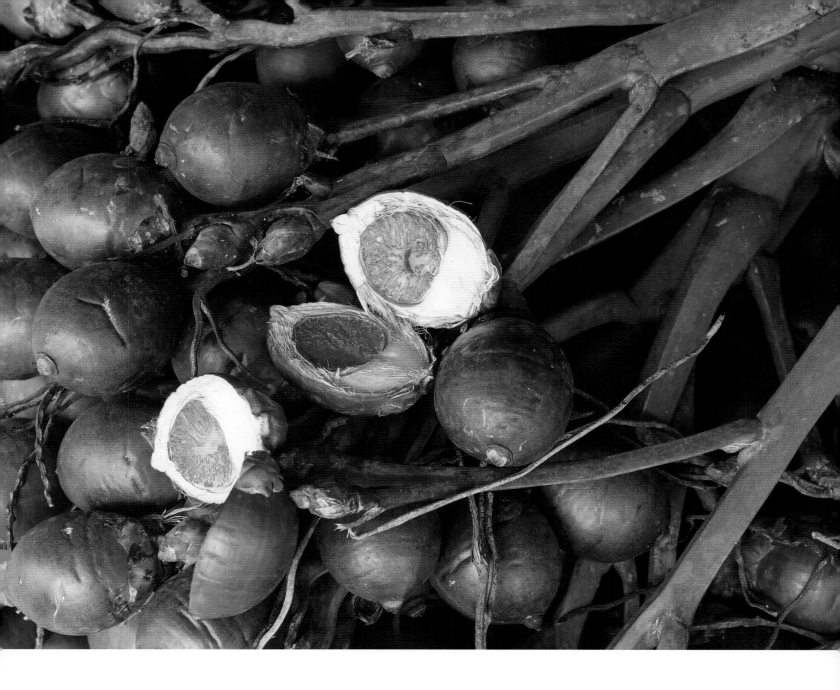

My Own Research and Discoveries

When you go to Bali, you may be offered a betel nut chew. It's a social habit and it's no wonder. Betel nut chew can leave you with a euphoric feeling, kind of like a buzz, and it helps you relax so you socialize more freely. It may have to do with some of the important medical effects the betel nut has on the nervous system.

In one study, Taiwanese doctors gave betel chews to a group of students. They discovered that chewing betel nut modulates the activity of part of your nervous system… the part that controls heartbeat and other "automatic" functions.[1]

In a recent animal study, researchers in Taiwan found areca nuts have anti-inflammatory and pain-relieving properties.[2]

Many countries that I have visited have the areca palm trees. And I noticed something during my travels: many of these cultures use the areca palms for teeth, gum and mouth conditions as well as for digestive problems.

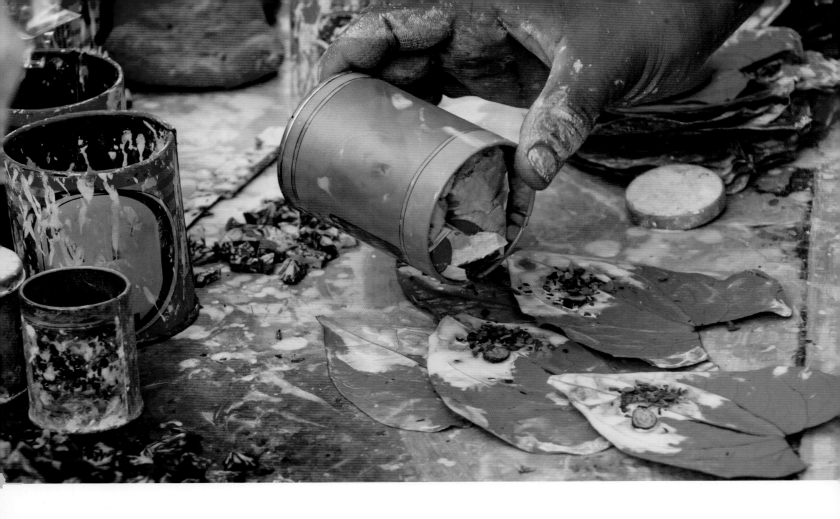

Not All Native Plants Are Good For You

In Taiwan and Papua New Guinea and other Asian countries where areca nut chewing, or "betel quid" chewing, is a regular habit, it can actually lead to problems. Not unlike smoking for many people, there are some risks involved with regular use. It may be the other ingredients mixed with the areca nut that are causing the potential problems. One of those ingredients often used is tobacco.

There are studies that have been done in the last 10 years that show the changes that take place in the mouth due to betel quid chewing. Those changes show that people are more susceptible to oral cancers. Often people add tobacco to the betel quid, speeding up that process.

They are also finding that it causes irregularities in the way the body deals with fats, so cholesterol levels and triglycerides are higher than they should be. It also interferes with the way the body deals with insulin release and glucose uptake in the cells, thereby increasing obesity and metabolic syndrome disorders.

I think limiting the use of the betel nut chewing is the best advice I can offer. With this emerging research showing possible oral cancer risks, diabetes and cardiovascular risks, along with increased obesity in regular betel nut chewing, it is better to limit its use.[3]

Now there is some good news for those that find it hard to break the habit of betel nut chewing. If one were to eat guava buds and use noni juice on a regular basis, it can help prevent the risk of diabetes associated with betel nut chewing.[4]

Here is What I Recommend

Areca Palms

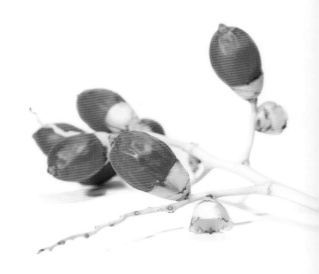

For Gum Disease: Boil 3 Tbsp powder of Areca nut root in 3 glasses of water until half of the water is boiled out. Swish and rinse in the mouth three times daily.

For Diarrhea: Add 2 pinches of powdered Areca nut to one tsp of sugar in a cup of water, stir and drink.

For Ascaris (roundworms): Boil 2 pinches of tender Areca nuts in one cup water. Cool and drink. Or, add the juice of one lime to 2 pinches of Areca nut powder. Mix with one glass of warm water and drink.

Since I mentioned Ketut Liyer, I'll also give you another natural remedy for pain...

Balians like Ketut often prescribe a special kind of meditative healing exercise called *Metta Bhavana*. It's designed to help improve your relationship with others and the world around you, and put you at harmony to relive pain and sickness.

You can try it for yourself:

• First, seat yourself however you feel comfortable.

• Stay completely silent throughout the exercise.

• Begin to focus around your solar plexus.

• Breathe in and out from that area, as if you are breathing from your center.

• Stay focused only on breathing and the sensations at your center.

• Concentrate on generating unconditional good feelings toward yourself and others. (It can help to think of a person who loves you unconditionally. Think of how that makes you feel and use that.)

• Try to notice any areas of your body that might resist you. Concentrate on soothing them and move on.

• If you want, you can repeat a traditional meditation phrase or one you choose yourself. Say or think it several times.

Practice this Balian meditation for 15 minutes every day and it will help you overcome pain and stress, achieve clarity and focus, strengthen your immune system, increase your energy and relieve worries.

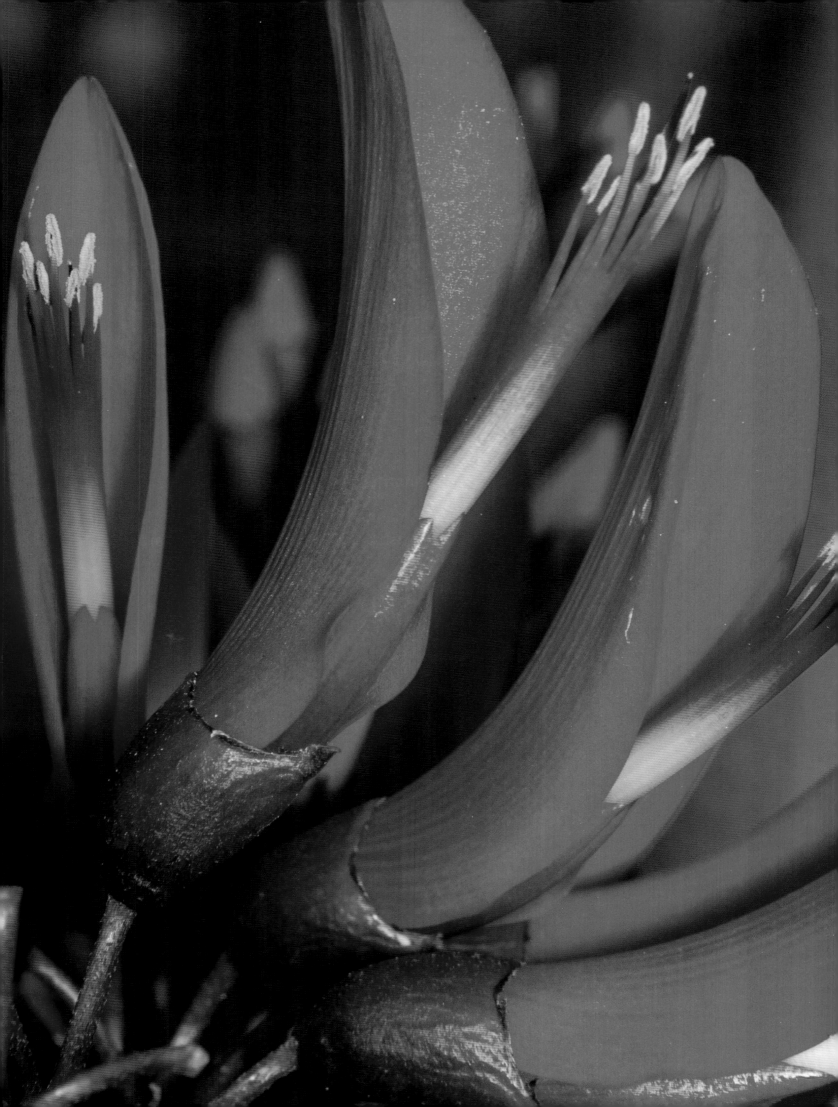

BALI'S BEAUTIFUL OFFERING OF HARMONY AND HEALING

Did you know they only use four names in Bali?

How that came to be, I have no idea.

The first born is called Wayan. The second born is called Madi. The third born is Nyoman. And the fourth born is called Ketut.

Can you guess the fifth born's name? They start all over again with Wayan.

I met a family with 12 people... they had three of each name!

To avoid confusion, what they do is use nicknames. But there aren't many nicknames, either. It can be a little strange if you're not from Bali, but when you meet people there, the nicknames and the confusion become a kind of endearing thing.

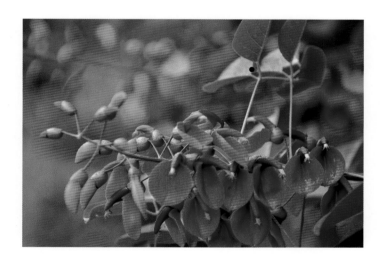

Take my friends Westi and Lelir. His name is Madi, and her name is Wayan... but if everyone called them that, it would be a mess. So they use their nicknames.

Still, no matter their names, they are the most humble and sweet people you will ever meet in your life.

The Julia Roberts Connection

As I mentioned earlier, Ketut Liyer is the healer who became famous because he was in the book and movie, *Eat, Pray, Love.*

But the star of the movie was Julia Roberts, one of the top-earning actresses of all time and quite famous herself.

I asked Ketut about her, what she was like and what it was like to know her. He laughed and said, "She very, very nice. Has great smile." He found her to be very genuine and very friendly.

The Balinese and Ketut are very much the same.

One thing you notice right away about Ketut Liyer is that he smiles all the time.

He wonders why people don't smile more. He says in *Eat, Pray, Love,* "Why they always look so serious in yoga? You make serious face like this, you scare away good energy. To meditate, only you must smile. Smile with face, smile with mind, and good energy will come to you and clear away dirty energy. *Even smile in your liver."*

It may sound strange to "smile in your liver." But Balians are taught that illnesses coming from inside the body are caused by disharmony.

Ketut Liyer and his healer brethren have a very strong relationship with nature. It's part of their form of Hinduism. That relationship is a source of harmony, which prevents illness.

So there are many ancient temples and sacred areas on Bali, full of spirit and life... and healing.

Westi described some of these temples and how they play into everyday Balinese life and healing practices.

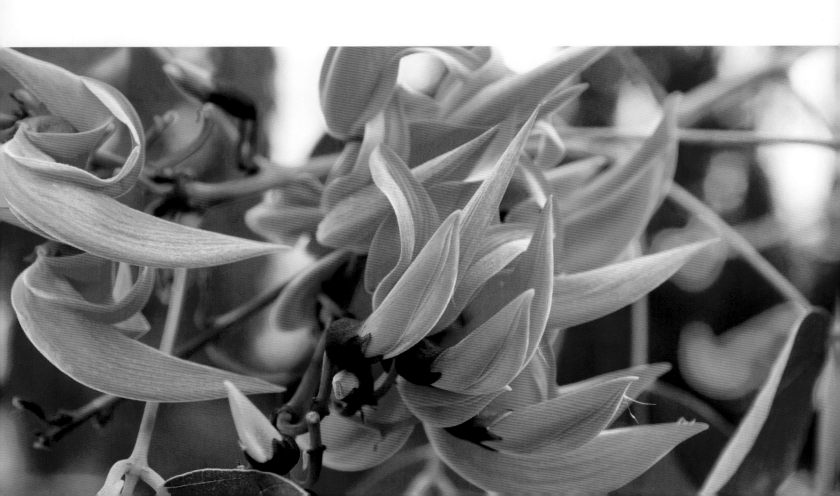

Cure for Fever and Pink Eye

(Erythrina variegata)

Balinese name: Dadap

Religion has always been at the center of Balinese village life. Every village has sacred areas. And most villages have three temples.

The first temple is called "Pura Puseh." This is the temple dedicated to the god Wisnu and is usually built at the upstream end of the village.

"Pura Desa," the village temple, is built near the center of the village. These temples are associated with Brahma.

Finally, there are the "Pura Dalem" – the temples of the dead. You'll find the Pura Dalem at the downstream end of a village. This is also where the village graveyard is located.

Many temples are surrounded by a sacred forest area. And just outside our city of Ubud there is a very special sacred forest surrounding a temple.

The Sacred Monkey Forest grows around the Pura Dalem of a village called Padangtegal. This forest – and temple – are special because more than 600 Balinese long-tailed macaques live there.

The monkeys feel quite at home on the temple grounds. And they've become quite a tourist attraction. Visitors love to wander around and watch the monkeys climbing on the statues and pagodas... chasing each other to steal food... or begging from the visitors.

But there's something equally amazing here that most people never really notice. The forest itself.

This one patch of forest – a speck in terms of Bali's vast jungles – contains 115 different kinds of trees.

With all this variety, it's easy to see how the plant life here became our natural "drug store." There are so many plants with so many different uses.

One of those plants – a tree that grows in the Sacred Monkey Forest – is called the coral tee. Or, as we call it in Balinese, dadap.

The coral tree spreads it branches wide, but doesn't grow very tall. It has broad, heart-shaped leaves and reddish-orange flowers. Because it's an important medicinal plant, many villagers grow dadap in their gardens.

It also helps support the piper betel vine, another important medicinal plant.

Because we are mostly Hindu on Bali, we don't eat meat often. But when we do, we sometimes use the dadap leaves to wrap around the meat for aging and flavoring.

Coral tree is very effective against bacteria. This may explain why it's so effective in cases of pink eye. The problem is often caused by bacteria.

When we apply mashed leaves to the (closed) eyes for a few minutes a day, the pink eye clears up quickly.

Like so many of our medicinal herbs, coral tree also has a spiritual use. When someone builds a new home in Bali, you'll find coral tree there. It's an important part of the ceremony we use to bless new homes.

The people of Bali traditionally believed that coral tree would keep illness and evil spirits away from a home. So having coral tree at the blessing ceremony ensures a happy and healthy home.

— Westi

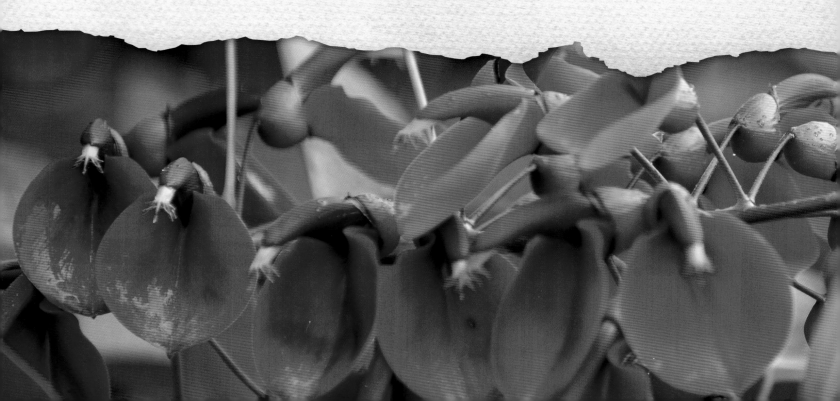

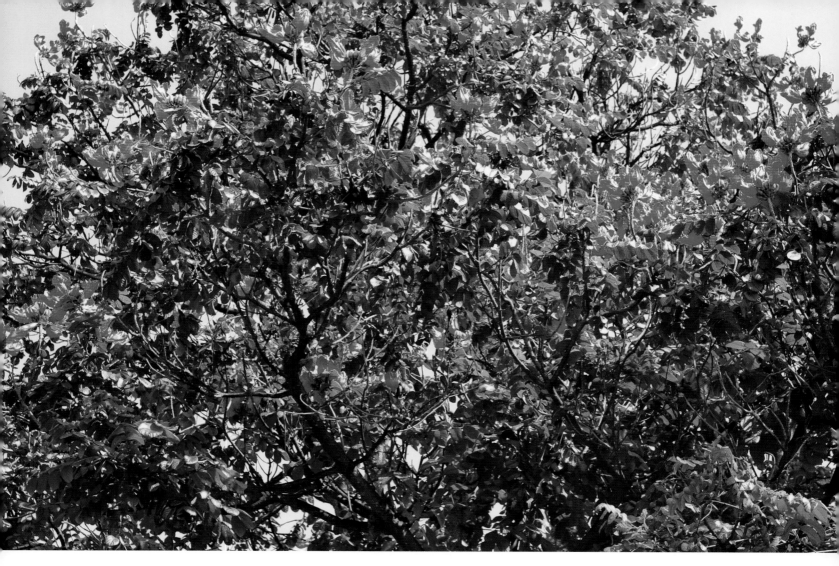

Extracts of the red and sometimes orange leaves of the coral tree are used to treat diabetes and to lower blood sugar.

My Own Research and Discoveries

In medicinal traditions around the world, the leaves and bark from the coral tree are revered.

In India, they use them in traditional mixtures to relieve joint pain, both internally and externally. Coral tree can also relieve coughs. And when they mix the juice from the leaves with honey, it can cure stomach pains and remove parasites.

Science also shows us that extracts of coral tree leaves contain compounds that treat diabetes and lower blood sugar.[1]

At Japan's Meijo University, a team discovered that coral tree contains a powerful compound. It's so strong, it kills MRSA — the incredibly tough-to-kill bacteria that's resistant to most antibiotics[2] and has health specialists around the world scared stiff. Yet here's a natural compound that can get rid of MRSA naturally that they don't even know about.

Extracts from the coral tree root also protect against bone loss.[3]

I broke open a coral tree seed pod and half a dozen or so kidney-bean-shaped seeds poured out. They weren't very tasty to me, but you can dry and eat them and they're very healthy. The seeds are over 30% protein, with 16 different amino acids, many essential to human health.[4]

On Bali, they use all parts of the coral tree for healing:

- Use the sap for chapped lips. Westi says to gently spread a little coral tree sap on dry, cracked lips. Within a few days, your lips will be fine again.

- Apply the mashed young leaves to relieve sores in the mouth.

- Use the older leaves as a fever remedy. Westi takes a few whole coral tree leaves and soaks them in water or arak (palm whiskey). Then he says to lay them across the fevered forehead. "I'm not sure why, but this always seems to cool a fever," he told me.

- Use coral tree leaves to remedy indigestion. Pick and wash a few young coral tree leaves. Mash them together with a red onion and some coconut oil. Apply the mixture on the stomach to relieve indigestion. (This is an external remedy only).

It's not very often you'll find the seeds or leaves of the coral available for sale.

But fortunately, you can grow a coral tree yourself if you live grow in a tropical or subtropical climate. They are very beautiful and ornamental. They are also very good for shade and good companions to other trees. If you'd like to learn more, the best places to go on the web that I've found are gardenweb.com, anniesannuals.com and davesgarden.com.

If you can't grow one yourself, one of my favorite sites, localharvest.org, can help you find out where someone might grow coral trees near you.

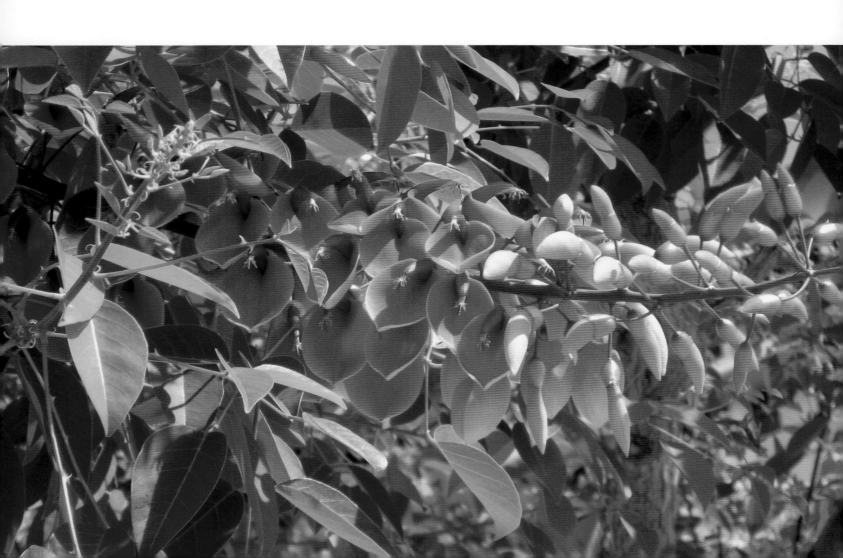

The Power of a Smile

Coral Tree

In Bali's temples, they do more than just decorate them with flowers.

Ketut's tradition teaches that in your work and daily routine you want to make sure you are doing something that helps other people. It's also important to maintain and strengthen your relationships so that you create harmony within the body to protect against illness.

To engender harmony, you begin by smiling.

Turns out there's more to smiling than you might think. Scientific studies consistently show that smiling boosts immunity, increases positive emotions, reduces stress and lowers blood pressure.

I want to share something simple from Ketut's Balian wisdom that is taught in temples around the island by Balian healers that you can use for yourself.

To help you get all the benefits of smiling more, here's a traditional Balinese exercise called "inner smile." You can do it sitting up or lying down.

1. Start by inhaling through your nose. Hold your breath for a moment, then exhale through your mouth. While you're doing this, feel your muscles start to unwind and simply visualize the word "smile."

2. As you continue to breathe slowly, focus your concentration on the muscles of your eyes. You tend to hold a lot of tension in the muscles of your face. Relax these muscles and focus on how they feel when you smile.

3. Now, imagine this feeling moving up towards your brow, around your ears and over your head. As your face starts to relax, bring the corners of your mouth up into a gentle smile.

4. Direct this inner smile into every part of your body. If you feel tension anywhere, just concentrate your smiling energy there until all your fear and worries drop away. Continue until your smile reaches all the way down to your toes.

5. Do this often enough and you'll promote healing in your body. You'll smile more like Ketut does... even in your liver.

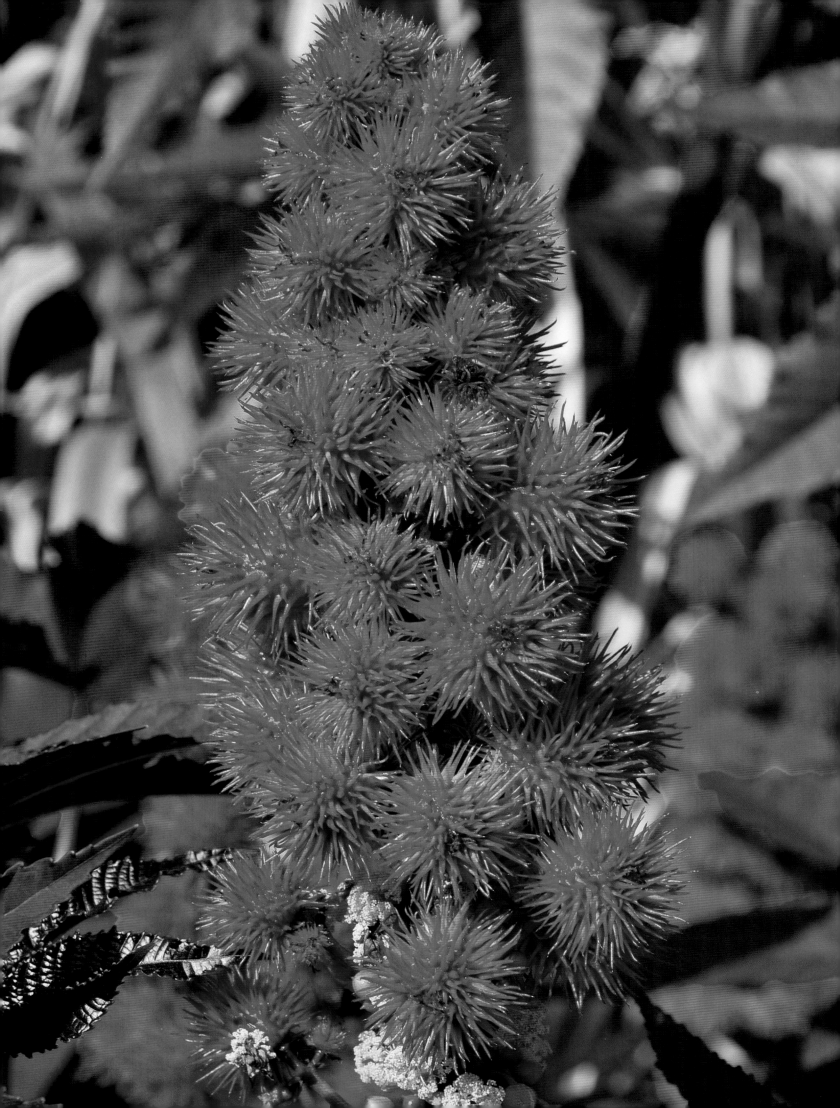

ANCIENT HEALING OIL

I get excited about traditional uses for plants that date over a thousand years. Would you use something that has proven effective for thousands of years?

Castor oil has been used for inducing labor for more than 6,000 years. It's estimated that the ancient Egyptians began using castor oil to induce labor around 4000 BC. They also used castor oil for their lamps and as ointment. In Bali, it is still being used this way today.

Cleopatra used castor oil on her eyes to brighten the whites. It was used by some Greeks to improve hair texture and growth, and also as a body ointment. In Ayurvedic medicine, castor oil is known for curing arthritis.

Castor oil has been successfully used for acne, moles, warts, liver spots, stretch marks, wrinkles, yeast and fungal infections, calloused skin and scars. When applied to the skin, it nourishes, cleanses, detoxifies, softens and soothes. Castor oil has even been used for hair growth, natural darkening, shine and as a mineral moisturizer.

In South Florida, we have one of the biggest horse shows in the world. These people really care for and keep their horses in top shape. In fact, there's a whole industry just for horse chiropractic care, massage and dentistry. And one of the ways people keep their horses healthy is by using castor oil in bathing and hoof-care regimes.

Recent studies have also shown that it's an effective and safe way to induce labor.[1] It's an amazingly versatile herb.

There's evidence behind its anti-inflammatory effect on dysentery. A research team in India tested the root extract on animals and found it had a strong anti-inflammatory effects.[2]

Castor oil also has potent antimicrobial, antifungal and antibacterial activities.[3,4]

Castor oil protects the liver,[5,6] is antidiabetic,[7] can be a laxative[8] and has free radical scavenging activities.[9]

Westi and I got to talking about castor oil, and he called it the "healing fence."

Castor Oil Plant – The Healing Fence

(Ricinus communis)

Balinese name: Daun Jarak

When I was very young, there were still many villages in Bali that didn't have electricity. The families in these villages used oil lamps for light. Looking down from the rice paddies on the hillside in the evening was quite a sight with lights flickering from every window...

This was lovely to see, but – believe me – those families are happy to have electricity today. But for some of them, this change has put their fences out of work.

This probably sounds strange, but let me explain. You see, many homes in Bali have "living fences." We often use plants for fencing. And most of these fences also provide spices or medicines. It's a wonderful way to save space.

Some families grew fences of castor oil plants. Or, as it's called in Bali, daun jarak. The shrub makes a good fence.... and it provides castor beans for oil.

For many generations, most families in Bali had castor oil lamps. The shrub grows wild here and does well in almost any moist, well-drained soil. To keep your house lit at night, you could just pick the beans from your "fence" and press them for oil.

Lamp oil is just one of many uses we have for the castor oil plant. But before I share some of them, I have a warning.

Do not attempt to use the castor oil plant unless you are an experienced herbalist. The seeds are very poisonous. And there is no antidote.

But don't worry. The commercial castor oil you can buy in stores is safe. And trained herbalists know how to use the castor oil plant safely. For medicine, we don't use the seeds – just the root and leaves.

And the leaves are very useful. If you have a blister on your lip, a young leaf is just what you need.

First, cut the stem from the leaf. A milky white sap will come out. Gently rub this sap on the blister. It should clear up in just a couple of days. We also use this sap to speed the healing of ulcers and wounds on the skin.

You can make a poultice from the young leaves to ease a fever and draw the infection out of wounds. And that's not all the leaves are good for.

Dysentery is a painful inflammation of the bowels that causes severe diarrhea, sometimes involving bloody stool. It can be caused by bacteria, a virus or even parasites.

Without modern medicine, our ancestors discovered how to fight this painful condition. They would juice a few young leaves of the castor oil plant. Then they'd strain the juice and give it to their patient to drink.

Long ago, dysentery could be fatal. But the juice from castor oil plants changed this. Now it is much less serious.

Castor oil — such as the type you buy in the store — is a powerful laxative. So it's very interesting to me that the juice from the plant's leaves would have the opposite effect.

Castor oil is also effective to ease childbirth. If a woman is past her due date, a little castor oil usually help bring on the birth.

The root of the castor oil plant also has healing properties. We make an extract from the root that speeds healing of all sorts of skin problems.

Castor root extract soothes herpes, eczema and ringworm. It's also used traditionally as an external antispasmodic for a painful stomach.

Of course, we also keep a castor oil lamp on hand... just in case a storm knocks our power out.

— Westi

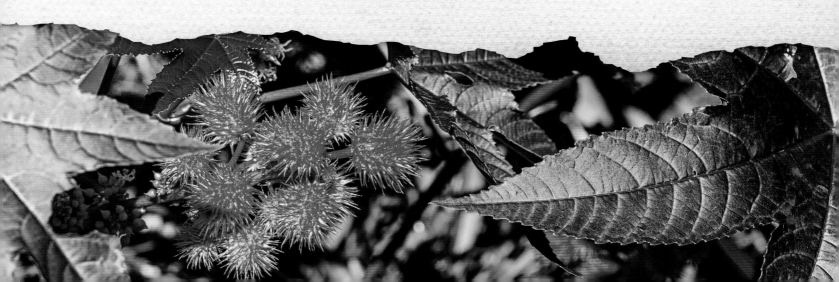

Using Castor Oil at Home

Westi also told me how they use castor oil to sooth burns and cuts.

One day when he was young, his mother suffered a bad burn in the kitchen. Westi's older sister had boiled some water and poured it into a jar. His mother accidentally knocked it off the counter.

It spilled on her leg and burned her badly. The wound also started swelling. "It looked really scary," Westi said. "My older brother asked me to take her to a doctor to get medicine, because my mother could not move her leg. It was horrible.

"We called the doctor and he said to cover the wound with Vaseline, but that made it worse. Then I recalled my herbal teaching and the benefits of castor sap. It stops bleeding and has great medicinal value. It is also an antiseptic and antibacterial. The treatment brought her great relief and really helped the burn."

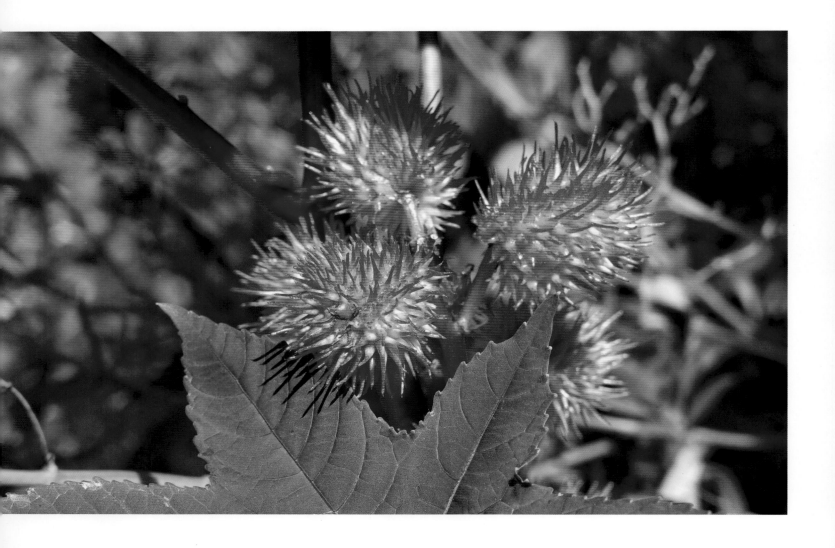

Castor oil plants grow in most yards on Bali.

In fact, this is how 80% of the world uses herbal remedies as medicine. Right from the local environment. You can use castor oil, too, to treat a number of ailments:

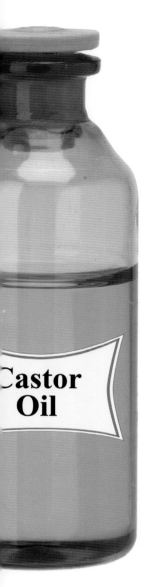

Lung congestion: Rub castor oil or dry mustard (mixed with water to make a poultice) on your chest, cover with muslin or flannel and lay a hot-water bottle on top to open up your airway and boost circulation in your lungs.[10]

Age Spots: The oil has been used for thousands of years as an anti-inflammatory and antioxidant. But the benefits don't stop there; castor oil can also help fade the age spots on your hands. (And the best part is you don't have to drink it!)

Simply apply castor oil with a cotton swab on the affected area when you first wake up, and then once more right before you go to bed. Be gentle and use circular motions when applying. You should notice the spots beginning to disappear within a month.

Yeast: Calcium undecylenate — castor oil — is one of the best things to take to inhibit the spread of Candida, and it is five times more powerful than other antifungal agents. Take 1 to 2 tablespoons a day.

Unhealthy nails: If your nails are peeling, dryness is probably the cause. Just as your skin loses moisture with each passing year, your nails lose natural oils. Exposure to harsh detergents and acetone nail polish remover can accelerate the effects. I tell my patients to hydrate their nails by soaking them in olive oil a few times a week. Before bed every night, apply a thin layer of castor oil to the nails and cuticles. You should see a difference within a week or two.

Castor oil is completely safe, even though some people worry that it might not be because the poison ricin is also made from the castor seed.

However, as the *International Journal of Toxicology* reports, ricin is not part of castor *oil*. It doesn't "partition" into the castor oil.[11]

As is true with many of the products from today's environment, you should be careful where you get your castor oil from.

If you buy it in a store, it's probably going to be from castor beans that were doused with pesticides. Then they probably used some sort of solvent like hexane, just like they do with soy, for example, and chemically processed it in some fashion.

These agents may seep into the castor oil, infusing it with toxic agents. And the processing might leach out the beneficial phytonutrients of the oil. Be sure to look for cold-processed, high-quality castor oil.

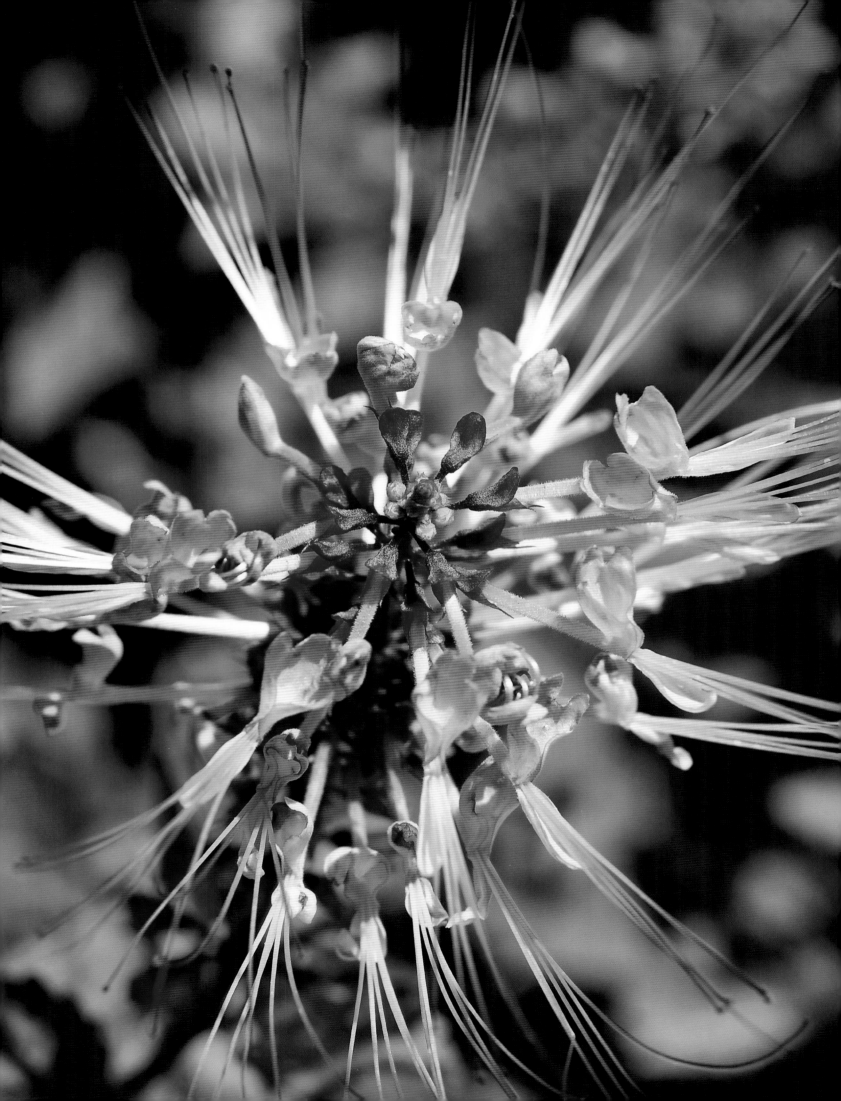

NATURAL CURE FOR KIDNEY STONES

Coca-Cola has seven storage and distribution centers on Bali. Soda is soon going to be everywhere on the island.

It's a problem because it can cause obesity, but also for another reason... something you don't see too much of on Bali yet, but will soon: kidney stones.

I've seen it a lot at my Wellness center in South Florida... people get kidney stones in Florida and other very hot places because people get dehydrated easily. Even though it's hot, they don't drink enough until they're thirsty. By then it's too late. So imagine what it will be like in the jungles of Bali when people start drinking soda instead of water.

How can soda lead to kidney stones?

You probably know that your body only functions well in a narrow range of body temperature. A temperature of 98.6 degrees

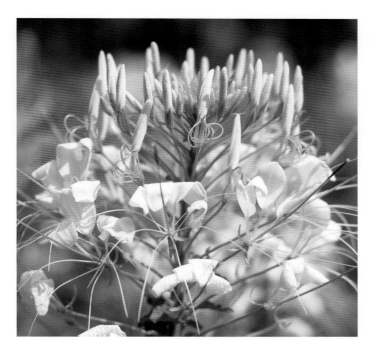

Cat's whiskers: A powerful remedy for kidney stones.

is normal. Any lower and you don't feel so good. If it goes higher you really don't feel well. Three or four degrees higher and you've got serious problems.

Your body also has another small range in which it can operate — your pH level. On this scale, less than 7 is acidic, 7 is neutral and between 7 and 14 is alkaline. Your body prefers a slightly alkaline pH level, between 7.365 and 7.390. Anything outside this range causes your body stress.

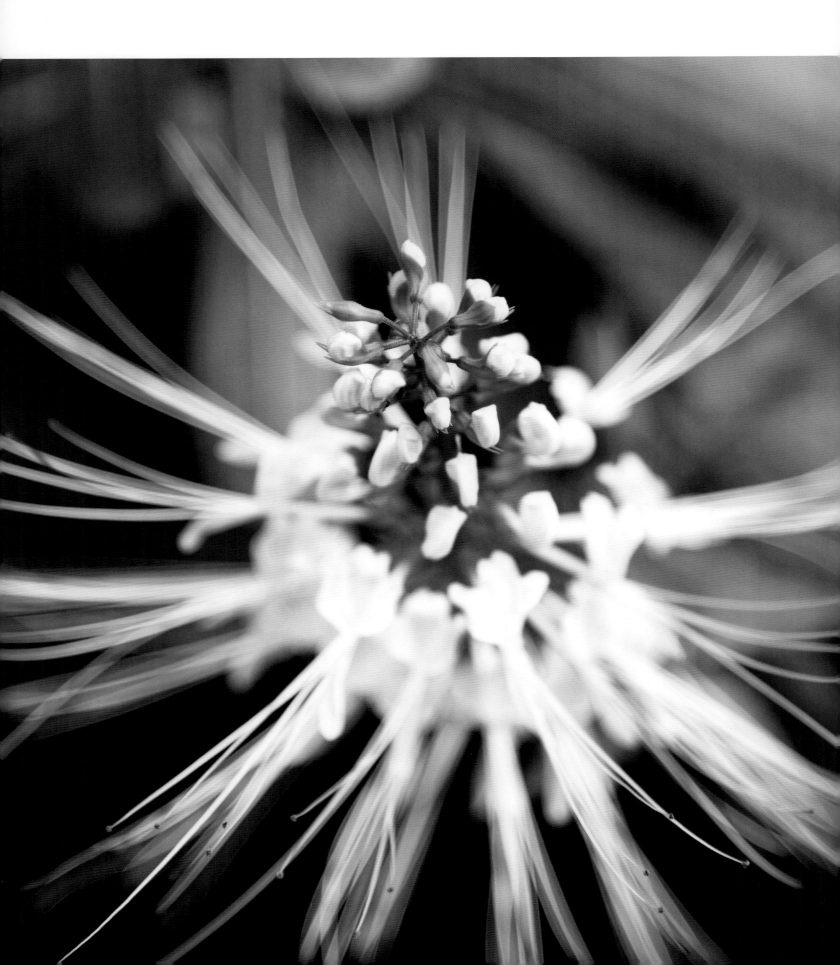

Bali's Time-Tested Remedy

To give you an idea of how acidic sodas are, pure distilled water has a pH of 7. Battery acid is a 1. Coke is around 2.5, and other sodas are not much better. That means your can of cola is tens of thousands of times more acidic than water.

When you consume these highly acidic drinks, it has a huge impact on your system. Your body will use its alkaline minerals, such as sodium, potassium, magnesium and calcium, to neutralize the acid and return your pH to normal.

Problem is, this upsets another balance — the one in your bloodstream.

Phosphoric acid helps keep your soda fizzy. But the shock of incoming phosphorus causes the calcium levels in your blood to decline. This triggers your body to dissolve calcium from your bones to restore this balance.

You almost always dissolve more calcium than is necessary, which can then form kidney stones. The high fructose corn syrup from soda also raises uric acid. If it crystallizes, it forms a different kind of stone.

To prevent these painful stones, it's obviously a good idea to stay away from soda.

But don't be fooled. Energy drinks, sports drinks, tea and coffee are not good substitutes. They are acid forming, too.

I didn't see many of these drinks in the stores around Westi's town of Ubud. But they're coming.

Fortunately, Bali's traditional herbal healers have a time-tested remedy... it's been handed down in Lelir's family for hundreds of years.

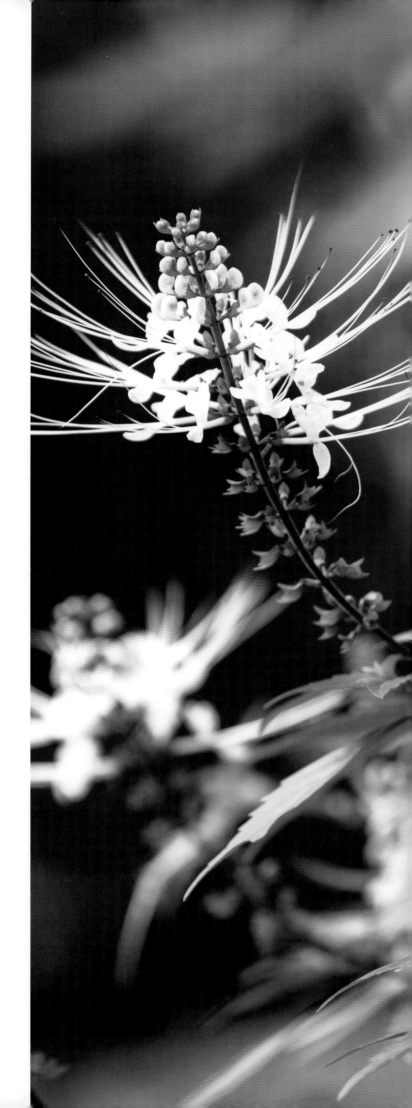

Natural Relief from Kidney Stones

(Orhosiphon spicatus)

Balinese name: Kumis Kucing

In Bali, it's usually considered an honor when a village leader visits your home. But this was obviously no social call.

As our village's headman inched his way toward our door, I could see he was in incredible pain. Every few steps he'd stop, wincing in pain. Westi rushed out to help him into the house.

Once we had him settled at our kitchen table, our guest explained the cause of his pain.

"I started to have terrible pain in my back and side," he said. "So I went to the doctor. The doctor told me I have stones in my kidney... and I may need surgery."

Our friend didn't want the doctor to "cut him open." In terrible pain and desperate, he had come to see us. "Please, do you have any medicine that can help me?" he begged.

Fortunately, we did.

We gathered some dandelion and the stems and leaves of a small flowering plant in our garden. We boiled what we call a "pull hand" – about 10 grams – in 3 glasses of water.

When the water was boiled down to two glasses, we let it cool. Then we strained out the herb and gave it to our village leader to drink.

We showed him how to make the tea, told him to drink a glass every day and sent him home.

Gradually, over the next few weeks, our friend's pain went away. In three months, his kidney stones were gone.

Many Asian cultures use this herb – called cat's whiskers – for urinary tract problems. My parents taught me about this herb. They called it "kumis kucing."

You can find cat's whiskers in many gardens in Bali. Its narrow serrated leaves and delicate white flowers make it a favorite decorative herb.

But we keep it on hand for its effect on urinary tract health. We often recommend a simple recipe to friends and visitors for maintaining urinary health.

We've seen it work time after time.

— *Lelir*

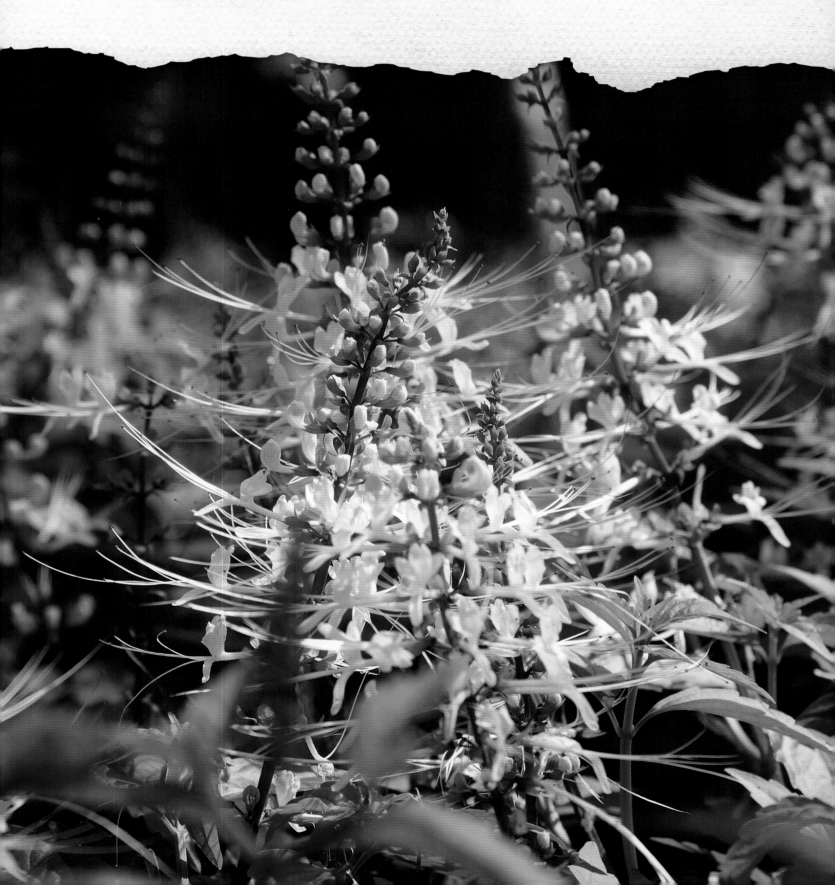

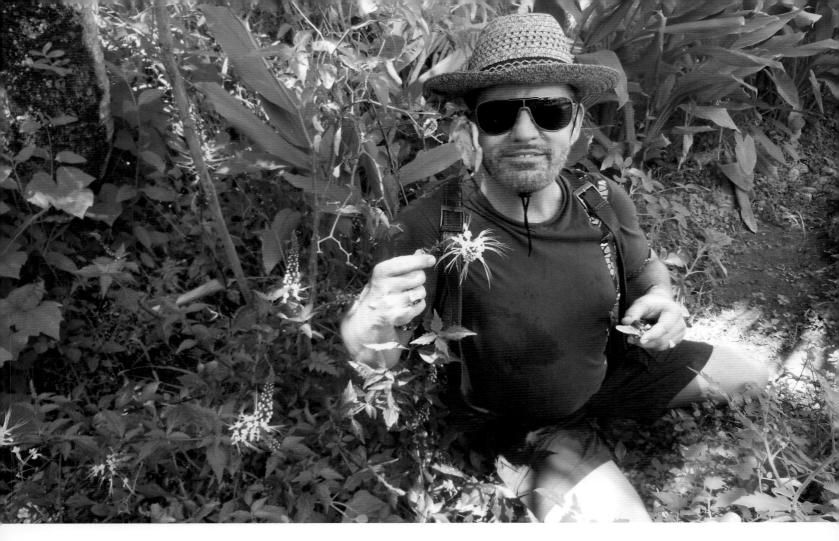

Westi showed me the cat's whiskers that grow on his property... it's used by traditional herbalists for urinary tract health, but it's also good for treating kidney stones.

My Own Research and Discoveries

Modern research on cat's whiskers is scarce. A couple of studies have found cat's whiskers are rich in flavonoids. These are chemicals that give color and flavor to many plants.

Flavonoids are powerful antioxidants. They also have anti-inflammatory effects. There is evidence they may help prevent heart disease and fight cancer. Other research hints that flavonoids may be useful against HIV.[1]

Though we haven't found much research on cat's whiskers, we did come across an interesting study from 2008. Scientists in Malaysia studied the effects of a close relative of cat's whiskers — called Orthosiphon stamineus.

They tested the effects of this plant on mice. And they discovered it had very strong effects on the urinary tract system.[2] This is the closest evidence we've found for the traditional use of cat's whiskers.

Researchers in the Department of Pharmacognosy at University of Oslo, Norway, discovered that cat's whiskers are a very effective anti-inflammatory.[3]

The flavonoids in cat's whiskers[4] are plant nutrients that have health-protecting qualities.

Preparation

Lelir makes a potent herbal tea for relief of kidney stones:

Cat's Whiskers

Take 30 grams of the stems, leaves and flowers of cat's whiskers.

Add it to a full teapot of boiling water and steep for several minutes.
Strain the herb out of the liquid.

For the best effect, drink several glasses of this tea daily for one month.

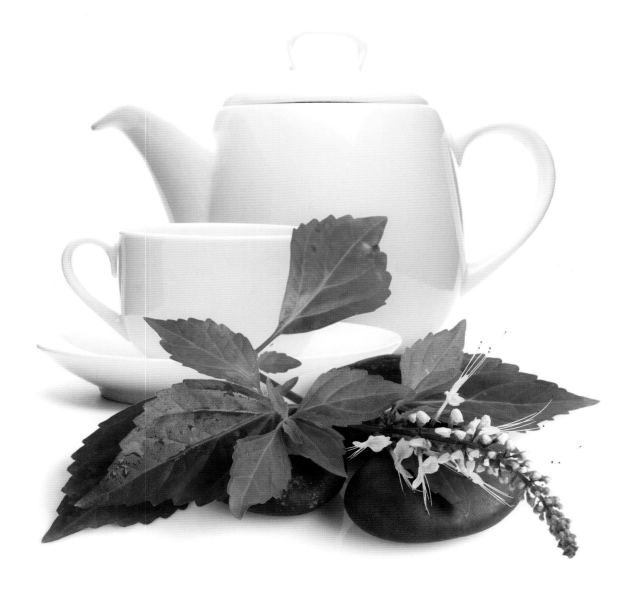

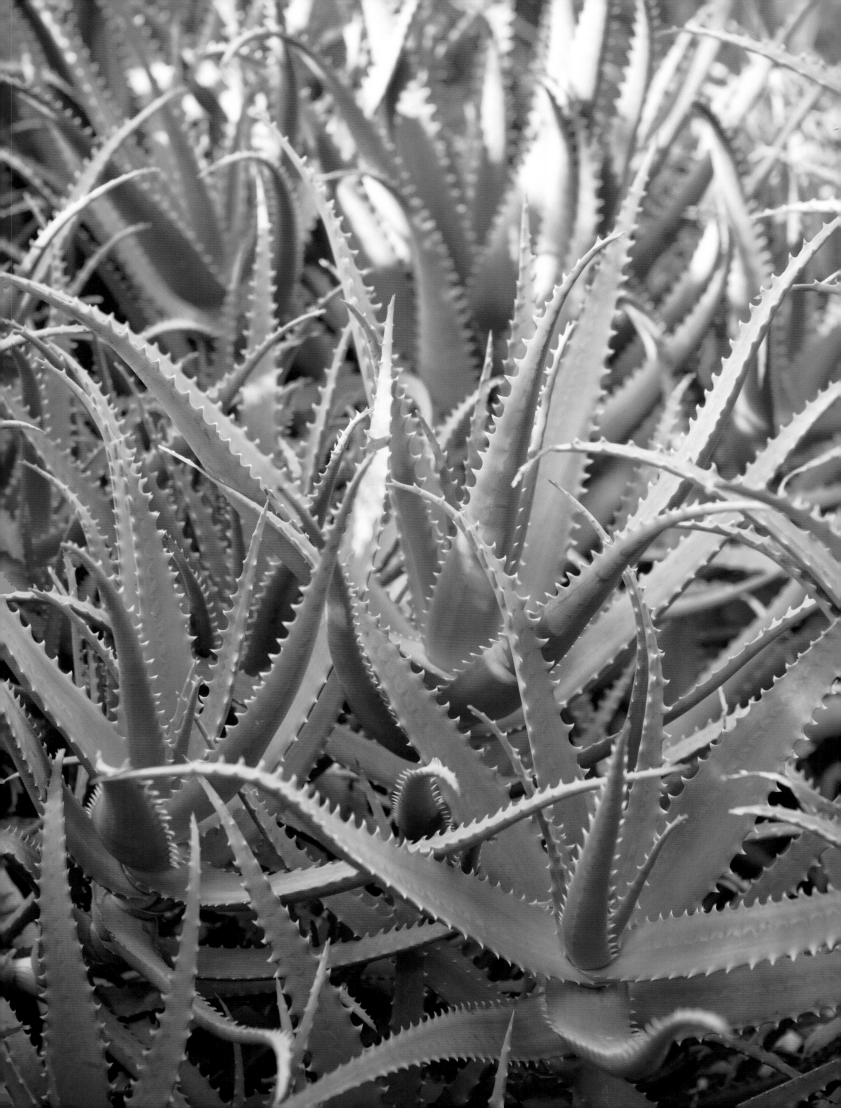

ANCIENT ADOPTED MIRACLE HEALER

Cornelis de Houtman — the man who started the entire Dutch spice trade — arrived on Bali in 1597. Legend tells us that his crew was so captivated by Bali's beauty that it took de Houtman a year to round them up so they could continue their voyage.

I don't know if that's true, but I can sympathize. Once you're in Bali, you don't want to leave.

Bali has a diverse landscape, rich culture and warm people. Its deep jungles, forests, lakes, hot springs, waterfalls, hills, cliffs, mountains and beaches with thousands of types of wildlife and plants make it a most alluring place.

Not only is it beautiful, but Bali is also located in a biodiversity hotspot. It's called the Sundaland hotspot. Much of Indonesia and Malaysia are also part of this hotspot of plant life, which is one of the richest on the planet.

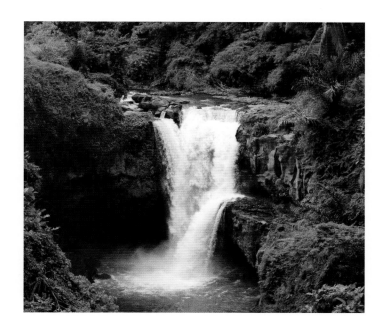

The first explorers on Bali were captivated by the islands astonishing natural beauty.

Biologists estimate that the Sundaland hotspot has over 25,000 species of vascular plants. And what was most incredible to me is that 60% of them are not found anywhere else on earth.

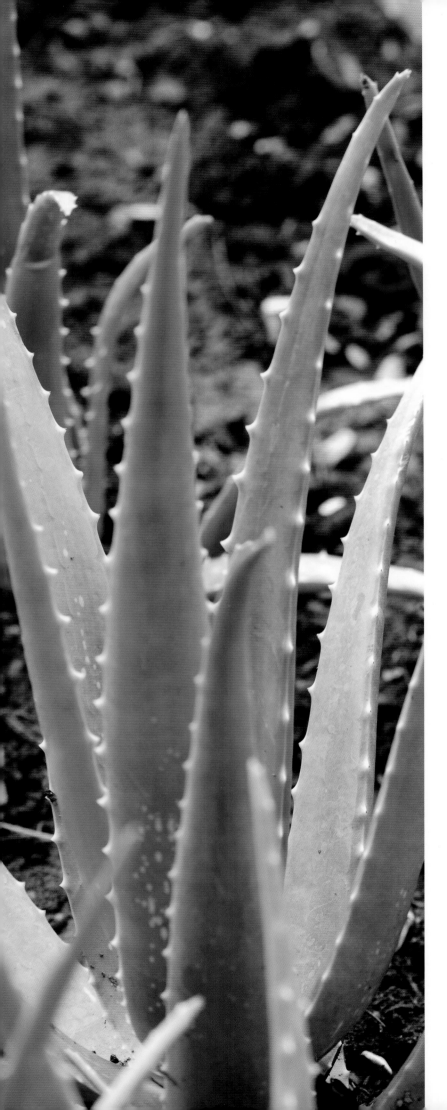

Gardening for Medicine

Bali has a few of these unique plants, to be sure. But one of the remarkable things about Balians is that they are so skilled as gardeners and so blessed with the fertile soil of the Sundaland, they can make plants seem uniquely their own.

This is what they've done with one of the oldest medicinal plants in the world: aloe vera.

Aloe has a very prominent place in herbal tradition, being possibly the first plant ever written about for its medicinal purposes on an ancient Mesopotamian clay tablet dated from 2000 BC.

Yet when you visit Bali, Westi and others like him cultivate and use plants like aloe in a way that makes it seem like they originated on Bali.

They have so many uses for aloe, it's grown and tended in every yard and landscape.

I have aloe in my yard and it's great because any time I have a burn or a cut, I can just take a leaf, break it open and squeeze the gel onto the burn. Instant relief and clean healing.

For Lelir and her family, aloe is a centuries-old healing tradition that seems even older. She told me about her family and how they use aloe.

The Free, Natural Cure-All

(Aloe vera)

Balinese name: Lidah buaya

Maybe it wasn't love at first sight, but I certainly became interested in my classmate pretty quickly.

We were both taking a tour-guide course at the university. But this young man wasn't like my other classmates.

He was friendly, but more serious. And he was serious about a subject that meant a lot to me: Bali's herbs.

It wasn't long before we were meeting after class and talking about our shared passion. Then, before I knew it, we were talking about starting a life together built around that passion.

My dream was to follow in my parents' footsteps. They were the 4th generation of herbalists in my family. Westi dreamed of bringing Bali's herbal knowledge back to our island.

I suppose that must sound a little strange. My family so involved in herbal medicine... yet Westi seeing a need to bring herbal knowledge back. But the truth is, most Balinese had forgotten many of our herbs.

Everyone still remembered the common "kitchen herbs." But Western medicine was rapidly replacing herbs for many illnesses.

Westi and I saw several reasons for returning to our herbal traditions.

To begin with, Western medicines were very expensive. Villagers often couldn't afford them. Or they would go heavily in debt to pay for them.

These drugs also have side effects that herbs don't. It seems odd to us that anyone would risk one sickness to cure another. But that's just what many modern drugs ask you to do.

Finally, we've found that herbs can be more effective than drugs. And they're very definitely more versatile. An herb you may know well is a perfect example of this.

My parents called it "lidah buaya," which means "crocodile tongue." You probably know it as aloe vera.

You may use aloe for your skin. Here in Bali, we do, too. My mother always had aloe on hand in case someone burned their hand on the stove.

I grew up in a typical Balinese family. That meant all the girls helped in the kitchen. The occasional burn was a fact of life. If one of us burned her hand moving a hot kettle or pot, Mother was always right there with the aloe.

She'd cut off a piece of aloe leaf, squeeze out the juice and rub it onto the burn. The cooling aloe quickly soothed the sting. And if we applied aloe to the spot a couple of times every day, the burn didn't even leave a mark.

Aloe also makes a fine moisturizer and I use it in my shop constantly. It's a powerful humectant — a substance that helps your skin hold moisture. It's especially helpful if you'll be out in the sun, or in a dry wind. Just rub on an aloe lotion before you go out to keep your skin soft and supple.

If my father suspected someone had an ulcer, he'd always recommend aloe. Purified juice from the aloe vera plant is very soothing and healing for your stomach lining.

Back then, my father didn't understand how aloe worked... he just knew that it did.

We have many other uses for aloe. For example, if a woman is having problems with her monthly cycle, aloe may help her cycle become more regular. It is also soothing for women who have painful menstruation.

Aloe helps heal the stomach as well, so we use it internally very often. It is known to stop harmful bacteria and to soothe people who have ulcers and stomach pain.

We also give it to those who have sugar problems. It's very helpful to those with diabetes, which is rare on Bali, but it is becoming worse as people eat more Western food instead of our traditional Hindu diet.

Aloe gel is a popular home remedy for conjunctivitis in Bali. It isn't as effective as some other herbs we use. But aloe is one of the herbs that's remained popular — even as Western drugs have taken hold. You'll find it in many kitchen gardens here.

Aloe is also a laxative. Mothers here like to use it with their children because it's gentle. Plus it does double duty, since it soothes the digestive system as it loosens the bowel. It's very healthy for the stomach.

I also use aloe for my Jamu body mask, which draws out toxins from a most important organ, your skin, while it soothes and heals at the same time.

— *Lelir*

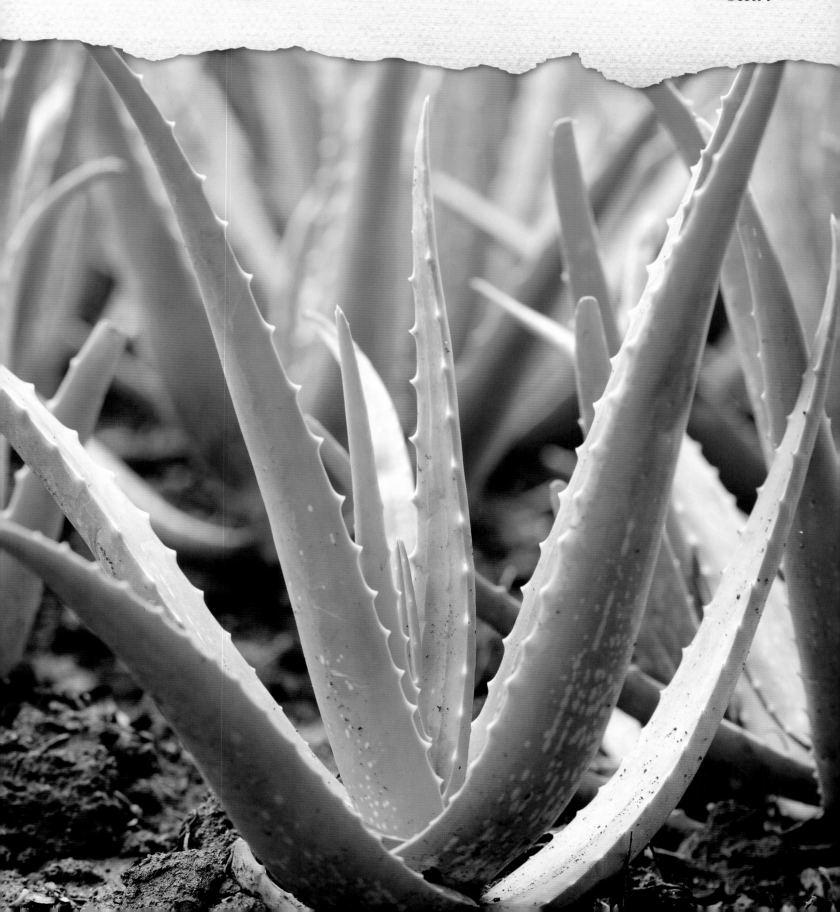

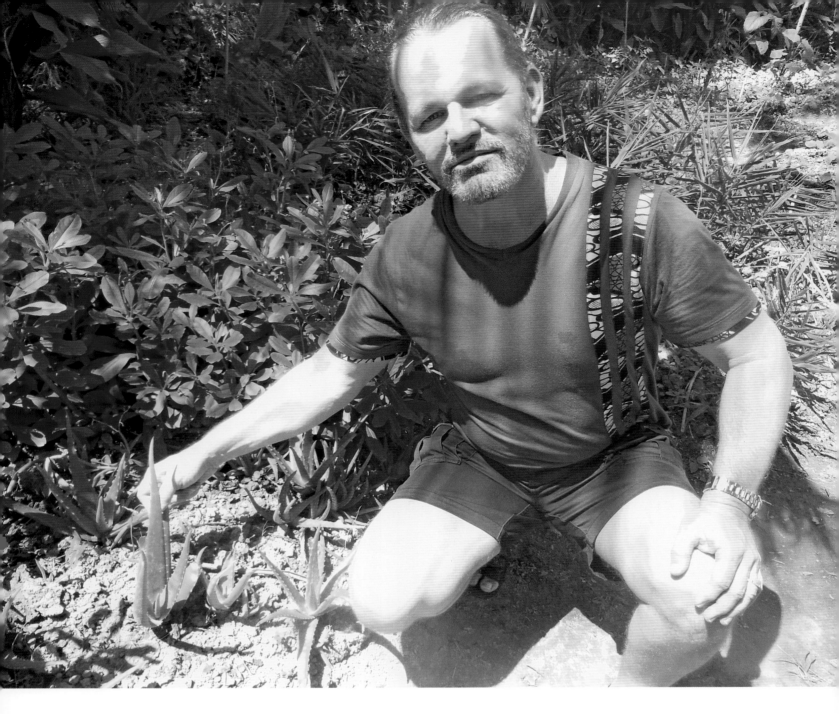

Westi showed me a few different kinds of aloe that he grows on his land in Bali.

My Own Research and Discoveries

You know aloe as the skin-soothing gel available at any supermarket or drugstore.

But aloe holds another secret...

Aloe has 23 polypeptides that stimulate the immune system and 20 polysaccharides that increase the action of white blood cells and compounds within the body to attack and fight viruses and cancer.

That means more "killer" T-cells and enhanced-strength "killer" T-cells. Research shows one of the aloe polysaccharides, acelated mannose, can double the number of both "killer" and "helper" T-cells within three weeks.

In fact, the Department of Agriculture approved aloe vera to treat soft tissue cancer in animals back in 1992.

Despite the power of aloe, there has been almost no study of aloe's anticancer effects in the U.S.

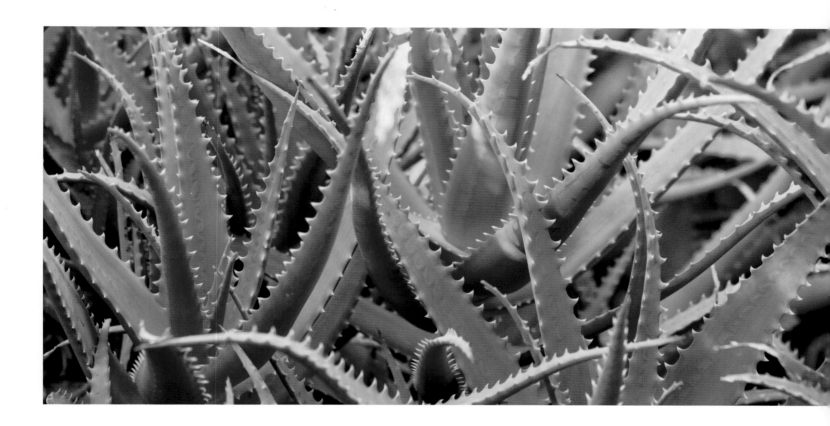

Straight From Leaves to Cure

We've been conditioned to think of medicine as something you buy. But in Bali and the other countries I've traveled to, they've used traditional medicines from plants all their lives.

For them, it's natural to get what you need right from your own backyard.

It's only after scientists get wind that something is effective that they begin to study it.

That's why there aren't many clinical trials on the effectiveness of aloe against cancer.

So I had to look deeper into aloe and I found some remarkable science to back up aloe's anticancer use.

For example, the Laboratories of Medical Research at the University of Verona in Italy list aloe vera specifically as one of the foods that can prevent the initiation and the progression of cancer formation in the digestive tract.[1]

A new study out of South Africa looked at aloe's ability to kill glandular cancer cells (adenocarcinoma), liver cancer cells and brain cancer cells.

They took aloe gel straight from the leaves and, at very small concentrations, aloe caused some cancer cells to die. At higher concentrations, even more cancer cells died.[2]

Aloe vera was especially good at causing liver cancer cells to die... all without causing any inflammation. And material from the aloe leaf stopped glandular cancer cells cold. The more they used, the more cancer cells died.

Another new study tested aloe's antioxidant strength to protect the heart. But what they found was an anticancer surprise...

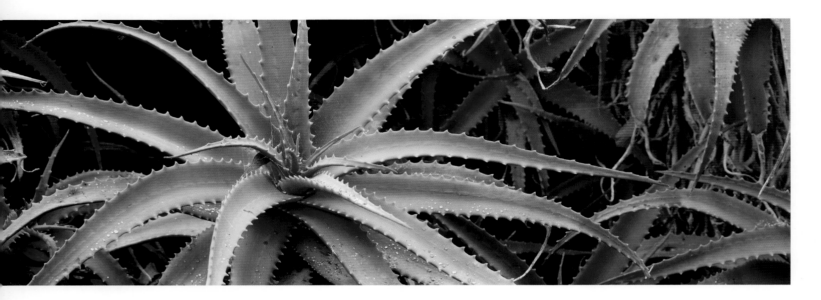

Aloe Turns On Your Body's Strongest Antioxidants and Uses Them to Stop Cancer

After only 14 days, the researchers saw that not only was aloe protective, but it also boosted two of the body's strongest antioxidants, SOD and glutathione.[3]

What do antioxidants have to do with cancer? Free radicals from oxidation can cause the DNA mutations that contribute to healthy cells converting to cancer cells. And high glutathione levels are known to prevent illness, slow aging and reduce cancer risk.

Lectins and emodines are two antitumor compounds in aloe vera that work alongside an aloe vera stimulated increase in the tumor necrosis factor.

One compound in particular, aloe-emodin, which is in the gel, sap and leaves of aloe vera, is both strongly antiviral AND can kill tumor cells all on its own. Aloe-emodin attacks many different kinds of tumors, such as lung cancer, liver cancer, breast cancer tumors and more.[4]

It's remarkable in that it does everything you want in a natural cancer killer: It disrupts cancer cells, causes them to die, stops the spread of cancer, cuts off the blood supply of tumors AND strengthens the body's immune system at the same time.[5]

Plus, aloe-emodin shows a high specificity for neuroectodermal tumor cells. These are very dangerous central nervous system tumors.[6]

It's so strong that the German Cancer Research Center is studying aloe-emodin for its anticancer effect. That's important because, unlike the U.S., where we have a government agency dedicated to stifling natural cures, Germany has set up the Federal Institute for Drugs and Medical Devices (Commission E) specifically for testing and approving natural cures. And aloe makes the list.

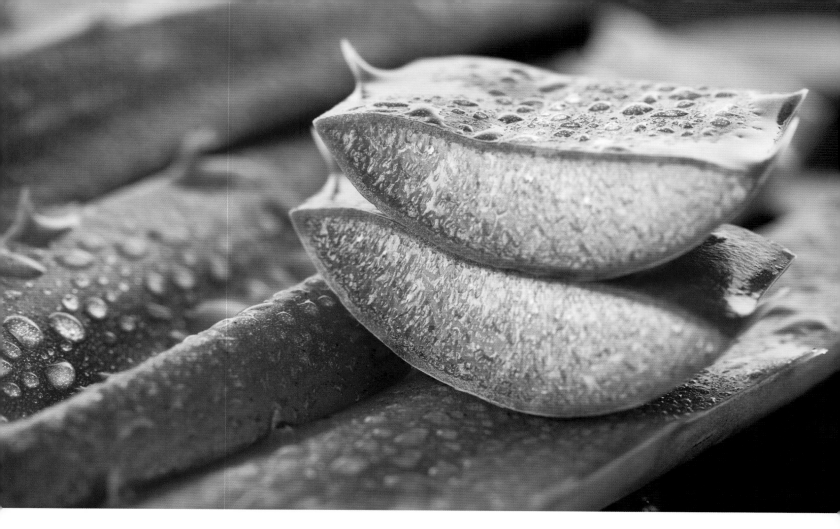

Aloe vera is best known in the West as a treatmant for sunburn, but it's also a natural cancer killer.

A Skin-Saving Secret

When you break open an aloe leaf, you notice right away that the gel is clear and pure. That's because the gel contains 96% water. This is aloe's skin-saving secret.

Water is the most important moisturizer for your skin. But water isn't the main reason why aloe vera is so powerful and effective in healing burns and even moisturizing skin. Aloe vera gel is a mixture of over 150 nutritional ingredients: vitamins, minerals, amino acids, enzymes, beta-sitosterol and healthy fatty acids.

The outer layer of your skin is partly made of fat. And keeping this layer of skin water-tight and healthy not only keeps your skin firm and smooth, but it's your best defense against pollutants the modern world produces. This slightly acidic layer is a barrier known as the "acid mantle."

Healthy skin pH should be between 4.5 and 5.0.[7] The gel of aloe vera has a pH value of 4.5. It aids in not only nutrient transportation to skin cells, but also in the health of the skin.

Aloe vera also makes your skin firm and supple by stimulating "fibroblasts." These are the cells that give rise to the connective tissue in your skin: collagen and elastin.

Aloe vera also has a class of long chain sugars called "Galactomannans."

Galactomannans have a variety of immune-stimulating and protective effects within the body. The gastrointestinal and immune systems are some of the most affected systems.

Aloe is also useful in stopping periodontal disease. Researchers gave an aloe mouthwash to 345 healthy people to use twice a day. Aloe stamped out plaque and gingivitis, and significantly lowered bleeding and inflammation compared to a placebo. Aloe worked just as well as the dangerous drug Chlorhexidine with no side effects.[8]

Researchers are also investigating aloe because its anti-inflammatory power may help ease osteoarthritis.[9]

Animal studies have revealed that aloe promotes healing of the stomach lining.[10] They also show aloe fights some of the effects of H. pylori — the bacteria linked to ulcers.[11] Taken internally, it also lowered blood sugar in people with diabetes.[12]

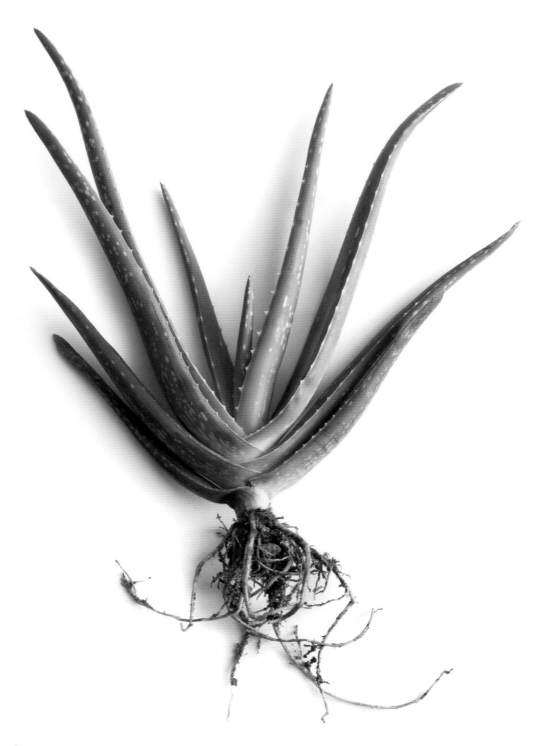

How to Use Aloe for a Healthy Body

If you live in the south, you may have aloe plants growing wild like I do in my yard. In that case, you can just cut open the ripe leaves and squeeze the gel into a glass container.

Fresh aloe will keep for a week in the fridge, or indefinitely in the freezer. But one of the ways you can increase the shelf life is to add vitamins. For every 1/4 cup of gel, add 500 mg of Vitamin C (ascorbic acid) and 400 IU of Vitamin E. Blend it and it will keep for many months in the refrigerator.

If you live in a colder climate and you want to purchase aloe, what you should know is that 95% of the aloe products on the market are either diluted or improperly processed. So you want to be careful when choosing an aloe product for internal use.

Most use only the inner gel of the aloe vera leaf, which has a lower concentration of beneficial components. The outer leaf and rind has 200% more than the inner gel. Processing the plant with high heat also destroys many of the beneficial ingredients of aloe.

The best products should be cold processed using the whole leaf with the aloin removed. Aloin is the irritating chemical in the plant that can cause diarrhea or intestinal cramping.

.... *Aloe Vera* ....

Nourishing Facial Mask

Ingredients:

½ teaspoon manuka honey

½ teaspoon aloe vera gel

½ teaspoon cold-pressed, organic coconut oil

½ teaspoon raw cacao powder

Please note: Do not purchase aloe vera gel from the pharmacy. It's synthetically thickened. Get the edible aloe vera gel from your local health-food store. Or use an aloe plant from home.

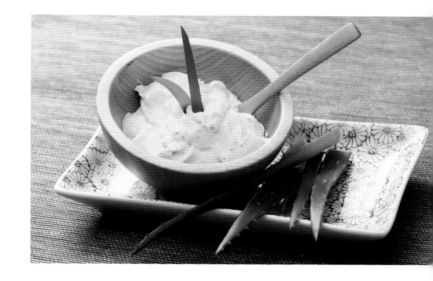

To make the mask, mix all the ingredients together in a medium-size bowl until a loose paste forms. Cleanse your face and place a hot towel over your skin for a few minutes to open your pores. Apply the mask using your fingertips. To help increase absorption and exfoliate your skin, lightly massage it in until the mask feels sticky. Leave the mask on your face for 5-10 minutes. Rinse well with warm (not hot) water. Pat dry with a clean towel.

Age spots and Burns

Simply break an aloe leaf and rub the gel on the affected area twice a day for at least a month. Be sure to leave it on your skin for at least 45 minutes before washing.

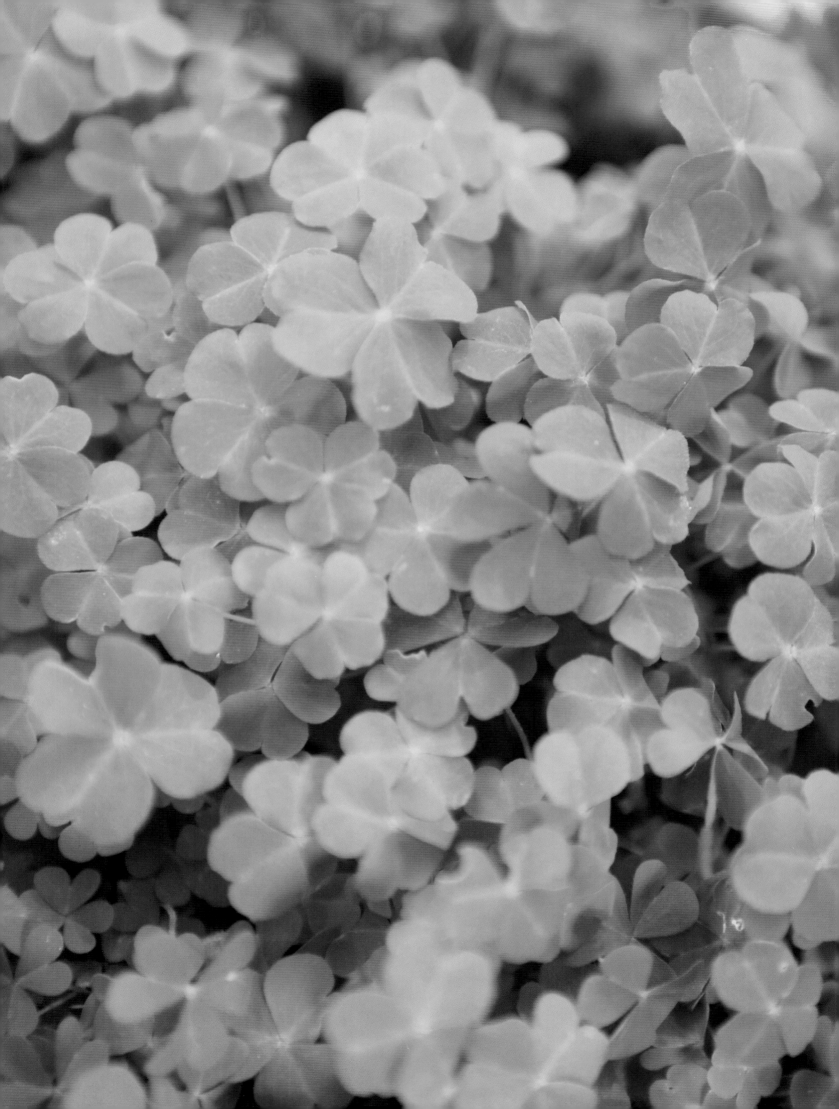

PREVENT HEART ATTACKS WITH HUMBLE "WEED"

Western scientists like to say, "A weed is a plant for which no useful purpose has yet been found."

If any of them visited Bali, they'd change their minds in a hurry.

The flowers I saw growing everywhere made Bali the lushest, most tropical paradise I'd ever visited. And many of them are considered "weeds" by Western standards.

Many of these weeds are not only ornamentally beautiful, but they have a lot of healing properties as well. Too bad Western science puts zero faith in what nature has provided for us... at least, not until they can make a synthetic drug out of it.

For example, I don't put any faith in any of the heart drugs out there... I've tried them all and stopped using each of them.

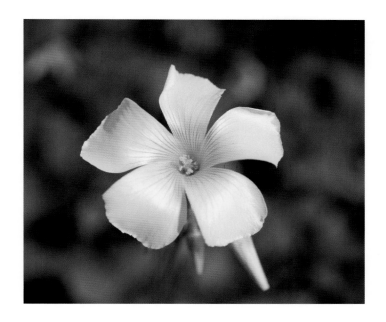

Wood sorrell is often regarded in the West as a weed, but in Bali it is a powerhouse heart healer.

Meanwhile, there's a plant that grows up and down the ancient walls around Bali that's a good example of a powerhouse heart healer ignored by the West.

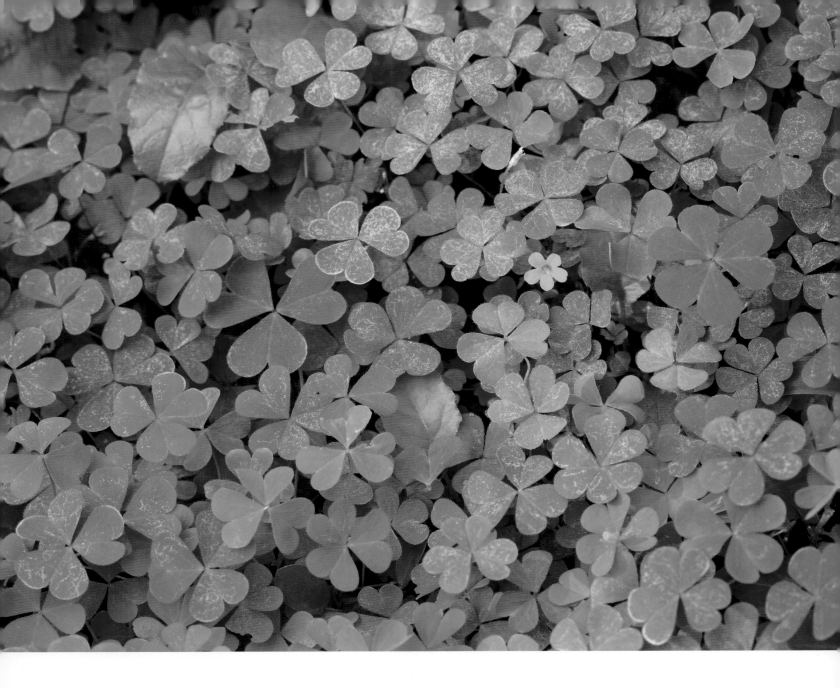

A Natural Heart Protector

A research team in India studied the effects of *Oxalis corniculata* — creeping wood sorrel — on animals' hearts. What they found was that an extract of the plant could prevent heart attacks.

First, they gave the animals a chemical that caused heart attacks. Then they pre-treated a second group of animals for 30 days with the plant extract. When they gave this second group the chemical, it didn't cause the heart attacks.[1]

Instead, the extract lowered their cholesterol levels, triggered greater antioxidant activity and lowered inflammation.

Creeping wood sorrel also raised the animals' vitamin C levels and their concentration of glutathione, one of the body's most powerful anti-inflammatory antioxidants.

Lelir told me about some other traditional uses for creeping wood sorrel, aside from its use as a heart tonic.

Wound Healing from the Walls

(Oxalis corniculata)

Balinese name: Semanggi

My introduction to herbs came early. Both my parents were herbalists. They used herbs to treat almost all our childhood problems. And our neighbors often depended on my parents for health advice and treatment.

When I was very young, my father sometimes took me along to visit patients. These were usually follow-up visits... non-emergencies where he would change dressings or check on a patient's progress.

One patient visit stands out in my mind because of a strange request my father made.

The patient had cut himself badly while working in the rice field, and my father was treating his wound to prevent infection and speed the healing process.

As he examined the wound's progress, my father turned to me. "Go pick some of the flowers growing on the wall outside," he said.

In those days, most homes in Bali were still built using traditional materials. Roofs were mostly made of thatch and walls were made of bamboo, stone or earth.

Sure enough, growing up — and out of — the man's earthen walls was a plant with vine-like stems, three-lobed leaves and delicate yellow blossoms. So I picked a few and brought them to my father.

He boiled the flowers — leaves, stems and all — in some water. Then he thoroughly washed the man's wound with the water when it had cooled. "This will help the cut stay clean and healthy, " he told the man. "It will also help it heal faster."

This was my introduction to semanggi, or creeping wood sorrel. In the years to come, I would see my parents use it for several complaints — both external and internal.

In fact, creeping wood sorrel is one of my favorite mild herbs. I use it to make an antiseptic wash... just the way my father did when I was a little girl.

This is what Westi and I used for our son when he was very young and got a rash. The sorrel wash is very soothing and kills any bacteria that may be causing the rash.

It's also effective for boils and other eruptions of the skin.

I also make a tea from creeping wood sorrel. It's really the same as the wash. I just wash a small handful of the flowers — including roots, leaves and stems — and boil them in a cup or two of water. Then I strain out the flowers. This tea is good for reducing fevers and soothing the urinary tract.

Because it's healing to the urinary tract, many women add small amounts of the leaves and flowers to salads as a preventative. The leaves have a pleasant lemony flavor and they're quite high in vitamin C.

Creeping wood sorrel grows easily in almost any shady wooded area. And it's quite widespread — even growing in North America. It grows so well, it's often considered a weed — overtaking gardens and lawns.

Historically, heart attacks have been rare in Bali. Perhaps creeping wood sorrel is one reason why.

— *Lelir*

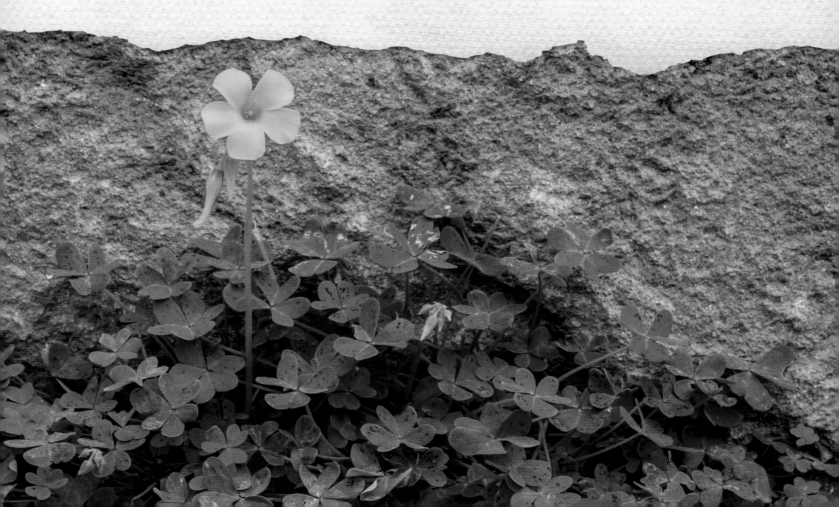

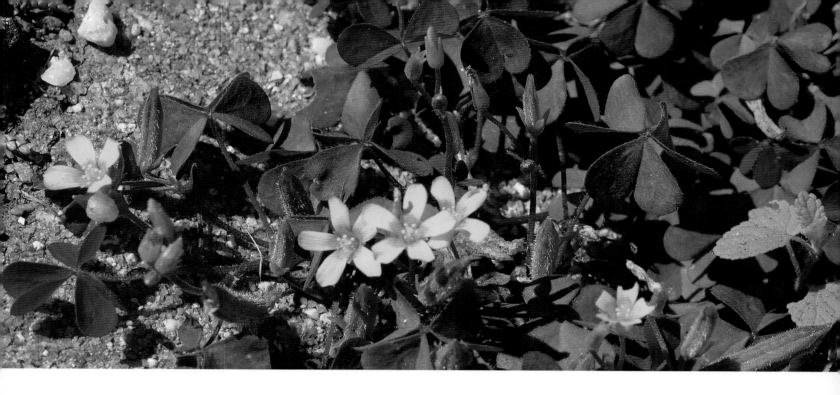

My Own Research and Discoveries

When visiting with Westi and Lelir, I often ate very fresh foods with the addition of herbs. In salads there was always a little wood sorrel added. This humble, little leaved plant grows very unassumingly. It creeps along the ground or on a wall, almost unnoticeable.

Often the humble little plants you barely take notice of have some very health-promoting qualities. Especially for people who live in the tropics.

Creeping wood sorrel has antimicrobial effects that are worth noting. For one thing, it has been shown to kill Giardia lamblia, which causes diarrhea in humans. Researchers were looking for natural compounds in the battle of giardia infections (giardiasis) and they found it in this unassuming little plant.[2]

People often get exposure to Giradia lamblia while traveling to foreign countries and drinking local water. It is associated with poor quality of the water.

The symptoms associated with giardiasis are feeling of cramps, bloating, nausea and bouts of watery, loose stools. Definitely not something you want to have while visiting a foreign country.

I think the locals are smart to put some creeping wood sorrel in many salad-type dishes. It can ensure that their visitors will be protected and have a more pleasant visit.

Along those same lines, it protects against amebiases,[3] which is a disease caused by the parasite *Entamoeba histolytica.* This is normally associated with poor sanitary conditions.

People don't always notice the symptoms of this disease, so prevention is important.

Gastric ulcers are another area where science is catching up with what the natives have known about this plant.[4] The old saying, "an ounce of prevention is worth a pound of cure" comes to mind when thinking of this plant.

A Powerful Enemy of Free Radicals

Creeping wood sorrel also has some powerful free radical scavenging effects. There was research done to see how an extract from wood sorrel protects lungs. What they found was that the extract prevented some serious alterations in a variety of enzyme systems in the lungs, in a dose-dependent manner.

The scientist noted that the reason it did this was because of the intrinsic properties within the extract that scavenges free radicals.[5]

Aging kidneys are becoming all too prevalent in our western society, but a study done on rats showed that an extract of creeping sorrel could have a powerful effect on preventing damage to kidneys.

They found that using an extract of creeping sorrel helped reverse the markers associated with the damage. The researchers concluded that the treatment caused a significant recovery. They believe that it was because of the antioxidant effects of the phenolic compounds in creeping wood sorrel.[6]

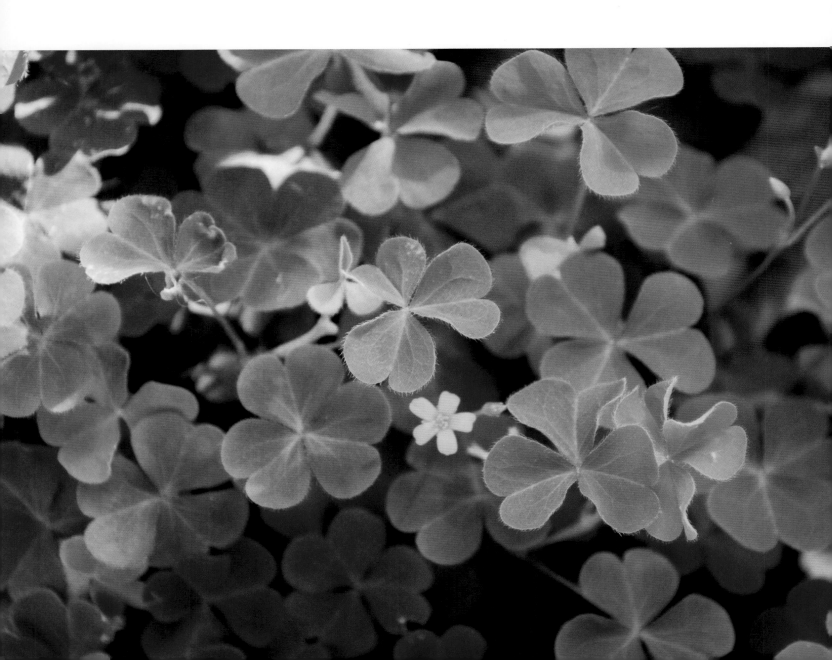

Preparations

Abscess

Grind fresh sorrel leaves and add a little hot water, just enough to turn into a paste.
Apply paste to area twice a day.

Diarrhea

Take one sorrel leaf, and boil it into buttermilk. Drink once a day.

Warts

Mix an equal quantity of sorrel leaf extract and onion juice. Apply to infected area once a day.

Insomnia

Mix an equal quantity of sorrel leaf extract and castor oil. Heat the mixture up to remove
moisture and then let it cool. Apply mixture onto the scalp at night.

Other Uses

• Boil leaves in water and apply wash over
  a cut or rash.

• Add leaves to salad.

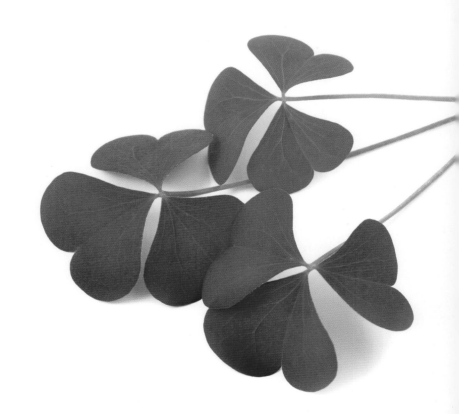

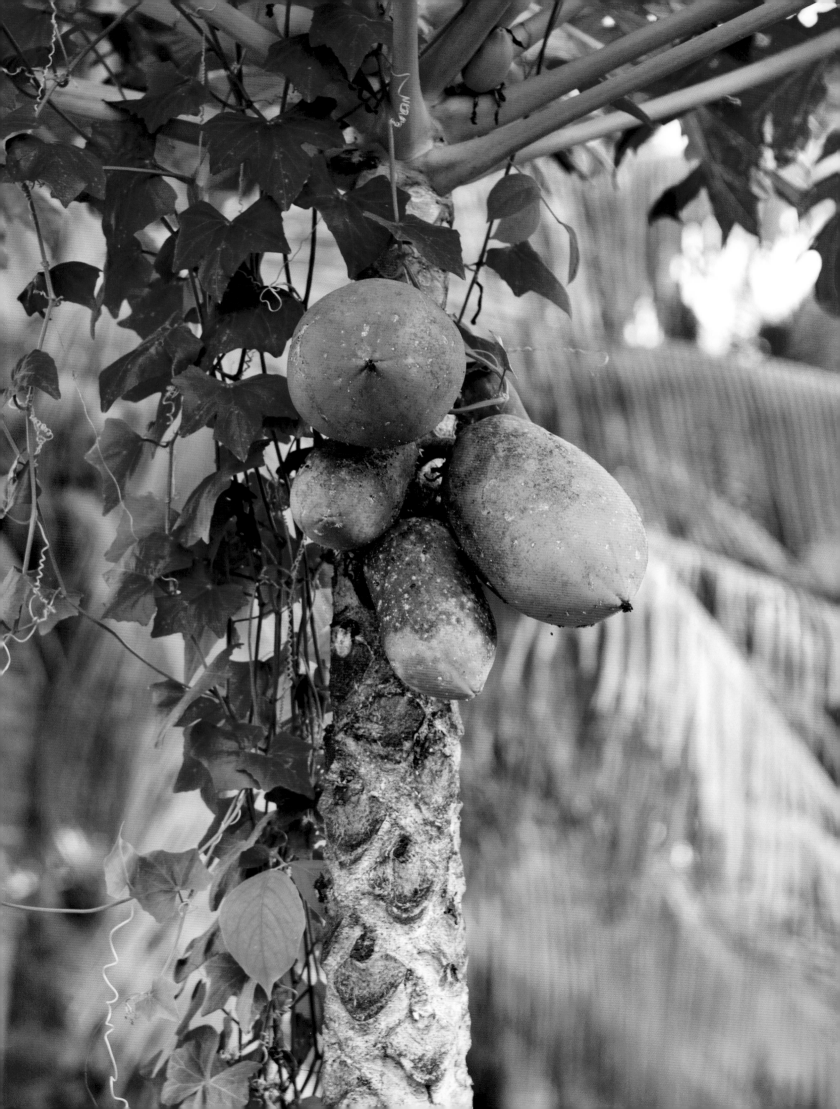

CAN THIS PAIN-KILLING FRUIT KEEP YOU YOUNG & CANCER-FREE?

Westi drove slowly, careful not to scrape the sides of his truck as we drove. The streets of his neighborhood are paved but narrow, with barely enough room to get by. Ancient stone walls topped with strange carvings pressed in from both sides. Wild cacao trees, the biggest I've ever seen, loomed overhead.

As we made our way toward his hidden garden, the roads narrowed even more, no wider than a sidewalk. Man-made walls gave way to thick foliage and immense trees. There were plants on top of plants as far down the road as you could see.

We drove into what looked like a tree tunnel, made a quick right and squeezed the truck through a tiny opening ... and what I saw amazed me.

A huge field with walking paths and more plants growing everywhere.

How could this be right here, with no hint of it from the road?

A Roadside Miracle

We got out of the truck and the first thing I saw was peppermint, just like I have growing in my yard in Florida. There was also tapioca, which grows so thick in Bali that the locals even use it for fences.

There was Ginkgo Biloba and ginger... teakwood trees and a jackfruit tree... and immensely huge palm trees so tall I could barely see the coconuts hanging near the top.

There was also the widest, tallest papaya tree I'd even seen. So big I couldn't get it into one photo. I had to take out my video camera and climb to the top of a hill to record it because I knew no one would believe me.

It didn't have any fruit on it yet, only flowers, but I could tell it would soon have papaya fruit all up and down its spine.

These are very important in Bali, not only because of the papaya fruit, but for the way the Balinese use all parts of the tree, especially the sap.

Papaya — Digestive Aid and Antimalarial

(Carica papaya)

Balinese name: Gedang

When you come to Bali, you'll discover that it's home to many beautiful butterflies. In fact, back in 1993, an International Conference on Butterflies was held in Indonesia. That's when some people in Bali decided to start Taman Kupu Kupu Bali – the Bali Butterfly Park.

As more and more Balinese move to cities, our children are beginning to lose touch with Nature. If the whole world was interested in Indonesia's butterflies, they thought our children should get to know them, too.

Today, hundreds of schoolchildren from Bali visit Taman Kupu Kupu each year. And so do many visitors to our island.

At the park, they discover Bali's many lovely butterflies – and even the giant Atlas moth, with wings almost as big as a man's hand. In the park's indoor rain forest, brightly colored butterflies will actually land on you. And park employees will introduce you to gentle stick insects as big as cigars and leaf insects that literally disappear into the foliage.

Taman Kupu Kupu Bali is one of our island's hidden little gems. It showcases some of our most beautiful and interesting creatures.

But not all the crawly things in Bali are quite as friendly as those at Taman Kupu Kupu. For instance, we have scorpions.

Our scorpions aren't as dangerous as those in some other places. And most visitors to Bali never see one. But I remember the first time our son was stung by a scorpion...

He was still very young and had been outside playing with some of his friends. Suddenly, he came running into the kitchen, crying and clutching his little arm.

From the red welt growing on his arm, he didn't need to tell me what had happened. Fortunately, though, I had an answer. Like so many other families in Bali, we had a papaya tree in our garden.

I picked a couple of fresh young leaves, broke them open, and applied the sap to the sting.

Pretty soon, my son was feeling much better. By the following day, the swelling and the pain were gone.

Papaya sap can also help you work out a stubborn splinter. Just be careful not to use too much – or leave it on too long. The sap can cause an itchy rash.

Papaya is native to South America. But it was brought to Bali many generations ago and our ancestors quickly added it to their list of healing herbs.

Today, papaya trees grow all over Bali. They're in practically every garden... and grow wild throughout the island.

Of course, the papaya fruit is delicious, which is why papaya has become so popular around the world. But it's more than delicious. Eaten in moderate amounts, papaya aids digestion. Eat a little more, and it's an effective laxative.

Interestingly, papaya seeds have the opposite effect. Travelers with diarrhea just have to thoroughly chew and swallow a few papaya seeds and their problem should clear up pretty quickly.

We even eat the leaves as a vegetable. We eat about 20 grams – ¾ ounce – of steamed papaya leaves to help prevent malaria. According to tradition, it works by making your blood unappetizing to mosquitoes.

– Lelir

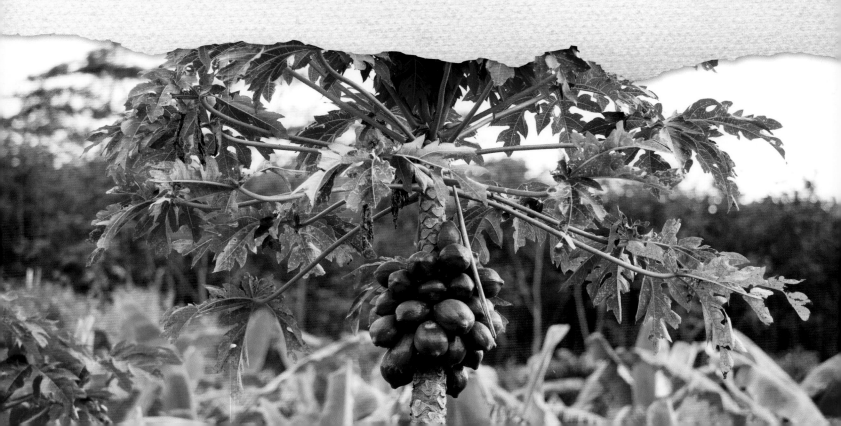

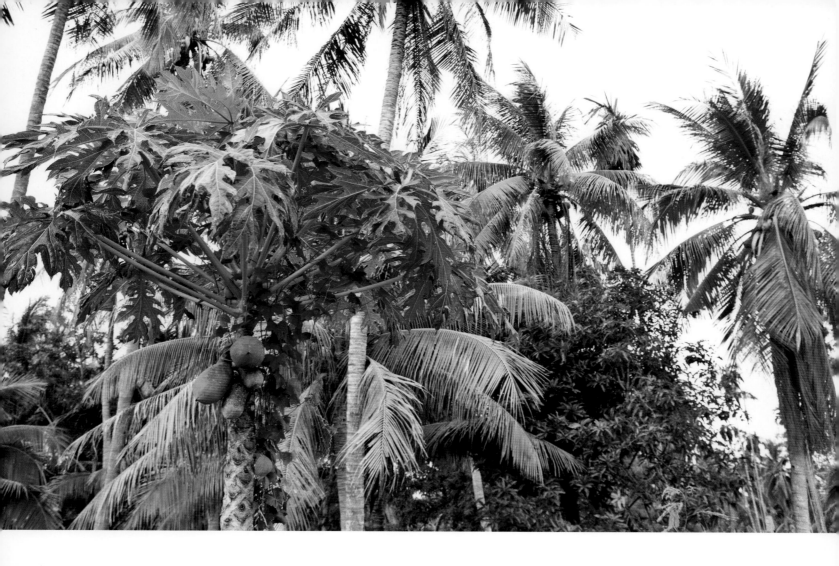

My Own Research and Discoveries

Like many of the plants that grow in Bali, the different parts of the papaya tree have different medicinal uses. The leaves of the papaya tree contain an anticancer extract.

Most of the research has been done in Asia. I found a clinical trial by a team at the University of Tokyo. They used an extract of the papaya leaves to kill cancer cells while enhancing healthy cells. Papaya leaf extract also increased the body's own cancer-suppressing genes. Plus, it suppressed tumor cell growth and stimulated antitumor effects within the body.[1]

Papaya seeds also have an effective anticancer compound. It's called *benzyl glucosinolate* (BG). It's in the pulp of the unripened fruit, and once the papaya fruit ripens, most of the BG is gone. However, it stays in the seeds. And studies show it stops cancer growth in many different well-known cancer cell lines.[2]

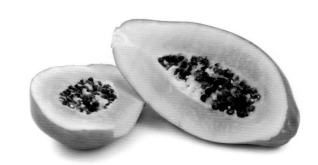

As Lelir told me, eating papaya may work by making the blood unappetizing to mosquitoes. However, papaya may have a stronger effect than just discouraging mosquitoes.

A Papaya a Day Keeps the Doctor Away

Scientists in India tested extracts from three tropical plants on blood infected with the malaria parasite. Two of the three plants had an obvious effect. And papaya was by far the stronger of the two.[3]

Studies also show why the seeds may be so effective against diarrhea. Japanese researchers discovered that compounds in papaya kill many bacteria — including E. coli and Salmonella.[4]

However, that's not what I usually use papaya for. Papayas are one of my favorite sources of vitamin C.

We now know that vitamin C guards the protective caps on the ends of your DNA, called telomeres. The shorter your telomeres, the older your cells act and the more susceptible your body is to diseases like heart disease and cancer.[5]

The new, exciting discovery about vitamin C is that it's very effective at stopping the oxidative stress that can shorten telomeres, keeping these tiny biological clocks ticking inside you for much longer, keeping you young.

A Japanese study tested vitamin C's effect on telomeres. It was found that raising the level of vitamin C in the cells could slow down the shortening of telomeres by up to 62%. Another study found that skin cells treated with vitamin C kept their young, firm shape because it slowed shortening of the cell DNA's telomeres. The telomeres also suffered less damage in the presence of vitamin C.[6]

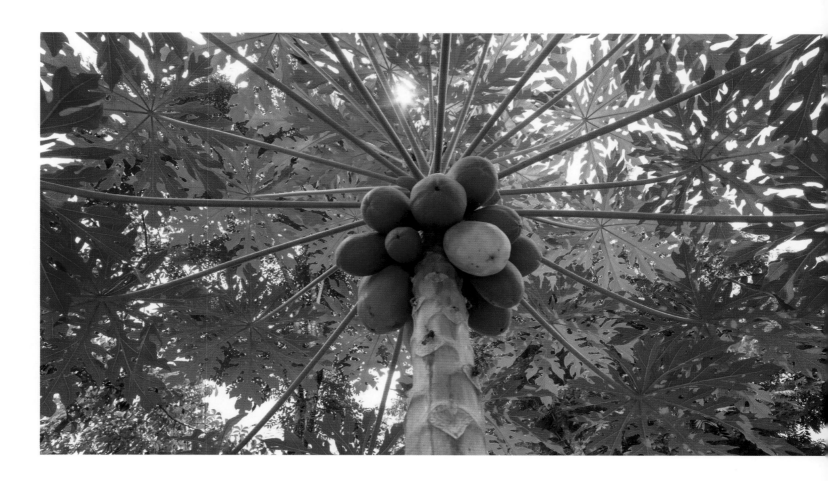

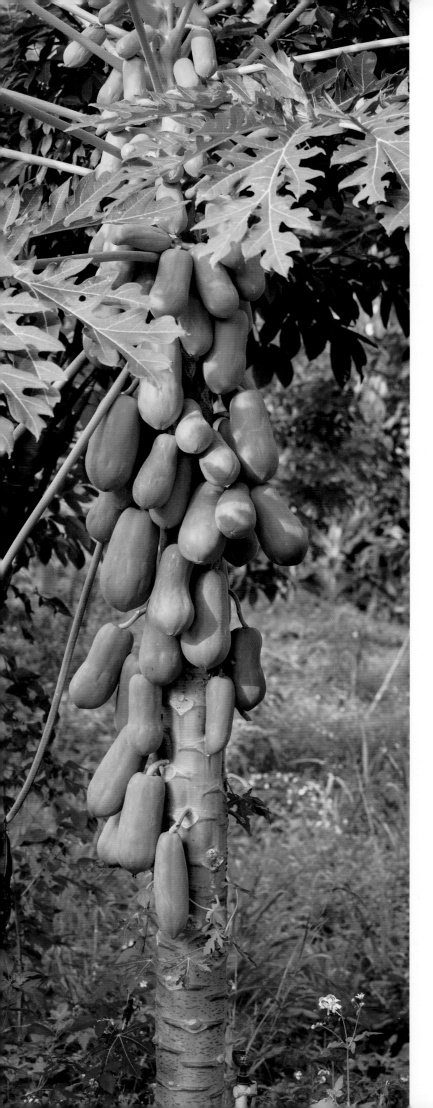

Papaya is also good for joint health. Your body uses vitamin C to make collagen, the building block of all your joints and connective tissue.

But, that's not all that papaya offers. There's an enzyme in papaya called "papain."

Papain is a proteolytic enzyme that can help if you suffer from excess inflammation and pain.

It helps increase your body's own pain threshold, helps you recover more quickly from injury and reduces circulating free radicals that lead to painful inflammation.

Papain helps relieve non-inflammatory pain, too, because it helps remove the cellular waste products that build up in the joints and cause pain. I recommend 250 mg a day of papain.

The good news is, papaya is one of the least contaminated fruits in terms of pesticides.[7] But, almost half of the papaya crops that come from Hawaii are genetically modified, so be sure you know where your papaya is coming from.

Preparations

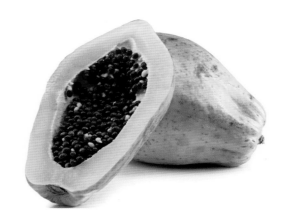

Papaya seeds have a kind of peppery flavor to them, so I encourage you to use them in salad dressings and to sprinkle them on foods you want to season.

I like the salad dressing option.

All you need is about a half of a papaya, 2 tablespoons of the fresh seeds, a half cup of some kind of nut oil (I like to use Sacha Inchi oil at home), and a tablespoon of vinegar. Westi and Lelir taught me to put it all in a blender and what you get is a nice, fruity, spicy, tangy dressing.

Of course, if you want something that's not sweet, you can just blend papaya and mustard seeds with oil and vinegar.

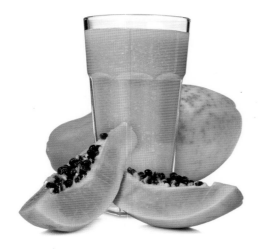

Papaya Smoothie

Makes 2 servings

1 papaya — peeled, seeded and diced

1 banana, peeled and sliced

1/2 cup sliced fresh strawberries

1/3 cup milk

1/4 cup sugar

15 ice cubes

Blend it all together until smooth.

Simple ways to add papaya to your diet:

Cut up a papaya and serve in small cubes on a salad;

Add it to fruit salad;

Sprinkle papaya with fresh lime juice and enjoy as is;

Slice a small papaya lengthwise, remove the seeds and fill it with fruit salad.

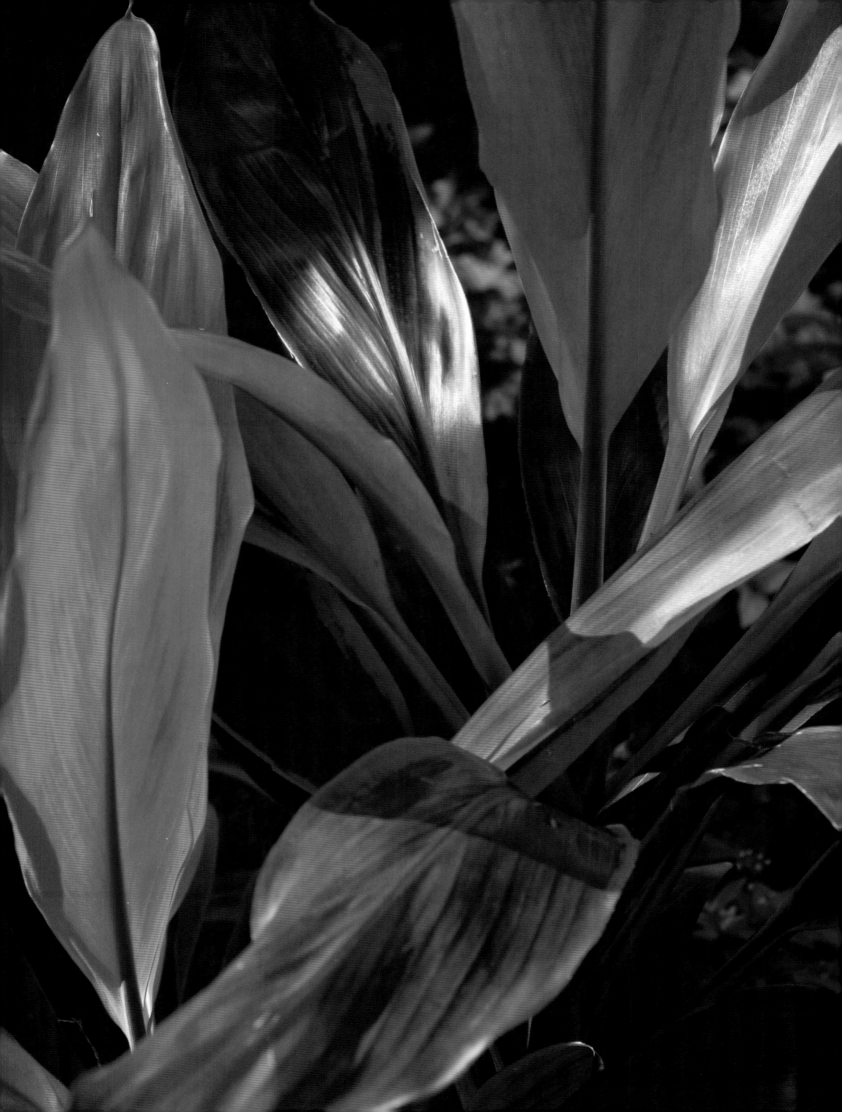

BALI'S SWEET HEALING TREAT

Many of the herbs Westi will grow at his dream health resort will be local and difficult to get when not on the island of Bali. In this book, I've shown you where to find and how to use some of these unique plants that have made their way slowly around the world.

But there's a plant you see everywhere on Bali that you can also find in the States.

...It's Called Cordyline

I'm sure you've seen these tall, pretty purplish beauties if you've visited anywhere in the Southern U.S., but they originate in the Pacific Islands.

Cordyline is so important and has such incredible material, nutritional, medicinal and religious importance that researchers at Cal Berkeley found you can use the spread of cordyline to trace human settlement around

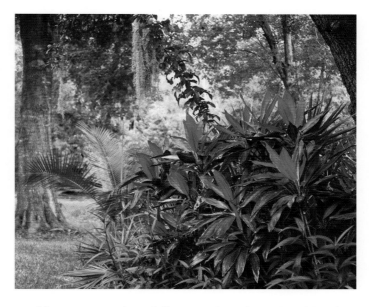

I have a row of cordyline growing along the side of my house in South Florida, but they don't have nearly as many giant leaves

the Pacific Islands.[1] That's how valuable it's been to human health.

If you've ever been to Hawaii, you saw these leaves in all the hula skirts. One of the adult leaves is plucked off and then torn

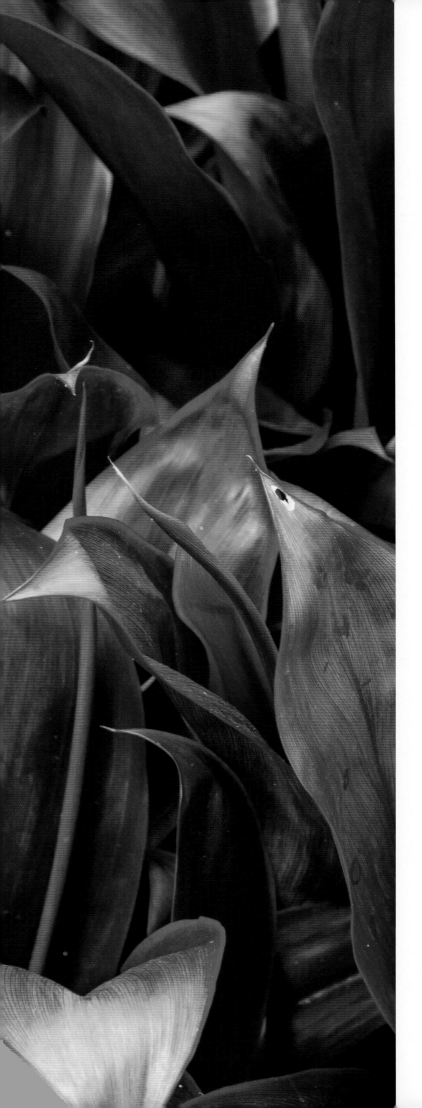

in half and tied to a string. After twenty minutes of plucking, tearing and tying, you have yourself an authentic Hawaiian Hula skirt.

The leaves produce a wax-like coating and were once used to make rain coats by people in the Pacific Islands. The water would slide right off and the coat could last nearly a lifetime. This coat would also be woven thick enough to protect from the occasional cold winds.

"DID YOU KNOW THAT CORDYLINE IS IN THE ASPARAGUS FAMILY?"

The leaves have been used as wrappings for cooking food and also for wrapping other herbs that needed to be steamed or boiled.

The young leaves are edible and can just be plucked off the plant and eaten. They have a sweet taste to them. The roots have been cooked and eaten by numerous cultures, some as a dessert and others as a good source of food during famine. They are beautiful, delicious and healthy.

On Bali, the Indonesians also use cordyline for decoration, but in quite a different way than the Polynesians.

Cordyline — From Decoration to Cure

(Cordyline fruticosa)

Balinese name: Andong

Lelir and I attended a friend's wedding recently. Weddings here — like weddings everywhere, I suppose — are a big affair. But on Bali, it takes several days to prepare all the offerings.

Weddings are one of the special times we eat meat and the groom's father, brothers and other men from the neighborhood slaughter animals both for food and for offerings. Meanwhile, the women prepare offerings of fruit, flowers and bright-colored cakes.

The wedding itself can last for three or four hours and involves many rituals. At one point, the bride holds up a small square of woven reeds in front of her. The groom then takes a kriss — a wavy-edged dagger — and pierces the mat.

There are blessings by the priest and many offerings. Some offerings are for the gods, others for what we call "butakala" — unseen spirits around us.

Our friend and his bride wore beautiful wedding clothes... though they weren't like the tuxedos and wedding dresses in an American wedding.

In Bali, the bride and groom wrap themselves in brightly colored and embroidered clothes, something like a sarong. The groom wears a sort of crown, while the bride wears a tall headdress. Our friend and his bride looked very much like a king and queen.

One of the most important plants in a traditional wedding is andong — red cordyline. We decorate the wedding with cordyline and include it in our offerings for spiritual protection. We use it to decorate our temples for the same reason.

You'll find cordyline growing all over Bali, because people here use it to create a "living fence" around their homes. They'll often plant cordyline close to the walls, because it acts as a natural air filter.

Like all plants, cordyline absorbs carbon dioxide and releases oxygen into the air. Our ancestors didn't understand this process. They just knew that planting cordyline near their homes made the air seem fresher... and the flowers added a lovely scent.

We use cordyline in our cooking, too, because it adds a lovely flavor to bland foods. Sometimes when she is cooking rice, Lelir will add a few tender, young leaves to the pot. This makes the rice smell and taste wonderful.

It's also very common to wrap rice, cakes or fish in cordyline. This gives these foods a delightful aroma. Fish that has been baked while wrapped in cordyline is a special treat. You can cook the young leaves as a vegetable, too.

Cordyline also has medicinal value. We use the rhizomes – spreading underground shoots – to treat diarrhea. But it is most popular as a decoration and in cooking.

The long, blade-like leaves make cordyline a striking decorative plant. You'll find it growing in the wild, but also in many Balinese gardens because, as I said before, it's very good at filtering the air around one's home.

— *Westi*

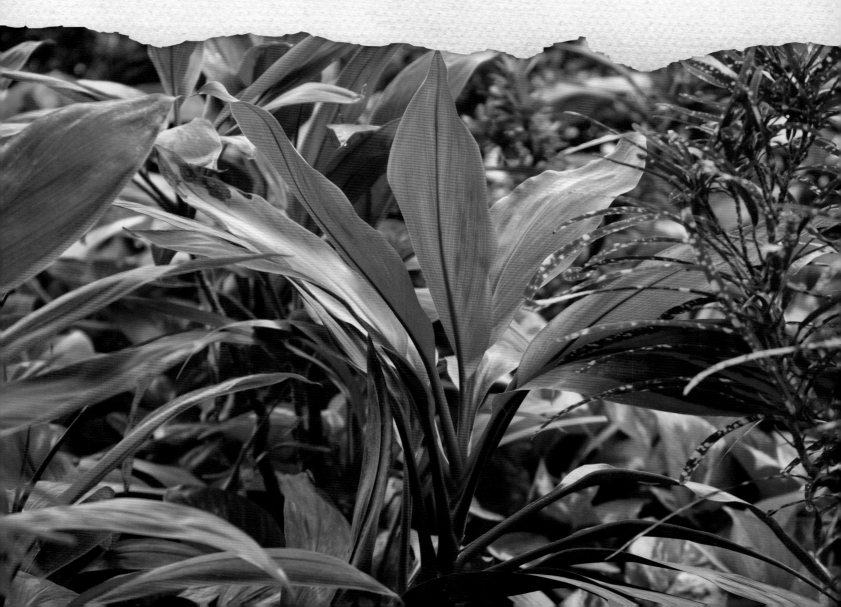

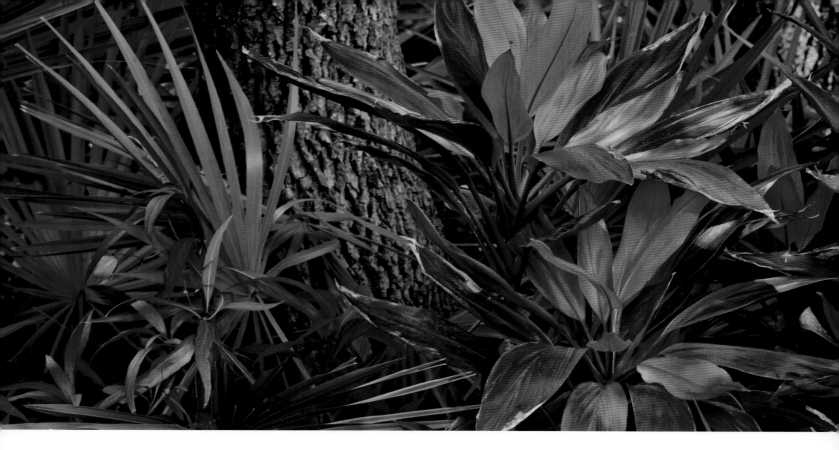

Cordyline fruticosa make a great office or house plant, because it captures toxic pollutants in the air.

My Own Research and Discoveries

Cordyline fruticosa make a great office or house plant. People often give them as gifts. Their red and reddish color brings life to a room.

Even better, modern science backs up their traditional use as air filters.

Researchers have found that cordyline is very good at absorbing toluene and ethylbenzene. Those are two of the toxic pollutants produced from gasoline and coal processing and from making plastics and foam.[2]

Cordyline captures pollutants through a fatty acid called hexadecanoic acid, which is the fat also found in palm oil and palm kernel oil. The toxins then travel into the roots and get removed from the plant.

That means these fats are very healthy for helping humans get rid of unwanted VOCs, or volatile organic chemicals, which are natural substances that are nonetheless still toxic to humans.

Did you know that cordyline is in the Asparagus family? You can find it under a wide variety of common names including Cabbage Palm, Good Luck Plant, Palm Lily and Ti Plant. You can grow them right in your house, as long as you have a room with full sun for at least a few hours a day.

Plant them in soil covered with 2-6 inches of mulch and they should grow from 2-6 feet. The more sun they get, the more variety of color you'll see.

You can eat the young green leaves and they are very sweet. If you want to eat the root, you can boil or cook it and add to a salad or stir fry.

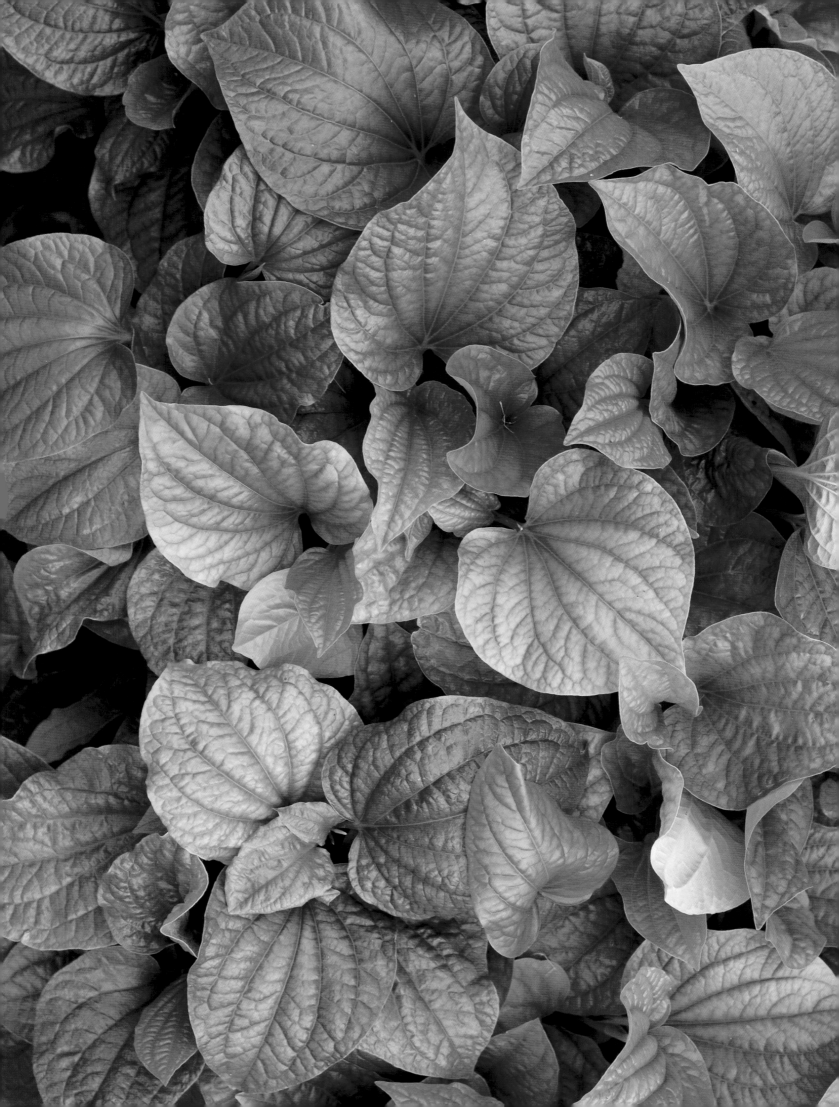

"RELAXING" VINE IS BALI'S ANTICANCER MIRACLE

Since antiquity, *piper betel Linn* has been crucial to traditional herbal medicine and healing throughout Southeast Asia. The leaves prevent bad breath, harden gums against gum disease, protect teeth and also prevent bronchitis, congestion, coughs and asthma.

It's gotten a bad reputation because some people chew the leaves while abusing tobacco and other cancer-causing agents like slaked lime.

But the reputation is undeserved. Researchers in India first discovered that betel leaves stop carcinogenic effects and even help prevent cancer, especially from carcinogens present in tobacco.[1]

Since then, there have been many studies into the cancer-preventing nature of piper betel leaves.

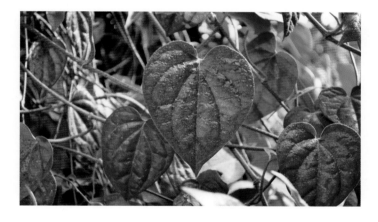

The heart-shaped leaves of the piper betel plant… maybe the best example of an under-the-radar cancer fighter on Bali.

Piper betel has an incredible range of "biophenolics," which are plant nutrients that stop and reverse disease. Compounds like hydroxychavicol, eugenol, chavibetol and piperols work together to put the brakes on free radical damage and help keep healthy cells alive while killing cancer cells.[2]

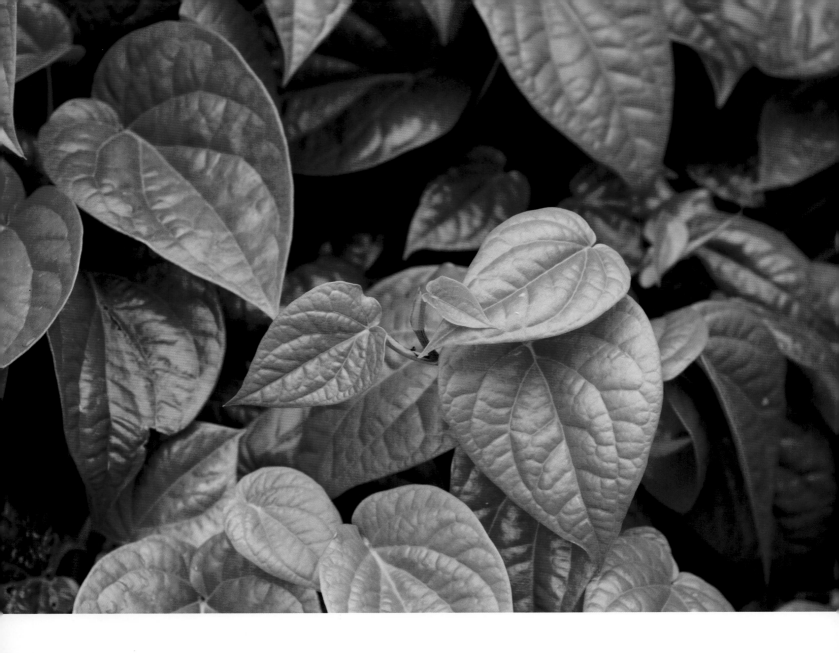

Causes Cancer Cells to "Self Destruct"

Piper betel seems to have a knack for pumping pre-cancerous cells with antioxidants to heal them and pumping up free radical levels in cancer cells so they self-destruct, sparing normal cells any damage.

The department of biology at Georgia State University has been looking into the anticancer properties of piper betel, even though most of the rest of the West seems to be ignoring its potential as a cancer treatment.

I found the small study they did on animals. They discovered that piper betel is quite good at killing prostate cancer cells. When they fed betel leaf extract to mice, it significantly inhibited the growth of human prostate cancer cells compared with those that got no piper betel.[3] The compound hydroxychavicol, which makes up more than 25% of the extract, seems to be the most powerful anticancer agent.

Maybe this helps explain why cancer is so rare in Bali. While they've been using piper betel to relax, take away pain and for other healing purposes, it's also been protecting them from cancer.

Holy Plant Fights Pain and Promotes Relaxation.

(Piper betel Linn)

Balinese name: Daun Base

The betel pepper – or Daun Base, as it's known in Bali – has been revered by Pacific islanders for centuries. According to tradition, the plant has the power to connect people with the divine and to remove curses.

At important meetings in Bali, you would always find betel pepper present. Our ancestors believed that the plant's divine power encouraged honest speech.

On the practical side, betel is a powerful, but gentle, pain reliever and tranquilizer. Here in Bali, we also use it for nausea and seasickness.

In India, betel pepper is called "pan patta." Traditional Indian healers use it for some of the same illnesses we do in Bali, such as pain relief and upset stomach.

The new health spas in Bali often use Daun Base in the way we have always used it traditionally... as a relaxant. Simply smelling the essential oil of the leaves will give you a calm feeling over your whole body. Chewing the leaves makes you feel relaxed.

Indians also believe betel is an aphrodisiac. For a long time, it was used in a common gift for newlyweds called "pan-supari." Taking this medicine was supposed to ensure a pleasurable wedding night.

I'm not sure if betel leaf is an aphrodisiac. But if it is, it may explain why we Balinese traditionally had such large families. Practically everyone here used to chew betel leaves.

The betel pepper is a perennial vine with dark green, heart-shaped leaves. Betel grows wild all over our island – as well as across much of the Pacific. It likes damp, shady gullies with rich soil. You'll often find it climbing on the trunks of trees.

— *Westi*

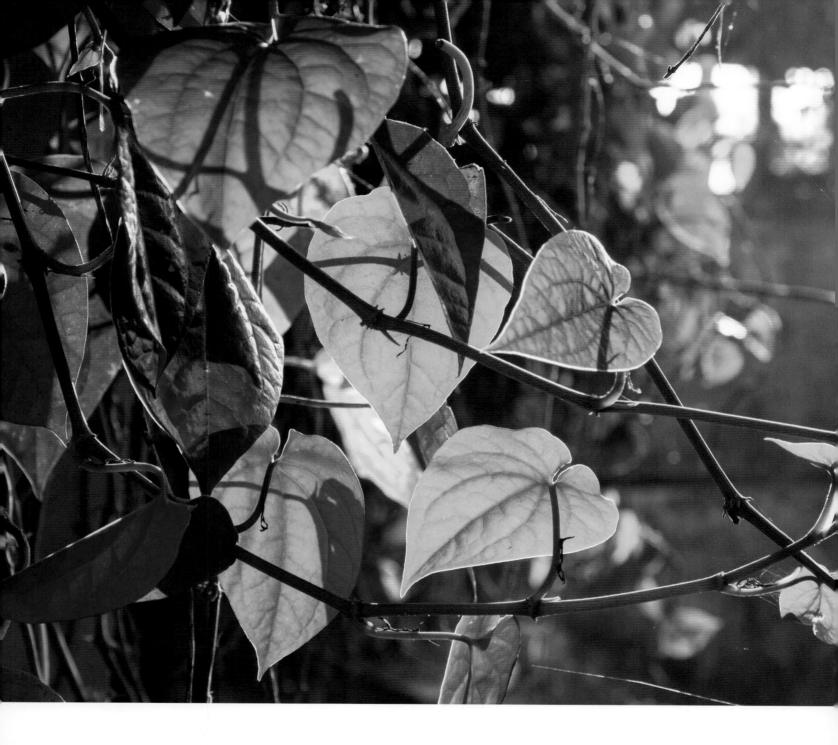

My Own Research and Discoveries

It doesn't surprise me that chewing betel leaves can help you feel relaxed.

The piper betel plant belongs to the genus piper of the Piperacea family, which has about 700 known species. One species, piper methysticum, known as kava kava, is well known as a relaxant around the world. And many studies show that kava eases anxiety[4] and promotes sleep.[5] It only makes sense that its close relatives might have some of the same properties.

Betel pepper isn't as well studied as kava kava. But I've come across an animal study that appears to back up its use for nausea and stomach upset.

In this study, doctors gave an extract of betel pepper to rats with stomach ulcers. After 7 days, the ulcers had healed.[6]

An animal study from Malaysia reveals another promising property of betel pepper.

You may know that diabetes slows the healing of wounds. So anything that speeds healing would be important news for anyone with diabetes.

In this study, scientists gave betel pepper extract to diabetic animals with wounds.

The scientists gave the betel pepper extract to some of the animals. The others got plain saline — salt water. After 10 days, the betel pepper group was far better off than the others. And get this...

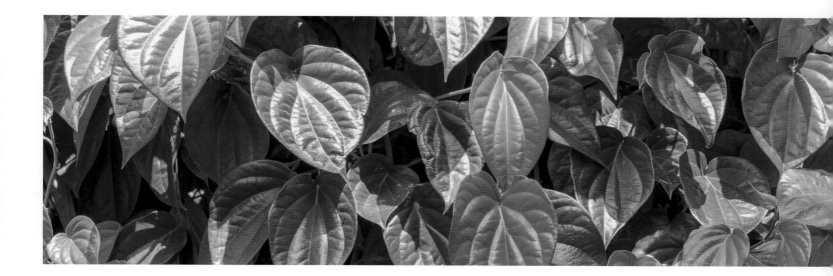

...Their Wounds Were Healing Almost Twice as Fast[7]

Science is finally beginning to reveal to the world what many cultures have recognized in piper betel. Its leaves contain antimicrobial activity, antifungal, insecticidal, antioxidant, pain numbing, antidiabetic, anti-inflammatory and gastro-protective activities. It has also been found to be safe in terms of liver, kidney and blood toxicity as well as organ weight.[8,9]

Piper betel has shown promising antioxidant activity against the group of free radicals and reactive molecules known as reactive oxygen species (ROS). ROS has been shown to be evident in higher amounts in people with thalassemia, a blood disorder resulting in anemia.[10]

In India, they use piper betel mixed with lime to rub on warts to remove them. Afterwards, a mixture with turmeric is applied to reduce scarring.[11]

Other areas of India have used the crushed-up leaves mixed with garlic to use on skin diseases, especially those related to a fungus or yeast.[12] The leaves are often chewed as a general tonic or an aid in digestion, and some cultures actually use the root, mixed with bamboo seeds, as a form of birth control.[13]

In Malaysia it has been used for joint pain and headaches. And it has been used as an infusion in Indonesia in order to aid in digestion, relieve constipation and to increase lactation.

In China, Indonesia, Philippines and Thailand they've used piper betel for toothaches.

Natural Bacteria Buster

This would make sense. Saliva is one of the main components in maintaining oral hygiene. Saliva contains peroxidase, lysozyme and secretory antibodies which fight against bacterial growth. Your mouth is one of the best places for microbial growth. Your saliva is battling daily to keep your mouth from being overtaken by bacterial growths.

This is why betel pepper is a great component in maintaining oral health. For one, chewing it causes an increase in salivation. This increase would also increase the levels of antimicrobials. But, since betel pepper also contains antimicrobials, this makes it a great option for oral health because now you are adding to an army of antimicrobials as you chew.

Studies showed that phenolic antibacterials from betel pepper cause suppression of bacterial activity in the oral cavity and prevent halitosis.

In Ayurvedic medicine, the shape of the plants parts is believed to affect the correlating body part. Because of the leaf's heart-like shape, it's been used in Ayurvedic medicine to treat the heart.

Studies now show that the leaf in fact does affect, within minutes, heart rate and other heart-health issues like irregular heart rhythm.

The Chinese have traditionally used piper betel to aid in fighting diabetes and studies show that the plant affects blood glucose metabolism.

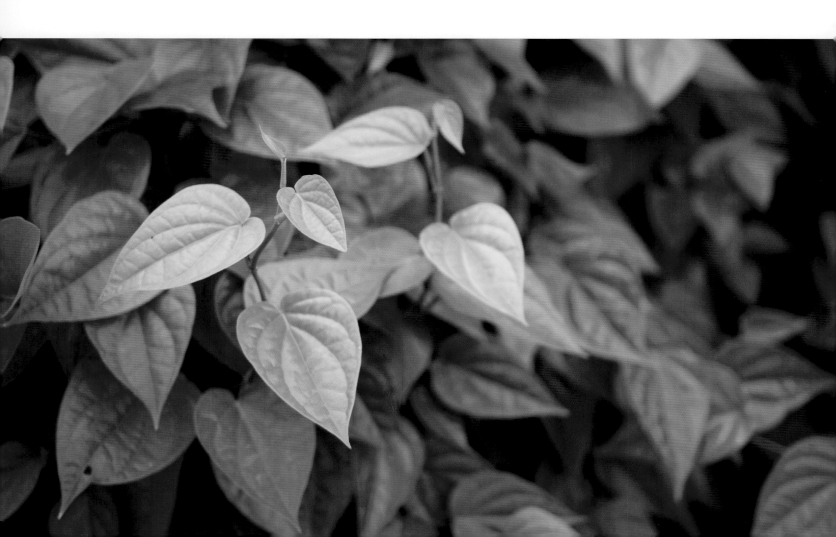

Preparations

You can get pure piper betel leaf extract in Asian specialty stores, but for the most part, the leaves are chewed to get piper betel's effect.

To relieve congestion, the traditional method Lelir taught me is to wrap a clove in a betel leaf and chew. The mucous will break up and your airways will clear in a short time.

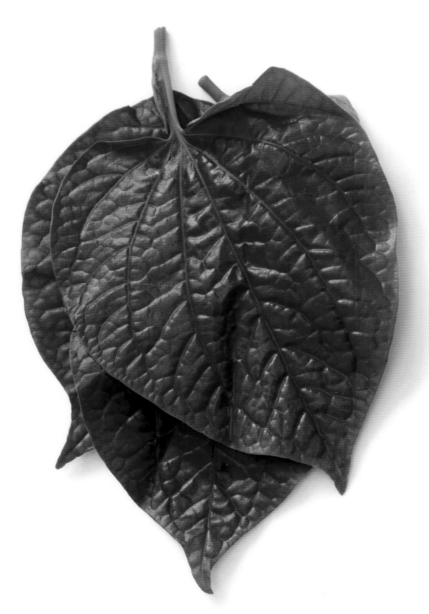

The betel leaf is a good source of calcium, carotene and iron and also helps in digestion. One of the favorite ways to chew the betel leaf in Bali is after a meal. They spread a bit of lime, sprinkle some coconut shavings, add a pinch or two of their favorite spices, then they fold it and savor each chew.

REFERENCES

Coconut Palm

1. Xue, C., et al, "Consumption of medium- and long-chain triacylglycerols decreases body fat and blood triglyceride in Chinese hypertriglyceridemic subjects," Eur J Clin Nutr. Jul 2009; 63(7): 879-886.

2. St-Onge, M.P. and Jones, P.J., "Greater rise in fat oxidation with medium-chain triglyceride consumption relative to long-chain triglyceride is associated with lower initial body weight and greater loss of subcutaneous adipose tissue," Int J Obes Relat Metab Disord. Dec 2003; 27(12): 1565-1571.

3. Saat M., et al. Rehydration after exercise with fresh young coconut water, carbohydrate-electrolyte beverage and plain water. *J Physiol Anthropol Appl Human Sci.* 2002;21(2):93-104

4. Nevin, K.G., Rajamohan, T., "Effect of topical application of virgin coconut oil on skin components and antioxidant status during dermal wound healing in young rats," *Skin Pharmacol.* Physiol. June 2010;23(6):290-7

5. "Coconut Oil: This cooking oil is a powerful virus-destroyer and antibiotic..." Mecola.com. October 22, 2010.

6. Kaunitz, H. 1986. Medium chain triglycerides (MCT) in aging and arteriosclerosis. J Environ Pathol Toxicol Oncol 6(3-4):115.

7. "Live Long & Well With Coconut Oil." Health Habits. January 6, 2010.

8. Hanne Müller et al. The Serum LDL/HDL Cholesterol Ratio Is Influenced More Favorably by Exchanging Saturated with Unsaturated Fat Than by Reducing Saturated Fat in the Diet of Women. J. Nutr. 133:78-83, Jan 2003

9. Nutrition Facts – Coconut Meat, Raw,"

10. "The Bad News about Magnesium Food Sources." Ancient Minerals by enviromedica.

11. The Bad News about Magnesium Food Sources." Ancient Minerals by enviromedica.

12. Jahnen-Dechent W, Ketteler M. "Magnesium Basics." Clinical Kidney Journal 2012;5(Suppl 1):i13-i14.

13. Reffelmann T, Ittermann T, Dörr M, et. al. "Low serum magnesium concentrations predict cardiovascular and all-cause..." *Atherosclerosis* June 12, 2011

14. "Magnesium: An invisible deficiency that could be harming your health." Mercola.com. January 19, 2015.

15. "The Truth About Coconut Water." WebMD. Food & Recipes.

16. Gunnars, K. "How coconut oil can help you lose weight and belly fat." Authority Nutrition. March 2016.

17. St-Onge, M.P. and Jones, P.J., "Greater rise in fat oxidation with medium-chain triglyceride consumption relative to long-chain triglyceride is associated with lower initial body weight and greater loss of subcutaneous adipose tissue." Int J Obes Relat Metab Disord. 2003; 27(12): 1565-1571.

18. Xue, C., et al, "Consumption of medium- and long-chain triacylglycerols decreases body fat and blood triglyceride in Chinese hypertriglyceridemic subjects," Eur J Clin Nutr. 2009; 63(7): 879-886.

Guava

1. Ryu N, et. al. "A hexane fraction of guava Leaves (Psidium guajava L.) induces anticancer activity by suppressing AKT/mammalian target of rapamycin/ribosomal p70 S6 kinase in human prostate cancer cells." *J Med Food.* 2012;15(3):231-41.

2. Gupta S, Phromnoi K, Aggarwal B. "Morin inhibits STAT3 tyrosine 705 phosphorylation in tumor cells through activation of protein tyrosine phosphatase SHP1." Biochem Pharmacol. 2013;85(7):898-912.

3. Karthik Kumar V, Vennila S, Nalini N. "Inhibitory effect of morin on DMH-induced biochemical changes and aberrant crypt foci formation in experimental colon carcinogenesis." Environ Toxicol Pharmacol. 2010;29(1):50-7.

4. Nandhakumar R, Salini K, Niranjali Devaraj S. "Morin augments anticarcinogenic and antiproliferative efficacy against 7,12-dimethylbenz(a)-anthracene induced experimental mammary carcinogenesis." Mol Cell Biochem. 2012;364(1-2):79-92.

5. Ibarretxe, G., Sánchez-Gómez, M.V., Campos-Esparza, M.R., et al, "Differential oxidative stress in

oligodendrocytes and neurons after excitotoxic insults and protection by natural polyphenols," *Glia* 2006;53(2):201-11.

6. Dhiman A. et al. In vitro antimicrobial activity of methanolic leaf extract of Psidium guajava L. *J Pharm Bioallied Sci.* 2011;3(2):226-9.

7. Sriwilaijaroen N, et al. Antiviral effects of Psidium guajava Linn. (guava) tea on the growth of clinical isolated H1N1 viruses: its role in viral hemagglutination and neuraminidase inhibition. *Antiviral Res.* 2012;94(2):139-46.

8. Kim SH, et al. Metabolic profiling and predicting the free radical scavenging activity of guava (Psidium guajava L.) leaves according to harvest time by 1H-nuclear magnetic resonance spectroscopy. *Biosci Biotechnol Biochem.* 2011;75(6):1090-7.

9. Rai PK. et al. Anti-hyperglycaemic potential of Psidium guajava raw fruit peel. *Indian J Med Res.* 2009;129(5):561-5.

10. Rai PK. et al. Anti-hyperglycaemic potential of Psidium guajava raw fruit peel. *Indian J Med Res.* 2009;129(5):561-5.

11. Rai PK. et al. Anti-hyperglycaemic potential of Psidium guajava raw fruit peel. *Indian J Med Res.* 2009;129(5):561-5.

12. Eidenberger T, et al. Inhibition of dipeptidyl peptidase activity by flavonol glycosides of guava (Psidium guajava L.): A key to the beneficial effects of guava in type II diabetes mellitus. *Fitoterapia.* 2013;89:74-9.

13. Siani AC, et al. Anti-inflammatory activity of essential oils from Syzygium cumini and Psidium guajava. *Pharm Biol.* 2013;51(7):881-7.

14. Dutta S, et al. A study of the anti-inflammatory effect of the leaves of Psidium guajava Linn. on experimental animal models. *Pharmacognosy Res.* 2010;2(5):313-7.

15. Lin CY, et al. Renal protective effects of extracts from guava fruit (Psidium guajava L.) in diabetic mice. *Plant Foods Hum Nutr.* 2012;67(3):303-8.

16. Soman S. et al. Beneficial effects of Psidium guajava leaf extract on diabetic myocardium. *Exp Toxicol Pathol.* 2013;65(1-2):91-5.

17. Lu W, et al. "Screening of anti-diarrhea effective fractions from guava leaf." *Zhong Yao Cai.* 2010;33(5):732-5.

18. Birdi T, et al. Newer insights into the mechanism of action of Psidium guajava L. leaves in infectious diarrhoea. *BMC Complement Altern Med.* 2010; 28;10:33

19. Birdi T, et al. Newer insights into the mechanism of action of Psidium guajava L. leaves in infectious diarrhoea. *BMC Complement Altern Med.* 2010; 28;10:33

20. Birdi T, et al. Newer insights into the mechanism of action of Psidium guajava L. leaves in infectious diarrhoea. *BMC Complement Altern Med.* 2010; 28;10:33

21. Livingston Raja NR, et al. Psidium guajava Linn confers gastro protective effects on rats. *Eur Rev Med Pharmacol Sci.* 2012;16(2):151-6.

22. Livingston Raja NR, et al. Psidium guajava Linn confers gastro protective effects on rats. *Eur Rev Med Pharmacol Sci.* 2012;16(2):151-6.

23. Adesida A, et al. Free radical scavenging activities of guava extract in vitro. *Afr J Med Med Sci.* 2012;41 Suppl:81-90.

Holy Basil

1. Mondal S, et. al. "Double-blinded randomized controlled trial for immunomodulatory effects of Tulsi (Ocimum sanctum Linn.) leaf extract on healthy volunteers." *J Ethnopharmacol.* 2011 Jul 14;136(3):452-6.

2. Ringbom T, et al. "Ursolicacid from Plantago major, a selective inhibitor of cyclooxygenase-2 catalyzed prostaglandin biosynthesis." *J Nat Prod.* 1998; 61:1212-15.

3. Chatterjee M, Verma P, Maurya R, Palit G. "Evaluation of ethanol leaf extract of Ocimum sanctum in experimental models of anxiety and depression." *Pharm Biol.* 2011 May;49(5):477-83.

4. Das, A., Banik, N.L., Ray, S.K., "Flavonoids activated caspases for apoptosis in human glioblastoma T98G and U87MG cells but not in human normal astrocytes," *Cancer* 2010;116(1):164-76

5. Liu, R., Zhang, T., Yang, H., et al, "The flavonoid apigenin protects brain neurovascular coupling against amyloid-β-induced toxicity in mice," *J. Alzheimers Dis.* 2011;24(1):85-100

6. Bharavi, K, et. al. "Prevention of cadmium bioaccumulation by herbal adaptogens." *Indian J Pharmacol.* 2011 February; 43(1): 45–49.

Frangipani

1. "Frangipani inhibit the development of TB germs." Herbal and Medicinal Plants. October 20, 2011.

2. Journal of Infectious Disease 2009 PP 151

3. Int J Health Res, June 2008; 1(2):79-85

Red Onion

1. Sugantha Priya E, Selvakumar K, Bavithra S, Elumalai P, Arunkumar R, Raja Singh P, Brindha Mercy A, Arunakaran J. "Anti-cancer activity of quercetin in neuroblastoma: an in vitro approach." *Neurol Sci.* 2013.

2. Lai WW, et al. Quercetin inhibits migration and invasion of SAS human oral cancer cells through inhibition of NF-κB and matrix metalloproteinase-2/-9 signaling pathways. *Anticancer Res.* 2013;33(5):1941-50.

3. Stoyanova S, Geuns J, Hideg E, Van Den Ende W. "The food additives inulin and stevioside counteract oxidative stress." *Int J Food Sci Nutr.* 2011 May;62(3):207-14.

4. Siddiq M, et al. "Total phenolics, antioxidant properties and quality of fresh-cut onions (Allium cepa L.) treated with mild-heat." *Food Chem.* 2013;136(2):803-6.

5. Lee B, et al. "Assessment of red onion on antioxidant activity in rat." *Food Chem Toxicol.* 2012;50(11):3912-9.

6. Matheson EM, et al. The association between onion consumption and bone density in perimenopausal and postmenopausal non-Hispanic white women 50 years and older. *Menopause.* 2009;16(4):756-9.

7. Taj Eldin I, Ahmed E, Elwahab H. "Preliminary Study of the Clinical Hypoglycemic Effects of Allium cepa (Red Onion) in Type 1 and Type 2 Diabetic Patients." Environ Health Insights. 2010;4:71-7.

8. Kim SH, et al. "Effects of Onion (Allium cepa L.) Extract Administration on Intestinal α-Glucosidases Activities and Spikes in Postprandial Blood Glucose Levels in SD Rats Model." *Int J Mol Sci.* 2011;12(6):3757-69.

9. Reddy RR, et al. Dietary fenugreek and onion attenuate cholesterol gallstone formation in lithogenic diet-fed mice. *Int J Exp Pathol.* 2011;92(5):308-19.

10. Ige S, et al. Common onion (Allium cepa) extract reverses cadmium-induced organ toxicity and dyslipidaemia via redox alteration in rats. *Pathophysiology.* 2013; pii: S0928-4680(13)00008-4.

11. Willital GH, et al. Efficacy of early initiation of a gel containing extractum cepae, heparin, and allantoin for scar treatment: an observational, noninterventional study of daily practice. *J Drugs Dermatol.* 2013;12(1):38-42.

12. Moon J, et al. Antiobesity effects of quercetin-rich onion peel extract on the differentiation of 3T3-L1 preadipocytes and the adipogenesis in high fat-fed rats. *Food Chem Toxicol.* 2013 Aug;58:347-54.

13. Yoshinari O, et al. Anti-obesity effects of onion extract in Zucker diabetic fatty rats. *Nutrients.* 2012 Oct 22;4(10):1518-26.

14. "What's New and Beneficial About Onions." The World's Healthiest Foods. www.whfoods.com. Retrieved Dec 5, 2013.

Beluntas

1. Sen, T., Dhara, A.K., Bhattacharjee, S., et al, "Antioxidant activity of the methanol fraction of Pluchea indica root extract," *Phytother. Res.* June 2002;16(4):331-5

2. Hong Y, Liao L, et. al. "Crude aqueous extracts of Pluchea indica (L.) Less. inhibit proliferation and migration of cancer cells through induction of p53-dependent cell death." *BMC Complementary and Alternative Medicine* 2012, 12:265.

3. "Chemical Constituent Investigation of Mangrove Plant Pluchea Indica (L.) Less." Master's Thesis from China Universities. mt.china-papers.com. Retrieved June 24, 2013.

4. Mahatoa S, et. al. "Potential antitumor agents from Lantana camara : Structures of flavonoid -, and phenylpropanoid glycosides." *Tetrahedron,* 1994;Volume 50, Issue 31, Pages 9439–9446.

5. Kleinová M, Hewitt M, Brezová V, Madden JC, Cronin MT, Valko M. "Antioxidant properties of carotenoids: QSAR prediction of their redox potentials." *Gen Physiol Biophys.* 2007 Jun;26(2):97-103.

6. Sugantha Priya E, Selvakumar K, Bavithra S, Elumalai P, Arunkumar R, Raja Singh P, Brindha Mercy A, Arunakaran J. "Anti-cancer activity of quercetin in neuroblastoma: an in vitro approach." *Neurol Sci.* 2013.

7. Berges R, et. al. "Treatment ... with b-sitosterol: an 18-month follow-up." *BJU International* 2000;85, 842±84.

8. Gorritti A. "Updating the Monograph – Sacha Inchi (Plukenetia volubilis L.)." Perúbiodiverso Project II, 2013.

9. Buapool D, et al. Molecular mechanism of anti-inflammatory activity of Pluchea indica leaves in macrophages RAW 264.7 and its action in animal models of inflammation. *J Ethnopharmacol.* 2013;146(2):495-504.

10. Sen, T., et al, Studies on the mechanism of anti-inflammatory and anti-ulcer activity of Pluchea indica-- probable involvement of 5-lipooxygenase pathway. *Life Sci.* 1993; 52(8): 737-743.

11. Mohamad, S., et al, Antituberculosis potential of some ethnobotanically selected Malaysian plants. *J Ethnopharmacol.* 2011; 133(3): 1021-1026.

12. Gomes, A., et al, "Viper and cobra venom neutralization by beta-sitosterol and stigmasterol isolated from the root extract of Pluchea indica Less. (Asteraceae)," *Phytomedicine.* 2007; 14(9): 637-643.

Turmeric

1. White B, Judkins D. "Clinical Inquiry. Does turmeric relieve inflammatory conditions?" *J Fam Pract.* 2011;60(3):155-6.

2. Negi P, et. al. "Antibacterial activity of turmeric oil: a byproduct from curcumin manufacture," *J Agric Food Chem.* 1999; 47(10): 4297-4300.

3. Panchatcharam M, et. al. "Curcumin improves wound healing by modulating collagen and decreasing reactive oxygen species." *Mol Cell Biochem.* 2006; 290(1-2): 87-96.

4. Jurenka S. "Anti-inflammatory Properties of Curcumin, a Major Constituent of Curcuma longa: A Review of Preclinical and Clinical Research." *Alternative Medicine Review* 2009; Volume 14, No. 2.

5. [1]Deodhar S. "Preliminary study on antirheumatic activity of curcumin (diferuloyl methane)." *Indian J Med Res.* 1980;71:632-4.

6. [1]Davis J. "Curcumin effects on inflammation and performance recovery following eccentric exercise-induced muscle damage." *Am J Physiol Regul Integr Comp Physiol.* 2007:R2168-73.

7. Grossman, A. "Turmeric Extract Suppresses Fat Tissue Growth in Rodent Models," Tufts University, news. tufts.edu 2009.

8. White B, Judkins D. "Clinical Inquiry. Does turmeric relieve inflammatory conditions?" *J Fam Pract.* 2011; 60(3): 155-156.

9. Teiten M, et. al. "Chemopreventive potential of curcumin in prostate cancer," *Genes Nutr.* 2010; 5(1): 61-74.

10. Kannappan R, et. al. "Neuroprotection by Spice-Derived Nutraceuticals: You Are What You Eat!" *Mol Neurobiol.* 2011; 44(2): 142-159.

11. Thangapazham R, et. al. "Beneficial role of curcumin in skin diseases," *Adv Exp Med Biol.* 2007; 595: 343-357.

12. Lee W, Loo C, Bebawy M, Luk F, Mason R, Rohanizadeh R. "Curcumin and its derivatives: their application in neuropharmacology and neuroscience in the 21st century." *Curr Neuropharmacol.* 2013;11(4):338-78.

13. Shytle R, et. al. "Optimized Turmeric Extract Reduces β-Amyloid and Phosphorylated Tau Protein Burden in Alzheimer's Transgenic Mice," *Curr. Alzheimer Res.* 2011.

14. Kumaraswamy P, Sethuraman S, Krishnan U. "Mechanistic insights of curcumin interactions with the core-recognition motif of β-amyloid peptide." *J Agric Food Chem.* 2013;61(13):3278-85.

15. Wang P, Su C, Li R, Wang H, Ren Y, Sun H, Yang J, Sun J, Shi J, Tian J, Jiang S. "Mechanisms and effects of curcumin on spatial learning and memory improvement in APPswe/PS1dE9 mice." *J Neurosci Res.* 2014 Feb;92(2):218-31.

Galangal

1. Middleton, E, Kandaswami, C. "The impact of plant flavonoids on mammalian biology: Implication for immunity, inflammation and cancer." In: Harborne J. "The flavonoids: Advances in Research since 1986." London. Chapman and Hall. 1993. pp.619-652.

2. Middleton, E, Kandaswami, C. "The impact of plant flavonoids on mammalian biology: Implication for immunity, inflammation and cancer." In: Harborne J. "The flavonoids: Advances in Research since 1986." London. Chapman and Hall. 1993. pp.619-652.

3. Sukhirun, N., et al, "Impact of Alpinia galanga rhizome extract on Bactrocera dorsalis population," *Commun Agric Appl Biol Sci.* 2010; 75(3): 399-403.

4. Rao, K., et al, "Antibacterial activity of Alpinia galanga (L) Willd crude extracts." *Appl Biochem Biotechnol.* 2010; 162(3): 871-884.

5. Al-Adhroey A, et. al. "Median lethal dose, antimalarial activity, phytochemical screening and radical scavenging of methanolic Languas galanga rhizome extract," *Molecules.* 2010; 15(11): 8366-8376.

6. Acharya S, et. al. "Analgesic effect of extracts of Alpinia galanga rhizome in mice," *Zhong Xi Yi Jie He Xue Bao.* 2011; 9(1): 100-104.

7. Singh H, et. al. "Neurotransmitter Metabolic Enzymes and Antioxidant Status on Alzheimer's Disease Induced Mice Treated with Alpinia galanga (L.) Willd." *Phytother Res.* 2011; (7):1061-7.

8. Halling K, Slotte J. "Membrane properties of plant sterols in phospholipid bilayers …." *Biochim Biophys Acta.* 2004;1664(2):161-171

9. Wilt T, Ishani A, MacDonald R, Stark G, Mulrow C, Lau J. "Beta-sitosterols for benign prostatic hyperplasia." *Cochrane Database Syst Rev.* 2000;(2):CD001043.

Ginger

1. Kikuzaki H and Nakatani N. "Antioxidant Effects of Some Ginger Constituents." *Journal of Food Science.* 2006;Volume 58 Issue 6, Pages 1407 – 1410.

2. Dugasani S, et al. "Comparative antioxidant . . .effects of [6]-gingerol, [8]-gingerol, [10]-gingerol and [6]-shogaol." *J Ethnopharmacol.* 2010;127(2):515-20.

3. Srivastava K, Mustafa T. "Ginger (Zingiber offincinale) in rheumatic and musculoskeletal disorders." *Med Hypotheses.* 1992;39(4):342-8.

4. Ozgoli G, Goli M, Moattar F. "Comparison of Effects of Ginger, Mefenamic Acid, and Ibuprofen on Pain in Women with Primary Dysmenorrhea," *J. Altern. Complement. Med.* 2009;15(2):129-32

5. Ernst E and Pittler MH. "Efficacy of ginger for nausea and vomiting: a systematic review of randomized clinical trials." *Br J Anaesth.* 2000;84(3):367-71.

6. Langner E, et al. "Ginger: history and use." *Adv Ther.* 1998;15(1):25-44.

7. Wu K, et al. "Effects of ginger on gastric emptying and motility in healthy humans." *Eur J Gastroenterol Hepatol.* 2008;20(5):436-40.

8. Ozgoli G, Goli M, Moattar F. "Comparison of effects of ginger, mefenamic acid, and ibuprofen on pain in women with primary dysmenorrhea." *J Altern Complement Med.* 2009;15(2):129-32.

Pineapple

1. Amini A, Ehteda A, Masoumi Moghaddam S, Akhter J, Pillai K, Morris D. "Cytotoxic effects of bromelain in human gastrointestinal carcinoma cell lines (MKN45, KATO-III, HT29-5F12, and HT29-5M21)." Onco Targets Ther. 2013;6:403-9.

2. Romano B, et. al. "The chemopreventive action of bromelain, from pineapple stem (Ananas comosus L.), on colon carcinogenesis is related to antiproliferative and proapoptotic effects." Mol Nutr Food Res. 2013. Epub ahead of print.

3. Fouz N, Amid A, Hashim Y. "Cytokinetic study of MCF-7 cells treated with commercial and recombinant bromelain." Asian Pac J Cancer Prev. 2013;14(11):6709-14.

4. [1]Maurer, H.R., et al. Bromelain: biochemistry, pharmacology and medical use. *Cell Mol Life Sci.* 2001; 58(9): 1234-1245.

5. Mahajan S, et al. Stem bromelain-induced macrophage apoptosis and activation curtail Mycobacterium tuberculosis persistence. *J Infect Dis.* 2012;206(3):366-76.

6. [1]Buford, T.W., et al. Protease supplementation improves muscle function after eccentric exercise. *Med. Sci. Sports Exerc.* Oct. 2009;41(10):1908-14

Salak

1. Leontowicz, M., et. al. "Two exotic fruits positively affect rat's plasma composition." Food Chemistry 2007; Volume 102, Issue 1, Pages 192-200.

2. Gorinstein S. "The comparative characteristics of snake and kiwi fruits." Food Chem Toxicol. 2009 Aug;47(8):1884-91.

Bitter Cucumber

1. Tabata K, Hamano A, Akihisa T, Suzuki T. "Kuguaglycoside C, A Constituent of Momordica Charantia, Induces Caspase-independent Cell Death of Neuroblastoma Cells." Cancer Sci. 2012;103(12):2153-8.

2. Weng J, Bai L, Chiu C, Hu J, Chiu S, Wu C. "Cucurbitane Triterpenoid from Momordica charantia Induces Apoptosis and Autophagy in Breast Cancer Cells..." *Evid Based Complement Alternat Med.* 2013;2013:935675.

3. Waiyaput W, Payungporn S, Issara-Amphorn J, Panjaworayan N. "Inhibitory Effects of Crude Extracts From Some Edible Thai Plants Against Replication of Hepatitis B Virus and Human Liver Cancer Cells." *BMC Complement Altern Med.* 2012;12:246.

4. Kobori M, Ohnishi-Kameyama M, Akimoto Y, Yukizaki C, Yoshida M. "Alpha-Eleostearic Acid and Its Dihydroxy Derivative Are Major Apoptosis-inducing Components of Bitter Gourd." *J Agric Food Chem.* 2008;56(22):10515-20.

5. Agrawal R, et. al. "Chemopreventive and anticarcinogenic effects of Momordica charantia extract." *Asian Pac J Cancer Prev.* 2010;11(2):371-5.

6. Teoh S, Latiff A, Das S. "The effect of topical extract of Momordica charantia (bitter gourd) on wound healing in nondiabetic rats and in rats with diabetes induced by streptozotocin." *Clin Exp Dermatol.* 2009;34(7):815-22.

7. "Tropical Plant Database" Retrieved Jul 12, 2013.

8. Bhujbal S, Hadawale S, Kulkarni P, Bidkar J, Thatte V, Providencia C, Yeola R. "A novel herbal formulation in the management of diabetes." *Int J Pharm Investig.* 2011;1(4):222-6.

9. Fuangchan A, et. al. "Hypoglycemic effect of bitter melon compared with metformin in newly diagnosed type 2 diabetes patients," *J Ethnopharmacol.* 2011; 134(2): 422-428.

10. Pongthanapisith V, Ikuta K, Puthavathana P. "Antiviral Protein of Momordica charantia L. Inhibits Different Subtypes of Influenza A." *Evid Based Complement Alternat Med.* 2013;2013:729081.

11. Huang T, et. al. "Studies on antiviral activity of the extract of Momordica charantia and its active principle." *Virologica.* 1990; 5(4): 367–73.

12. Yesilada E, et. al. "Screening of Turkish anti-ulcerogenic folk remedies for anti-Helicobacter pylori activity." *J. Ethnopharmacol.* 1999; 66(3): 289–93.

Chastetree

1. Tanner C, et. al. "Occupation and Risk of Parkinsonism." *Arch. Neurol.* 2009;66(9):1106-1113

2. Costello S, et. al. "Parkinson's Disease and Residential Exposure to Maneb..." *Am. J. Epidemiol.* 2009; 169(8): 919–926

3. Tanner C, et. al. "Rotenone, Paraquat and Parkinson's Disease." *Environ. Health Perspec,* 2011.

4. Kannathasan K, et. al. "Larvicidal activity of fatty acid methyl esters of Vitex species against Culex quinquefasciatus." *Parasitol Res.* 2008; 103(4): 999-1001.

5. Hossain M, et. al. "Atibacterial activity of Vitex trifolia." *Fitoterapia.* 2001; 72(6): 695-697.

6. Kannathasan K, Senthilkumar A, Venkatesalu V. "In vitro antibacterial potential of some Vitex species against human pathogenic bacteria." *Asian Pac J Trop Med.* 2011;4(8):645-8.

7. Geetha V, Doss A, Doss AP. "Antimicrobial potential of vitex trifolia linn." *Anc Sci Life.* 2004;23(4):30-2.

8. Matsui M, et. al. "Characterisation of the anti-inflammatory potential of Vitex trifolia L. (Labiatae), a multipurpose plant of the Pacific traditional medicine." *J Ethnopharmacol.* 2009; 126(3): 427-433.

9. Manjunatha B, et. al. "Comparative evaluation of wound healing potency of Vitex trifolia L. and Vitex altissima L." *Phytother Res.* 2007; 21(5): 457-461.

10. Li W, Cui C, Cai B, Wang H, Yao X. "Flavonoids from Vitex trifolia L. inhibit cell cycle progression at G2/M phase and induce apoptosis in mammalian cancer cells." *J Asian Nat Prod Res.* 2005;7(4):615-26.

11. Wu J, Zhou T, Zhang S, Zhang X, Xuan L. "Cytotoxic terpenoids from the fruits of Vitex trifolia L." *Planta Med.* 2009;75(4):367-70.

Cloves

1. Basu N, et. al. "Gastrointestinally Distributed UDP-glucuronosyltransferase 1A10, Which Metabolizes Estrogens and Nonsteroidal Anti-inflammatory Drugs, Depends upon Phosphorylation." *J Bio Chem* 2004;279, 28320-28329.

2. Trongtokit Y, et al. "Comparative repellency of 38 essential oils against mosquito bites." Phytother Res. 2005 Apr;19(4):303-9.

3. Fouz N, Amid A, Hashim Y. "Cytokinetic study of MCF-7 cells treated with commercial and recombinant bromelain." *Asian Pac J Cancer Prev.* 2013;14(11):6709-14.

4. Habu D, Shiomi S, Tamori A, et al. Role of vitamin K2 in the development of hepatocellular carcinoma in women with viral cirrhosis of the liver. JAMA. 2004 Jul 21;292(3):358-61.

5. Shibayama-Imazu T, et. al. "Vitamin K(2) selectively induced apoptosis in ovarian TYK-nu and pancreatic MIA PaCa-2 cells out of eight solid tumor cell lines through a mechanism different geranylgeraniol." *J Cancer Res Clin Oncol.* 2003;129(1):1-11.

6. Miyazawa K, Yaguchi M, Funato K, et al. "Apoptosis/differentiation-inducing effects of vitamin K2 on HL-60 cells: dichotomous nature of vitamin K2 in leukemia cells." *Leukemia.* 2001;15(7):1111-7.

7. Yoshida, Makiko, Booth, Sarah, Meigs, James, et al, "Phylloquinone intake, insulin sensitivity, and glycemic status in men and women." *Am. J. of Clinical Nutr,* July 2008;88(1):210-215

8. "Spices, cloves, ground." Self Nutrition Data. nutritiondata.self.com. Retrieved Feb 18, 2014.

9. "Top 100 High ORAC Value Antioxidant Foods." Source: US Dept. of Agriculture. Retrieved from Mar 5, 2014.

Moringa

1. Gupta R, Mathur M, Katariya P, Yadav S, Kamal R, Gupta R. "Evaluation of antidiabetic and antioxidant activity of Moringa oleifera in experimental diabetes." J Diabetes. 2011.

2. Sreelatha S, Jeyachitra A, Padma P. "Antiproliferation and induction of apoptosis by Moringa oleifera leaf extract on human cancer cells." Food Chem Toxicol. 2011 Jun;49(6):1270-5.

3. Calderón-Montaño JM, et al. A review on the dietary flavonoid kaempferol. *Mini Rev Med Chem.* 2011;11(4):298-344.

4. Berkovich L, et al. Moringa Oleifera aqueous leaf extract down-regulates nuclear factor-kappaB and increases cytotoxic effect of chemotherapy in pancreatic cancer cells. *BMC Complement Altern Med.* 2013;13(1):212.

5. Atawodi SE. Nigerian foodstuffs with prostate cancer chemopreventive polyphenols. *Infect Agent Cancer.* 2011;6 Suppl 2:S9.

6. Manaheji, H., et al, Analgesic effects of methanolic extracts of the leaf or root of Moringa oleifera on complete Freund's adjuvant-induced arthritis in rats. *Zhong Xi Yi Jie He Xue Bao.* Feb 2011; 9(2): 216-222.

Butterfly Pea

1. Sen Z, Zhan X, Jing J, Yi Z, Wanqi Z. "Chemosensitizing activities of cyclotides from Clitoria ternatea in paclitaxel-resistant lung cancer cells." Oncol Lett. 2013;5(2):641-644.

2. Jain N, Ohal C, Shroff S, Bhutada R, Somani R, Kasture V, Kasture S. "Clitoria ternatea and the CNS." *Pharmacol Biochem Behav.* 2003;75(3):529-36.

3. Rai K, Murthy K, Karanth K, Nalini K, Rao M, Srinivasan K. "Clitoria ternatea root extract enhances acetylcholine content in rat hippocampus." *Fitoterapia.* 2002;73(7-8):685-9.

Champak

1. Kapoor S, Jaggi, R. "Chemical Studies On Flowers Of Michelia Champaca." *IJPS.* 2004; 66:4: 403-406.

2. Kumar R, Kumar S, Shashidhara S, Anitha S, Manjula M. "Antioxidant and Antimicrobial Activities of Various Extracts of Michelia champaca Linn flowers." *World Applied Sci Journal* 2011;12 (4): 413-418.

3. Khan M. "Antimicrobial activity of Michelia champaca." Fitoterapia. 2002; 73(7-8): 744-748.

4. Shanbhag T, Kodidela S, Shenoy S, Amuthan A, Kurra S. "Effect of Michelia champaca Linn flowers on burn wound healing in Wistar rats." *Intl J Pharm Sci Rev and Research* 2011;7:112-5.

5. Jarald E. "Antidiabetic activity of flower buds of Michelia champaca." *Indian J Pharmacol.* 2008; 40(6): 256-260.

6. Taprial S, et. al. "Antifertility effect of hydroalcoholic leaves extract of Michelia champaca L.: an ethnomedicine used by Bhatra women in Chhattisgarh state of India." J Ethnopharmacol. 2013;147(3):671-5.

7. Yeh Y, et. al. "Bioactive constituents from Michelia champaca." *Nat Prod Commun.* 2011;6(9):1251-2.

Rice

1. Abe M, et. al. "A rice-based soluble form of a murine TNF-specific llama variable domain of heavy-chain antibody suppresses collagen-induced arthritis in mice." *J Biotechnol.* 2014. pii: S0168-1656(14)00078-9.

2. Lee A, et. al. "Hypolipidemic effect of Goami-3 rice on C57BL/6J mice is mediated by the regulation of peroxisome proliferator-activated receptor-α and -γ." *J Nutr Biochem.* 2013;24(11):1991-2000.

3. Wang D, et. al. "Joint Association of Dietary Pattern and Physical Activity Level with Cardiovascular Disease Risk Factors among Chinese Men." *PLoS One.* 2013;8(6):e66210.

Gotu Kola

1. Soumyanath A, Zhong Y, Gold S, Yu X, Koop D, Bourdette D, Gold B. "Centella asiatica accelerates nerve regeneration upon oral administration and contains multiple active fractions increasing neurite elongation in-vitro." J Pharm Pharmacol. 2005;57(9):1221-9.

2. Garcia-Alloza M, Dodwell S, Meyer-Leuhmann M, Hyman B, Bacskai B. "Plaque-derived oxidative stress mediates distorted neurite trajectories in the Alzheimer mouse model." *J Neuropathol Exp Neuro.* 2006;65(11): 1082-9.

3. Wanakhachornkrai O, Pongrakhananon V, Chunhacha P, Wanasuntronwong A, Vattanajun A, Tantisira B, Chanvorachote P, Tantisira M. "Neuritogenic effect of standardized extract of Centella asiatica ECa233 on human neuroblastoma cells." BMC Complement Altern Med. 2013;13(1):204.

4. Wang L, et al. "Antiproliferative, cell-cycle dysregulation effects of novel asiatic acid derivatives on hum an non-small cell lung cancer cells." *Chem Pharm Bull (Tokyo).* 2013. Epub ahead of print.

Sacred Lotus

1. Bin X, et al. "Nelumbo nucifera alkaloid inhibits 3T3-L1 preadipocyte differentiation and improves high-fat diet induced obesity and body fat accumulating in rats." *Journal of Medicinal Plants Research.* 2011; 5(10):2021–28.

2. Ono Y, et al. "Anti-obesity effect of Nelumbo nucifera leaves extract in mice and rats." *J Ethnopharmacol.* 2006;106(2):238-44.

3. You J, Lee Y, Kim K, Kim S, Chang K. "Anti-obesity and hypolipidaemic effects of Nelumbo nucifera seed ethanol extract in human pre-adipocytes and rats fed a high-fat diet." *J Sci Food Agric.* 2014;94(3):568-75.

4. Kashiwada Y, et al. "Anti-HIV benzylisoquinoline alkaloids and flavonoids from the leaves of Nelumbo nucifera, and structure-activity correlations with related alkaloids." *Bioorg Med Chem.* 2005;13(2):443-8.

5. Liao C, Lin J. "Lotus plumule polysaccharide ameliorates pancreatic islets loss and serum lipid profiles in non-obese diabetic mice." *Food Chem Toxicol.* 2013 Aug;58:416-22.

6. Shad M, et. al. "Phytochemical composition and antioxidant properties of rhizomes of *Nilumbo nucifera.*" *J Med Plant Res.* 2012 Feb 16;6(6):972-980

7. Peng Z, et. al. "Protective effect of neferine on endothelial cell nitric oxide production induced by lysophosphatidylcholine..." *Can J Physiol Pharmacol.* 2011;89(4):289-94.

8. Nakamura S, et. al. "Alkaloid constituents from flower buds and leaves of sacred lotus with melanogenesis inhibitory activity in B16 melanoma cells." *Bioorg Med Chem.* 2013;21(3):779-87.

9. Zhao X, Shen J, Chang K, Kim S. "Analysis of fatty acids and phytosterols in ethanol extracts of Nelumbo nucifera seeds and rhizomes by GC-MS." *J Agric Food Chem.* 2013;61(28):6841-7.

10. Poornima P, Weng C, Padma V. "Neferine, an alkaloid from lotus seed embryo, inhibits human lung cancer cell growth by MAPK activation and cell cycle arrest." *Biofactors.* 2013. Epub ahead of print.

11. Yoon J, Kim H, Yadunandam A, Kim N, Jung H, Choi J, Kim C, Kim G. "Neferine isolated from Nelumbo nucifera enhances anti-cancer activities in Hep3B cells..." *Phytomedicine.* 2013;20(11):1013-22.

12. Ahn Y, Park S, Woo H, Lee H, Kim H, Kwon G, Gao Q, Jang D, Ryu J. "Effects of allantoin on cognitive function and hippocampal neurogenesis." *Food Chem Toxicol.* 2014;64:210-6.

Indian Mulberry

1. Devore E, Kang J, Breteler M, Grodstein F. "Dietary intakes of berries and flavonoids in relation to cognitive decline." *Ann Neurol.* 2012.

2. Jäger A, Saaby L. "Flavonoids and the CNS." *Molecules.* 2011;16(2):1471-85.

3. Wang M, et. al. "Cancer preventive effect of Morinda citrifolia." *Ann NY Acad Sci.* 2001;952:161-8.

4. Letawe C, et. al. "Digital image analysis of the effect of topically applied linoleic acid on acne microcomedones." *Clin Exp Dermatol.* 1998; 23(2): 56-58.

5. Prapaitrakool S. and Itharat A. "Morinda citrifolia Linn. for prevention of postoperative nausea and vomiting." *J Med Assoc Thai.* 2010; 93 Suppl 7: S204-209.

6. Mahattanadul S, et. al. "Effects of Morinda citrifolia aqueous fruit extract and its biomarker scopoletin on reflux esophagitis and gastric ulcer in rats." *J Ethnopharmacol.* 2011; 134(2): 243-250.

Java Cardamom

1. Agnihotri S, Wakode S. "Antimicrobial activity of essential oil and various extracts of fruits of greater cardamom." *Indian J Pharm Sci.* 2010 Sep;72(5):657-9.

2. Lee, J.-H., et al, "Anti-Asthmatic Effects of an Amomum compactum Extract on an Ovalbumin (OVA)-Induced Murine Asthma Model," Bioscience, Biotechnology, and Biochemistry. 2010; 74(9): 1814-1818.

3. Moteki H, Hibasami H, Yamada Y, Katsuzaki H, Imai K, Komiya T. "Specific induction of apoptosis by 1,8-cineole in two human leukemia cell lines, but not a in human stomach cancer cell line." *Oncol Rep.* 2002;9(4):757-60.

4. Wang W, Li N, Luo M, Zu Y, Efferth T. "Antibacterial activity and anticancer activity of Rosmarinus officinalis L. essential oil compared to that of its main components." *Molecules.* 2012;17(3):2704-13.

5. Choi H, Lee J, Jung Y. "Nootkatone inhibits tumor necrosis factor α/interferon γ-induced production of chemokines in HaCaT cells." Biochem Biophys Res Commun. 2014 May 2;447(2):278-84.

Globe Amaranth

1. Lans C. "Ethnomedicines used in Trinidad and Tobago for urinary problems and diabetes mellitus." J Ethnobiol Ethnomed. 2006;2:45.

2. Silva L, et. al. "Phytochemical investigations and biological potential screening with cellular and non-cellular models of globe amaranth inflorescences." *Food Chem.* 2012;135(2):756-63.

3. Wang C, et. al. "Betacyanins from Portulaca oleracea L. ameliorate cognition deficits and attenuate oxidative damage induced by D-galactose in the brains of senescent mice." *Phytomedicine.* 2010; 17(7): 527-532.

4. Sreekanth D, et. al. "Betanin a betacyanin pigment purified from fruits of Opuntia ficus-indica induces apoptosis in human chronic myeloid leukemia Cell line-K562." *Phytomedicine.* 2007; 14(11): 739-746.

5. Lee, K.M, et al, Kaempferol inhibits UVB-induced COX-2 expression by suppressing Src kinase activity," *Biochem. Pharmacol.* 2010; 80(12):2042-9

6. Arcanjo D, et. al. "Phytochemical screening and evaluation of cytotoxic, antimicrobial and cardiovascular effects of Gomphrena globosa L." *Journal of Medicinal Plants Research* 2011;Vol. 5(10), pp. 2006-2010.

Canaga Flower

1. Cha J, Lee S, Yoo Y. "Effects of aromatherapy on changes in the autonomic nervous system, aortic pulse wave velocity and aortic augmentation index in patients with essential hypertension." *J Korean Acad Nurs.* 2010;40(5):705-13.

2. Hsieh T, Chang F, Chia Y, Chen C, Chiu H, Wu Y. "Cytotoxic constituents of the fruits of Cananga odorata." *J Nat Prod.* 2001;64(5):616-9.

3. Matsumoto T, et. al. "Structure of constituents isolated from the flower buds of Cananga odorata and their inhibitory effects on aldose reductase." *J Nat Med.* 2014 May 11. Epub ahead of print.

4. Rahman M, Lopa S, Sadik G, Harun-Or-Rashid, Islam R, Khondkar P, Alam A, Rashid M. "Antibacterial and cytotoxic compounds from the bark of Cananga odorata." *Fitoterapia.* 2005;76(7-8):758-61.

5. Quintans-Júnior L, et. al. "Antinociceptive Activity and Redox Profile of the Monoterpenes (+)-Camphene, p-Cymene, and Geranyl Acetate in Experimental Models." *ISRN Toxicol.* 2013;2013:459530.

Indian Long Pepper

1. Vinjay S, et. al. "Pharmacognostical and phytochemical study of piper longum l. and piper retrofractum vahl." JPSI 2012;62-66.

2. Kubo M, Ishii R, Ishino Y, Harada K, Matsui N, Akagi M, Kato E, Hosoda S, Fukuyama Y. "Evaluation of constituents of Piper retrofractum fruits on neurotrophic activity." *J Nat Prod.* 2013;76(4):769-73.

3. Nakatani N, Inatani R, Ohta H, Nishioka A. "Chemical constituents of peppers (Piper spp.) and application to food preservation: naturally occurring antioxidative compounds." *Environ Health Perspect.* 1986;67:135-42.

4. Hlavackova L, Urbanova A, Ulicna O, Janega P, Cerna A, Babal P. "Piperine, active substance of black pepper, alleviates hypertension induced by NO synthase inhibition." *Bratisl Lek Listy.* 2010;111(8):426-31.

5. Diwan V, Poudyal H, Brown L. "Piperine attenuates cardiovascular, liver and metabolic changes in high carbohydrate, high fat-fed rats." *Cell Biochem Biophys.* 2013;67(2):297-304.

6. Kim K, Lee M, Jo K, Hwang J. "Piperidine alkaloids from Piper retrofractum Vahl. protect against high-fat diet-induced obesity by regulating lipid metabolism and activating AMP-activated protein kinase." *Biochem Biophys Res Commun.* 2011;411(1):219-25.

7. Wilt T, Ishani A, MacDonald R, Stark G, Mulrow C, Lau J. "Beta-sitosterols for benign prostatic hyperplasia." Cochrane Database Syst Rev. 2000;(2):CD001043.

Hibiscus

1. Adhirajan N, et. al. "In vivo and in vitro evaluation of hair growth potential of Hibiscus rosa-sinensis Linn." *J Ethnopharmacol.* 2003;88(2-3):235-9.

2. Nadkarni A. "Indian Materia Medica." Bombay, 1954, 631.

3. Kumar S, Kumar V, Sharma A, Shukla Y, Singh A. "Traditional Medicinal Plants in Skin Care," Central Institute of Medicinal and Aromatic Plants, 103.

4. Cheng Y, Lee S, Harn H, Huang H, Chang W. "The extract of Hibiscus syriacus inducing apoptosis by activating p53 and AIF in human lung cancer cells." Am J Chin Med. 2008;36(1):171-84.

5. Chang Y, Huang H, Hsu J, Yang S, Wang C. "Hibiscus anthocyanins rich extract-induced apoptotic cell death in human promyelocytic leukemia cells." Toxicol Appl Pharmacol. 2005;205(3):201-12.

6. Lin H, Huang H, Huang C, Chen J, Wang C. "Hibiscus polyphenol-rich extract induces apoptosis in human gastric carcinoma cells via p53 phosphorylation and p38 MAPK/FasL cascade pathway." *Mol Carcinog.* 2005;43(2):86-99.

7. Sarkar B, Kumar D, Sasmal D, Mukhopadhyay K. "Antioxidant and DNA damage protective properties of anthocyanin-rich extracts from Hibiscus and Ocimum: a comparative study." *Nat Prod Res.* 2014;14:1-6.

8. Nevade S, Lokapure S, Kalyane N. "Study on anti-solar activity of ethanolic extract of flower of Hibiscus rosa-sinensis Linn." *Research Journal of Pharmacy and Technology.* 2011;4(3): 472–473

Lemongrass

1. Baldacchino F, et al. "The repellency of lemongrass oil against stable flies, tested using video tracking." *Parasite.* 2013;20:21.

2. Tyagi A, Malik A. "Liquid and vapour-phase antifungal activities of selected essential oils against Candida albicans: microscopic observations and chemical characterization of Cymbopogon citratus." *BMC Complement Altern Med.* 2010;10:65.

3. Carmo E, Pereira Fde O, Cavalcante N, Gayoso C, Lima Ede O. "Treatment of pityriasis versicolor with topical application of essential oil of Cymbopogon citratus (DC) Stapf - therapeutic pilot study." *An Bras Dermatol.* 2013;88(3):381-5.

4. Viana G, Vale T, Pinho R, Matos F. "Antinociceptive effect of the essential oil from Cymbopogon citratus in mice." *J Ethnopharmacol.* 2000;70(3):323-7.

5. Francisco V, Figueirinha A, Neves B, García-Rodríguez C, Lopes M, Cruz M, Batista M. "Cymbopogon citratus as source of new and safe anti-inflammatory drugs: bio-guided assay using lipopolysaccharide-stimulated macrophages." J Ethnopharmacol. 2011 Jan 27;133(2):818-27.

6. Francisco V, et. al. "Anti-inflammatory activity of Cymbopogon citratus leaves infusion via proteasome and nuclear factor-κB pathway inhibition: contribution of chlorogenic acid." J Ethnopharmacol. 2013;148(1):126-34.

7. Gayathri K, Jayachandran K, Vasanthi H, Rajamanickam G. "Cardioprotective effect of lemon grass as evidenced by biochemical and histopathological changes in experimentally induced cardiotoxicity." Hum Exp Toxicol. 2011 Aug;30(8):1073-82.

8. Adeneye A, Agbaje E. "Hypoglycemic and hypolipidemic effects of fresh leaf aqueous extract of Cymbopogon citratus Stapf. in rats." J Ethnopharmacol. 2007;112(3):440-4.

9. Adeneye A, Agbaje E. "Hypoglycemic and hypolipidemic effects of fresh leaf aqueous extract of Cymbopogon citratus Stapf. in rats." J Ethnopharmacol. 2007;112(3):440-4.

10. Tyagi AK, et al. Liquid and vapour-phase antifungal activities of selected essential oils against Candida albicans: microscopic observations and chemical characterization of Cymbopogon citratus. *BMC Complement Altern Med.* 2010 Nov 10;10:65.

11. Shah G, et al. Scientific basis for the therapeutic use of Cymbopogon citratus, stapf (Lemon grass). *J Adv Pharm Technol Res.* 2011;2(1):3-8.

12. Costa C, Kohn D, de Lima V, Gargano A, Flório J, Costa M. "The GABAergic system contributes to the anxiolytic-like effect of essential oil from Cymbopogon citratus (lemongrass)." *J Ethnopharmacol.* 2011;137(1):828-36.

13. Fernandes C, De Souza H, De Oliveria G, Costa J, Kerntopf M, Campos A. "Investigation of the mechanisms underlying the gastroprotective effect of cymbopogon citratus essential oil." *J Young Pharm.* 2012;4(1):28-32.

14. Khan M, Ahmad I. "Biofilm inhibition by Cymbopogon citratus and Syzygium aromaticum essential oils in the strains of Candida albicans." J Ethnopharmacol. 2012;140(2):416-23.

15. Grice I, Rogers K, Griffiths L. "Isolation of bioactive compounds that relate to the anti-platelet activity of Cymbopogon ambiguus." Evid Based Complement Alternat Med. 2010 Jan 4. [Epub ahead of print].

16. Basu N, et. al. "Gastrointestinally Distributed UDP-glucuronosyltransferase 1A10, Which Metabolizes Estrogens and Nonsteroidal Anti-inflammatory Drugs, Depends upon Phosphorylation." *J Bio Chem,* July 2004;279, 28320-28329.

17. Basu N, et. al. "Gastrointestinally Distributed UDP-glucuronosyltransferase 1A10, Which Metabolizes Estrogens and Nonsteroidal Anti-inflammatory Drugs, Depends upon Phosphorylation." *J Bio Chem,* July 2004;279, 28320-28329.

Areca Catechu

1. Chiou, S.S. et al. Effect of chewing a single betel-quid on autonomic nervous modulation in healthy young adults. *J Psychopharmacol.* Nov 2008; 22(8): 910-917.

2. Bhandare, A.M., et al, Potential analgesic, anti-inflammatory and antioxidant activities of hydroalcoholic extract of Areca catechu L. nut. *Food Chem Toxicol.* Dec 2010; 48(12): 3412-3417.

3. Javed F, et al. Areca-nut chewing habit is a significant risk factor for metabolic syndrome: a systematic review. *J Nutr Health Aging.* 2012 May;16(5):445-8.

4. Owen P. Asia Pac Consumption of guava (Psidium guajava L) and noni (Morinda citrifolia L) may protect betel quid-chewing Papua New Guineans against diabetes. J Clin Nutr. 2008;17(4):635-43.

Coral Tree

1. Kumar A. et. al. "Hypoglycemic activity of Erythrina variegata leaf in streptozotocin-induced diabetic rats," *Pharm Biol.* 2011; 49(6): 577-582.

2. Tanaka H, et. al. "Three new constituents from the roots of Erythrina variegata and their antibacterial activity against methicillin-resistant Staphylococcus aureus." *Chem Biodivers.* 2011; 8(3): 476-482.

3. Zhang Y, et. al. "Erythrina variegata extract exerts osteoprotective effects by suppression of the process of bone resorption," *Br J Nutr.* 2010; 104(7): 965-971.

4. Kumar A, Lingadurai S, Jain A, Barman N. "Erythrina variegata Linn: A review on morphology, phytochemistry, and pharmacological aspects." Pharmacogn Rev. 2010; 4(8): 147–152.

Castor Plant

1. Davis, L., "The use of castor oil to stimulate labor in patients with premature rupture of membranes." *Journal of Nurse-Midwifery.* 1984; 29(6): 366-370.

2. Ilavarasan, R, et al. "Anti-inflammatory and free radical scavenging activity of Ricinus communis root extract." *J Ethnopharmacol.* 2006; 103(3): 478-480.

3. Rabia Naz* and Asghari Bano. "Antimicrobial potential of Ricinus communis leaf extracts in different solvents against pathogenic bacterial and fungal strains." *Asian Pac J Trop Biomed.* 2012; 2(12): 944–947.

4. Jeyaseelan E, Jashothan P. "In vitro control of Staphylococcus aureus (NCTC 6571) and Escherichia coli (ATCC 25922) by Ricinus communis L." *Asian Pac J Trop Biomed.* 2012;2(9):717-21.

5. Yanfg L, Yen K, Kiso Y, Hikino H. "Antihepatotoxic actions of Formosan plant drugs." *J Ethnopharmacol.* 1987;19:103–10.

6. Yanfg L, Yen K, Kiso Y, Hikino H. "Antihepatotoxic actions of Formosan plant drugs." *J Ethnopharmacol.* 1987;19:103–10.

7. Shokeen P, Anand P, Murali Y, Tandon V. "Antidiabetic activity of 50% ethanolic extract of Ricinus communisand its purified fractions." *Food Chem Toxicol.* 2008;46:3458–66.

8. Capasso F, Mascolo N, Izzo A, Gaginella T. "Dissociation of castor oil-induced diarrhea and intestinal mucosal injury in rat: effect of NG-nitro-L-arginine methyl ester." *Br J Pharmacol.* 1994;113:1127–30.

9. Ilavarasan R, Mallika M, Venkataraman S. "Anti-inflammatory and free radical scavenging activity of Ricinus communisroot extract." *J Ethnopharmacol.* 2006;103:478–80.

10. Grimes M. "Kitchen Wisdom: Alternative treatments for Common Ailments." Health News. healthnews.com. Dec. 4, 2010. Retrieved June 20, 2014.

11. "Final Report on the Safety Assessment of Ricinus Communis (Castor) Seed Oil..." International Journal of Toxicology 2007;vol. 26 no. 3 suppl 31-77.

Cat's Whiskers

1. Yao, L.H., et al, "Flavonoids in food and their health benefits." *Plant Foods Hum Nutr. Sum* 2004; 59(3): 113-122.

2. Arafata, O.M., et al, "Studies on diuretic and hypouricemic effects of Orthosiphon stamineus methanol extracts in rats," *Journal of Ethnopharmacology.* 2008; 118(3): 354-360.

3. Lyckander I, Malterud K. "Lipophilic flavonoids from Orthosiphon spicatus prevent oxidative inactivation of 15-lipoxygenase." *Prostaglandins Leukot Essent Fatty Acids.* 1996;54(4):239-46.

4. Malterud K, Hanche-Olsen I, Smith-Kielland I. "Flavonoids from Orthosiphon spicatus." *Planta Med.* 1989;55(6):569-70.

Aloe Vera

1. Zanini S, Marzotto M, Giovinazzo F, Bassi C, Bellavite P. "Effects of Dietary Components on Cancer of the Digestive System." Crit Rev Food Sci Nutr. 2014. Epub ahead of print.

2. du Plessis L, Hamman J. "In vitro evaluation of the cytotoxic and apoptogenic properties of Aloe whole leaf and gel materials." Drug Chem Toxicol. 2014;37(2):169-77.

3. Kaithwas G, Singh P, Bhatia D. "Evaluation of in vitro and in vivo antioxidant potential of polysaccharides from Aloe vera (Aloe barbadensis Miller) gel." Drug Chem Toxicol. 2014;37(2):135-43.

4. Chen R, Wang S, Zhang J, Chen M, Wang Y. "Aloe-emodin loaded solid lipid nanoparticles: formulation design and in vitro anti-cancer study." Drug Deliv. 2014. Epub ahead of print.

5. Chen R, Zhang J, Hu Y, Wang S, Chen M, Wang Y. "Potential antineoplastic effects of Aloe-emodin: a comprehensive review." Am J Chin Med. 2014;42(2):275-88.

6. Ahirwar K, Jain S. "Aloe-emodin novel anticancer Herbal Drug." *International Journal of Phytomedicine* 2011;3, 27-31.

7. Lambers H, et al. Natural skin surface pH is on average below 5, which is beneficial for its resident flora. *Int J Cosmet Sci.* 2006;28(5):359-70.

8. Karim B, Bhaskar D, Agali C, Gupta D, Gupta R, Jain A, Kanwar A. "Effect of Aloe vera Mouthwash on Periodontal Health: Triple Blind Randomized Control Trial." *Oral Health Dent Manag.* 2014;13(1):14-9.

9. Cowan D. "Oral Aloe vera as a treatment for osteoarthritis: a summary." *Br J Community Nurs.* 2010;15(6):280-2.

10. Park C, et. al. "Polymer fraction of Aloe vera exhibits a protective activity on ethanol-induced gastric lesions." *Int J Mol Med.* 2011; 27(4): 511-518.

11. Prabjone R, et. al. "Anti-inflammatory effects of Aloe vera on leukocyte-endothelium interaction in the gastric microcirculation of Helicobacter pylori-infected rats." *Clin Hemor Microcirc.* 2006; 35(3): 359-366.

12. Huseini H, et. al. "Anti-hyperglycemic and anti-hypercholesterolemic effects of Aloe vera leaf gel in hyperlipidemic type 2 diabetic patients: a randomized double-blind placebo-controlled clinical trial." *Planta Med.* 2012; 78(4): 311-316.

Wood Sorrell

1. Abhilash P, et al. "Cardioprotective effects of aqueous extract of Oxalis corniculata in experimental myocardial infarction." *Exp Toxicol Pathol.* 2011;63(6):535-40.

2. Manna D, et al. "A novel galacto-glycerolipid from Oxalis corniculata kills Entamoeba histolytica and Giardia lamblia." *Antimicrob Agents Chemother.* 2010;54(11):4825-32.

3. Manna D, et al. "Polyunsaturated fatty acids induce polarized submembranous F-actin aggregates and kill Entamoeba histolytica." *Cytoskeleton* (Hoboken). 2013;70(5):260-8.

4. Sakat S, et al. "Gastroprotective Effect of Oxalis corniculata (Whole Plant) on Experimentally Induced Gastric Ulceration in Wistar Rats." *Indian J Pharm Sci.* 2012;74(1):48-53.

5. Ahmad B, et al. "Amelioration of carbon tetrachloride-induced pulmonary toxicity with Oxalis corniculata." *Toxicol Ind Health.* 2013. Epub ahead of print.

6. Khan MR, Zehra H. "Amelioration of CCl(4)-induced nephrotoxicity by Oxalis corniculata in rat. *Exp Toxicol Pathol.*" 2013;65(3):327-34.

Papaya Tree

1. Otsuki N, Dang NH, Kumagai E, Kondo A, Iwata S, Morimoto C. "Aqueous extract of Carica papaya leaves exhibits anti-tumor activity and immunomodulatory effects." *J Ethnopharma.* 2010;127(3):760-7.

2. Li ZY, Wang Y, Shen WT, Zhou P. "Content determination of benzyl glucosinolate and anti-cancer activity of its hydrolysis product in Carica papaya L." *Asian Pac J Trop Med.* 2012;5(3):231-3.

3. Bhat, G.P. and Surolia, N. In vitro antimalarial activity of extracts of three plants used in the traditional medicine of India. *Am J Trop Med Hyg.* 2001; 65(4): 304-308.

4. Osato, J.A., et al. « Antimicrobial and antioxidant activities of unripe papaya." *Life Sci.* 1993; 53(17): 1383-1389.

5. Furumoto K. et al. "Age-dependent telomere shortening is slowed down by enrichment of intracellular vitamin C via suppression of oxidative stress." *Life Science* 1998; vol. 63, no. 11 pp. 935-48

6. Yokoo S, et al. "Slow-down of age-dependent telomere shortening is executed in human skin keratinocytes by hormesis-like-effects of trace hydrogen peroxide or by anti-oxidative effects of pro-vitamin C in common concurrently with reduction of intracellular oxidative stress." *J Cell Biochem.* 2004;93(3):588-97.

7. "EWG's 2013 Shopper's Guide to Pesticides in Produce." Environmental Working Group.

Cordyline

1. Hinkle A. "Population structure of Pacific Cordyline fruticosa (Laxmanniaceae) with implications for human settlement of Polynesia." Am J Bot. 2007;94(5):828-39.

2. Sriprapat W, Suksabye P, Areephak S, Klantup P, Waraha A, Sawattan A, Thiravetyan P. "Uptake of toluene and ethylbenzene by plants: removal of volatile indoor air contaminants." *Ecotoxicol Environ Saf.* 2014;102:147-51.

Piper Betel

1. Rai M, Thilakchand K, Palatty P, Rao P, Rao S, Bhat H, Baliga M. "Piper betel Linn (betel vine), the maligned Southeast Asian medicinal plant possesses cancer preventive effects: time to reconsider the wronged opinion." *Asian Pac J Cancer Prev.* 2011;12(9):2149-56.

2. Gundala S, Aneja R. "Piper betel leaf: a reservoir of potential xenohormetic nutraceuticals with cancer-fighting properties." Cancer Prev Res (Phila). 2014;7(5):477-86.

3. Paranjpe R, Gundala S, Lakshminarayana N, Sagwal A, Asif G, Pandey A, Aneja R. "Piper betel leaf extract: anticancer benefits and bio-guided fractionation to identify active principles for prostate cancer management." Carcinogenesis. 2013 Jul;34(7):1558-66.

4. Sarris, J., et al, "Kava: a comprehensive review of efficacy, safety, and psychopharmacology." *Aust N Z J Psychiatry.* 2011; 45(1): 27- 35.

5. Lehrl S. "Clinical efficacy of kava extract WS 1490 in sleep disturbances associated with anxiety disorders. Results of a multicenter, randomized, placebo-controlled, double-blind clinical trial." *J Affect Disord.* 2004; 78(2): 101-110.

6. Bhattacharya S, et al. "Healing property of the Piper betel phenol, allylpyrocatechol against indomethacin-induced stomach ulceration and mechanism of action." *World J Gastroenterol.* 2007; 13(27): 3705-3713.

7. Keat, E.C., et al, "The effect of Piper betel extract on the wound healing process in experimentally induced diabetic rats," *Clin Ter.* 2010; 161(2): 117-120.

8. Arambewela L, et al. "Investigations on Piper betel grown in Sri Lanka." *Pharmacogn Rev.* 2011; 5(10): 159–163.

9. Suprapta D. "Anti-fungal activities of selected tropical plants from Bali Island." *Phytopharmacology* 2012, 2 (2) 265-270.

10. Srimani P., et al. Antioxiant effect of ethanolic extract of Piper betel Lin (Paan) on erythrocytes from patients with HbE-beta thalassemia. *Indian J Biochem & Biophys* 2009;vol 46, pp. 241-246.

11. Shekhawat D. "Household remedies of Keshavraipatan tehsil in Bundi district." *Rajasthan Indian Journal of Traditional Knowledge* 2006;Vol 5(3), pp 362-367.

12. Jeeva G. "Traditional treatment of skin diseases in South Travancore, southern peninsular India." *Indian Journal of Traditional Knowledge* 2007;Vol 6(3), pp 498-501.

13. Chandra R. "Ethnomedicinal formulations used by traditional herbal prectisioners of Ranchi, Jharkhand." *Indian Journal of Traditional Knowledge* 2007;Vol 6(4), pp 599-601.

14. Kumar N. "Piper betel Linn. a maligned Pan-Asiatic plantwith an array of pharmacological activities and prospects for drug discovery." *Current Science,* 2010; Vol. 99, No. 7.

INDEX

Thyroid, 9, 14

TNF-alpha inflammatory compound, 144

Toluene, 283

Toxin-absorbing properties
    cordyline, 283

Toxins, 10, 49, 108, 255, 283

Traditional Chinese Medicine, 185

Tranquilizing properties
    piper betel, 287

Triglycerides, 9, 17, 23, 76, 144, 160, 199, 226

Triterpenoids, 152

Tufts University (USA), 61

Tumors, 38, 50, 51, 61, 68, 83, 85, 96, 149, 258

Tumor cells, 22, 50, 95, 104, 116, 258

Turmeric, 57-63. *Also see* Curcumin

U

University of Calcutta (India), 54

University of California, Berkeley (USA), 103, 279

University of Florence (Italy), 112

University of Miami, 95

University of North Carolina (USA), 59

University of Oslo (Norway), 248

University of Verona (Italy), 257

V

Virus/viruses, 9, 10, 11, 23, 38, 71, 239, 256

Vitamins, 13, 15, 21, 42, 45, 68, 85, 112, 115, 117, 201, 218, 259, 261

W

Wood Sorrel (*Semanggi*; *Oxalis corniculata*), 263-269

Y

Yellow Hibiscus. *See* Hibiscus

Ylang-ylang. *Also see* Cananga

Z

Zinc, 13

INDEX OF AILMENTS

red onion, 46

Body odor
beluntas, 55

Boils
Indian mulberry, 166, 168
wood sorrel, 266

Bone health
coconut water, 14
long pepper, 199
soda pop and, 245

Brain aging, protection against
acetylcholine, 129-130
butterfly pea, 130
gotu kola, 148-149
long pepper, 199
sacred lotus, 160

Brain boosters
butterfly pea, 125
gotu kola, 148
guava, 22
Shanka Pushpi mixture, 130

Brain cells, rejuvenating compounds
gotu kola, 148-149
long pepper, 199
sacred lotus, 160

Brain health
choline, 7
coconut, 7
mcts, 9
sacred lotus, 160

Brain tumors
turmeric, 61

Breast cancer. *See under* Cancer, by type

Breastfeeding. *See* Lactation, increasing

Bronchitis
pineapple, 85
piper betel, 285

Bug bites
gotu kola, 151
red onion, 43-44

Bug repellent. *See* Insect repellent

Burns
aloe vera, 259
castor oil, 240
gotu kola, 152
pineapple, 85

C

Cancer, by type. *See* individual types below

Breast

aloe vera, 258
bitter cucumber, 95
champak, 137
guava leaves, 22

Cervical
beluntas, 50
red onion, 42

Colon
bitter cucumber, 95
cardamom, 176
galangal, 68
guava, 22

Endocrine
red onion, 42

Leukemia
beluntas, 50
bitter cucumber, 95
globe amaranth, 183
guava leaves, 21
hibiscus, 208

Liver
aloe vera, 258
beluntas, 50
bitter cucumber, 95
cananga, 191
cloves, 112
hibiscus, 209
sacred lotus, 160

Lung
aloe vera, 258
butterfly pea, 129
champak, 137
gotu kola, 149
hibiscus, 208
red onion, 42
sacred lotus, 160
salak, 89

Neuroblastoma (nerve cells)
bitter cucumber, 95

Ovarian
red onion, 42

Pancreatic
moringa, 119
red onion, 42

Prostate
champak, 136
guava leaves, 21
piper betel, 286
turmeric, 61

Stomach
beluntas, 50
hibiscus, 208
salak, 89

moringa (horseradish tree), 118
piper betel, 289
red onion, 46
quercetin, 41
rice seeds, 143
turmeric, 58
wood sorrel, 264
ylang-ylang, 192

Inflammatory bowel disease
turmeric, 61

Injury, soft tissue. *See* Soft tissue injury

Injury, wounds. *See* Wounds

Insect repellent
chastetree, 100-102, 104
clove oil, 111
lemongrass, 216-217
red onion, 44

Insomnia
kava kava, 288
wood sorrel, 269

Itching
butterfly pea, 127
long pepper, 195
red onion, 44

J

Joint health
papaya, 276

Joint pain
coral tree, 233
ginger, 77
piper betel, 289
pineapple, 84

Joint stiffness/swelling
turmeric, 61

K

Kidney stones
cat's whiskers, 243

L

Lactation, increasing
piper betel, 289

Leukemia. *See under* Cancer, by type

Libido, low
aphrodisiac properties
betel nut, 224
long pepper, 195
piper betel (reputed), 287
sacred lotus, 158
ylang-ylang, 188

Liver cancer. *See under* Cancer, by type

Liver protection
castor oil, 237
hibiscus, 209

Liver spots
castor oil, 237

Lung cancer. *See under* Cancer, by type

Lung protection
quercetin, 42
wood sorrel, 268

M

Memory, protecting
butterfly pea, 130
gotu kola, 147
holy basil, 31
sacred lotus, 160

Menopause. *Also see* Perimenopause
coconut oil, 9
bone fractures and, 46
red onion, 46

Menstrual cycle, irregular
aloe vera, 254
pineapple, 85

Menstrual pain
aloe vera, 254
pineapple, 85

Moles
castor oil, 237

Morning sickness, remedies for
coconut water, 16
galangal, 67
ginger, 71

Mosquito repellent. *Also see* Insect repellent
chasteree, 100-104
cloves, 107, 112
holy basil, 31
lemongrass, 105, 213, 217
papaya leaves, 273-274

Motion sickness
ginger, 76

Muscle pain
ginger, 73, 76
Lelir's boreh, 113
pineapple, 83
smiling exercise, 235

N

Nails, dry and cracked
castor oil, 241
olive oil, 241

MORE UNDISCOVERED CURES — BEFORE THEY'RE LOST FOR GOOD!

I've hacked my way through jungles and swam through pristine, untouched waters in more than 30 countries around the world in search of natural cures.

With a native guide at my side and the freshest air in my lungs, I've rediscovered natural cures that were almost lost forever. And with the increasing industrialization and Westernization of the world, more and more cures are in danger of being lost.

Which is why I'm sharing my monthly newsletter, *Confidential Cures.* And it's changing lives.

> **"Dr. Sears has an amazing knack for sorting the winners from the losers in the very rapidly developing technology of anti-aging medicine."**
> — Dr. Ron Klatz, MD, President and Founder of the American Academy of Anti-Aging (A4M)

Every month, I'll write to you. So you can have the latest research on natural cures available. Things like...

- The **cancer killer** found in an East African tree leaf;

- The "tiger herb" that can **restore your memory and repair your brain;**

- How to **fight congestive heart failure** with one simple antioxidant;

- Natural, <u>no side-effect</u> ways to **beat depression** — without antidepressants;

- And much, much more!

But don't expect to hear about these cures from your doctor. Big Pharma keeps your doctor in the dark. That way they can profit off you for years to come.

I don't want that for you. I want you to be disease-free. For good. There are already thousands of people benefiting from the research in *Confidential Cures.*

> **"I've watched Dr. Sears transform my own health and the lives of dozens of my friends. I've made Dr. Sears my doctor for life. I recommend you do the same."**
> — Michael Masterson; Delray Beach, FL; Founder, Early to Rise; Author of *Power and Persuasion*

And when you subscribe today, you'll get an immediate FREE download of my special report, *The 8th Element: Nature's Universal Cancer Killer.* In it, you'll learn exactly how a special element can help prevent and cure cancer. And how to get it into your system.

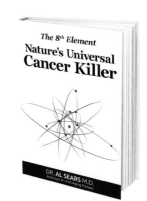

Your subscription will automatically renew after one year for $39.00 USD. You can cancel at any time by calling Customer Support (toll free) at 866.792.1035, or email support@alsearsmd.com.

Item: CONFCURES
Price: $39.00

Call 866.792.1035 or use the order form at the end of this book to subscribe today!

Anti-aging pioneering MD, Dr. Al Sears, offers new hope to help you...
AVOID THE MODERN "TOXIC MENOPAUSE" NIGHTMARE

American women are suffering.

They feel betrayed by their bodies... out of control. I hear it from my patients every day.

These symptoms affect so many women today... and your age doesn't matter. You can suffer just as much in your mid-thirties as someone who is 20 years older. Worse yet... this suffering can drag on for years... even decades.

But let me assure you... this is not normal.

There is a reason why you feel this way... and a reason why you feel betrayed by your body and the doctors who should support you. You are *not* losing your mind, no matter what you might think... or what your doctor might suggest.

Truth is, there's an overall lack of attention, research, and resources put into women's health.

I've made it my mission to make sure women know their options, and get the targeted attention they deserve. That's why I launched *Anti-Aging Confidential for Women.*

It's a monthly newsletter dedicated to empowering you with practical solutions, sound advice, and cutting-edge therapies to right mainstream medicine's wrongs regarding women's health care. I've spent years doing research on a core platform of women's health issues, and I've developed specific therapies to address women's unique health concerns.

I bring them to you every month in *Anti-Aging Confidential for Women*. You'll learn...

- How to free your body of the dangerous hormone disrupters in the air you breathe, the water you drink and the food you eat — even everyday things you touch — that often trigger the development of chronic disease

- The most important thing you can do to prevent breast cancer, cervical and ovarian cancers

- The most natural and beneficial way to replace the hormones your body loses with age

- A 5-step "de-stressing" plan to increase your DHEA. It's all natural, easy-to-follow and effective

- What 4 things women need to stay happy and strong for life...

You can understand what your body is trying to tell you... and take simple steps to help your body to detoxify and heal — in ways that nature intended.

Most importantly, you can feel good again — and enjoy life with your spouse and family on your terms. And you can start... right now... with your risk-free membership in *Anti-Aging Confidential for Women.*

Your subscription will automatically renew after one year for $39.00 USD. You can cancel at any time by calling Customer Support (toll free) at 866.792.1035, or email support@alsearsmd.com.

Item: AACW
Price: $39.00
Call 866.792.1035 or use the order form at the end of this book.

FORGET CARDIO AND BUILD HEART STRENGTH

Dr. Sears shocked the fitness world by revealing the dangers of aerobics, "cardio" and long-distance running and developed a fast, simple solution to restore muscle strength, guard against heart attack, and burn excess fat. Today, **PACE** is practiced by thousands of people worldwide.

P.A.C.E.: The 12-Minute Fitness Revolution shatters all the myths and misconceptions about health, aging, and fitness.

So throw away your jogging shoes, cancel your aerobics class, and say goodbye to hours of long, tiresome workouts. Then round up all your "diet" books and toss them in the garbage...

Now YOU can get your hands on the same patented, easy-to-learn program that:

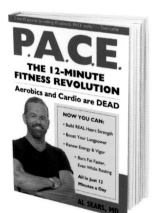

- Boosts Your Lungpower
- Rebuilds Your Lungs — Even If You're an Ex-Smoker!
- Burns Fat Faster, Even While Resting
- Builds REAL Heart Strength
- Adds Years — Even Decades — of Healthy Living to Your Life
- Pumps Up Your Immune System — Making You Virtually Disease-Proof!
- Builds Pounds of New Muscle — Without Lifting Weights!

Item: PACE2H
Price: $39.95

Call 866.792.1035 or use the order form at the end of this book.

BURN FAT WITHOUT DIETING OR COUNTING CALORIES

Dr. Sears busts the biggest fat-loss lies in *High-Speed Fat Loss in 7 Easy Steps.*

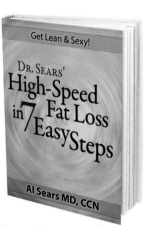

Learn why:
- Counting calories won't help you lose weight
- Eating fat won't make you fat
- Traditional exercise won't keep you lean and trim

High-Speed Fat Loss in 7 Easy Steps returns you to your native diet and makes hitting your ideal weight a sure thing.

Dr. Sears uses these same techniques to slim down his patients. With amazing results... Many patients make double-digit drops in their first month: 12, 18, even 22 lbs. of fat loss in the first 30 days!

Within minutes you'll put these easy-to-understand principles to work and effectively burn fat — even if nothing has worked for you in the past.

Item: FLBHC
Price: $37.95

Call 866.792.1035 or use the order form at the end of this book.

CLINICALLY-PROVEN PLAN OF BREAKTHROUGH HEALTH SECRETS HELPS YOU BUILD A POWERFUL, DISEASE-FREE HEART

Dr. Sears' bestselling book, *The Doctor's Heart Cure,* shows you how to stop heart attacks and strokes in a way that's easy to understand and simple to follow. You'll learn how to determine your own risk and put together a program that fits your own needs.

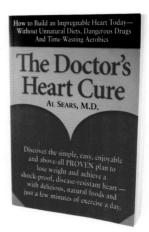

Don't leave yourself vulnerable to the lightning fast and deadly strike of a heart attack or stroke. *The Doctor's Heart Cure* lowers your risk to zero.

Item: DHCB
Price: $24.00

Call 866.792.1035 or use the order form at the end of this book.

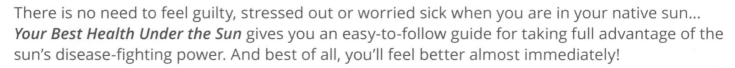

PUT ONE OF THE MOST DANGEROUS MYTHS OF OUR TIME TO REST

Your Best Health Under the Sun gives you everything you need to enjoy the sun safely, while using its power to prevent disease, burn fat and power up your sex life...

Here's a glimpse of what you'll discover:

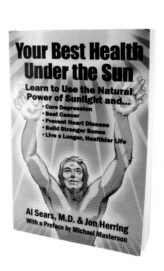

- How 20 minutes in the sun can prevent 17 deadly cancers

- The 7 dangerous chemicals in sunscreen that increase your risk of skin cancer

- Why skin cancer rates are skyrocketing in cities that get the least amount of sunshine

- The little-known secret that powers-up your sex drive and boosts your sex hormones by an amazing 200%...

How sunlight controls your blood sugar, improves your response to insulin and helps you burn fat...

There is no need to feel guilty, stressed out or worried sick when you are in your native sun... *Your Best Health Under the Sun* gives you an easy-to-follow guide for taking full advantage of the sun's disease-fighting power. And best of all, you'll feel better almost immediately!

Item: FSUNE
Price: $34.95

Call 866.792.1035 or use the order form at the end of this book.

RESET YOUR BIOLOGICAL CLOCK:

Stay Active, Vital & Energized As You Age

Work hard, play hard and keep doing what you love well into your 80s, 90s or 100s.

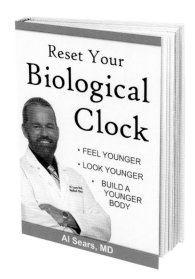

That's not wishful thinking — it's a medical reality. With new breakthrough technology, you can tinker with the aging process, so you can not only keep looking fresh and vibrant, you'll stay active and keep moving like a 50-year-old right through the age of 100.

You'll find the keys to this rejuvenation in *Reset Your Biological Clock,* the revolutionary new book from renowned integrative physician and natural health expert Dr. Al Sears.

A leading authority in anti-aging medicine, Dr. Sears has helped thousands of people like you look, feel and live younger.

Now, with the publication of *Reset Your Biological Clock,* Dr. Sears has taken alternative medicine and natural health to a new level.

He explains step-by-step how you can live younger as the years go by — and how working from the inside out, you can regain maximum vitality and keep your independence well into "old" age.

He reveals an exciting breakthrough that can enable you to turn on your anti-aging genes and reduce the effects of 10 to 20 years of aging.

He also dispels misconceptions about cardio exercise, weight training and aerobics. And, instead, offers an alternative that can get your body into the best shape of your life.

You'll learn:

- How to get your body to work like a well-oiled machine;

- Which vitamins can help you reverse your genetic clock;

- What to do to reduce your skin's age by 30%;

- How to recreate the body of your 20s.

If you want to stay independent, keep moving and do more than you ever thought you could.

Item: BIOCLOCK
Price: $24.97

Call 866.792.1035 or use the order form at the end of this book.

ATTENTION MEN: HAVE MORE SEX... MORE AMBITION... MORE GUSTO... STRONGER MUSCLES... BIGGER DREAMS...

When men come to my clinic for help, I introduce them to my *12 Secrets to Virility,* a program I developed to help guys overcome the loss of power and potency that comes with age.

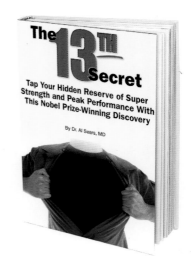

But after years of research, I discovered a new, more powerful way of giving men the lift they need to be more competitive, more dominant and more in control of their own game.

The 13th Secret is the chemical messenger that opens up your blood vessels, allowing a rush of oxygen when you need it most.

This is the same idea that makes Viagra work. But Viagra is limited to a specific area.

What I discovered is a way to give your whole body the same rush of energy and readiness.

"Open up the pipes" and you get a body-wide surge that includes:

- Bigger, harder and more frequent erections

- Fatigue-busting energy and a feeling of clarity and alertness

- Pumping, well-defined muscles

- Increased stamina, strength and mobility

- A stronger heart and bigger lung capacity

- This kind of power is not a fantasy. It's a reality you make your own.

Never again will you have to listen to a doctor tell you, "It's just part of the aging process..." *12 Secrets to Virility* will reveal the real truth about male health and aging.

More importantly, the secrets you will learn will transform you. You'll lose your gut, strengthen your body and regain youthful sexuality.

When you order *The 13th Secret,* I'll send you a **FREE** copy of *12 Secrets to Virility.*

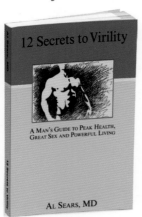

In my 198-page best seller, you'll find the man-building strategies I use with my male patients to help them reclaim the energy, drive and muscle of their younger days.

Item: 13SECRET
Price: $19.95

Call 866.792.1035 or use the order form at the end of this book.

REPAIR YOUR AGING BRAIN

As you age, your mental functions slow down. Both your thinking and your reaction time is slow. It's probably natural. But is it unavoidable?

Despite what you may have heard, cognitive decline is not inevitable. What's more, maintaining your memory has little to do with genetics, and even less to do with drugs.

In this report, you'll discover a different approach. It's the best way to improve your mental performance and stave off age-associated cognitive decline. And, it's free!

Many of these simple exercises take just minutes a day. They're easy to understand and easy to do.

You'll find:

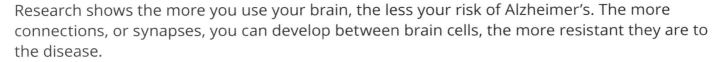

1. Tools you can use to reverse cognitive decline

2. How to beat the brain-destroying effects of cortisol

3. The best way to protect yourself from dreaded Alzheimer's disease

Think of your brain as a dynamic system. The neurons respond to environmental factors and mental stimulation. By stimulating your mind, you preserve your memory, and can even restore the clarity you had in your youth!

Research shows the more you use your brain, the less your risk of Alzheimer's. The more connections, or synapses, you can develop between brain cells, the more resistant they are to the disease.

How do you create these connections?

Discover now in Dr. Sears' Free Report — *Repair Your Aging Brain... in Just 15 Minutes a Day!* Get your FREE report INSTANTLY... along with the latest health news and little-known health solutions that really work.

Simply sign up to receive Dr. Al Sears' FREE *Doctor's House Call* e-letter, (published 5x per week), plus access to over 420 articles on the HOT topics that affect YOUR health, and we'll immediately send you his exclusive research report... Absolutely FREE!

To claim your free report go to www.repairyouragingbrain.com

BREAKTHROUGH CURES FROM 13 WORLD-RENOWNED ANTI-AGING EXPERTS YOU CAN USE RIGHT NOW!

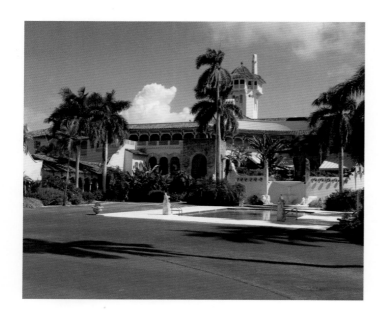

During my private, closed-door *Palm Beach Anti-Aging Summit,* 13 of the world's leading researchers revealed their little-known, anti-aging breakthroughs.

It was held at the exclusive Mar-a-Lago Club, a member-only resort on exotic Palm Beach Island. Two hundred and sixty-eight people from all over the world — including England, Malaysia, Ghana and Lebanon — paid up to $500 to attend.

The intense demand for this summit was unlike anything I've experienced before. And I understand why...

I hand-picked each member of this anti-aging "dream team" because of their stellar contributions to anti-aging medicine... and the practical, actionable advice they have to offer.

I managed to get all of them in one room over the course of two days... *and got them to reveal their secrets.*

I'm talking about the world's leading-edge therapies and technologies that can actually make you decades younger biologically and defeat age-related diseases — including cancer, heart disease, diabetes, rheumatoid arthritis and Alzheimer's disease.

These discoveries are so new and innovative they haven't been discussed outside of an elite group of alternative medicine doctors. And to gain access to them, you'd have to pay thousands upon thousands of dollars to become their patients.

Fortunately, I caught the whole event on video. Every miraculous story. Every amazing breakthrough. *And every bit of life-changing advice.*

And you can see for yourself the miraculous difference these breakthroughs will make to your life and your health right now.

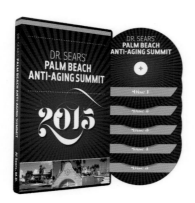

Get these anti-aging secrets today!

Palm Beach Anti-Aging Summit Recording — $199

Includes 13 Informative Presentations on 5 DVDs

Item: SUMMITDVD
Price: $199.00

Call 866.792.1035 or use the order form at the end of this book.

WELLNESS RESEARCH FOUNDATION

OUR MISSION: Our mission is to research natural and alternative health care methods and educate the public with truthful information about these alternative methods. With a stockpile of health information, research, studies, opinions, ideas, blogs, websites, and companies that exist today, it can be difficult to make a well-informed decision on health matters. Our aim is to tell the truth, give facts, and aid in opening eyes to see the broader scope of what one health decision can do to a person as a whole.

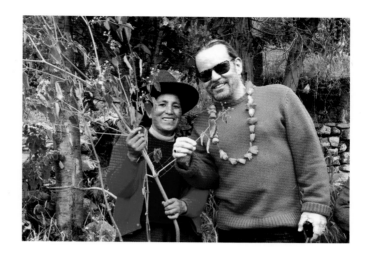

KIMBRA FOUNDATION

Together We Can Make a Difference in the Life of an African Child

The focus of the **Kimbra Foundation,** a 501(c)3 non-profit organization, is to nurture and support underserved children in Uganda by providing them with basic necessities including food, shelter and clothing, as well as a solid educational base.

KIMBRA KIDS **benefit from...**

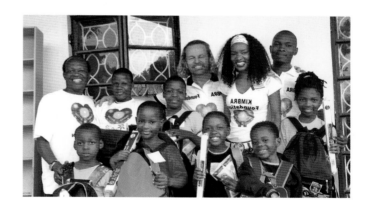

- Access to Educational Books

- Services of a Health Clinic and Medical Supplies

- Clean Water and Sanitation

- Feminine Hygiene Products and Toiletries

- Nutritious Meals

- Shoes and Uniforms... and much more!

How the Sponsorship Program Works
Your tax-deductible contribution will help provide basic necessities listed above, as well as education for your sponsored child. We will mail you a packet that includes your child's name, photo and personal story. You will learn about their community, family, activities and the education they are receiving.

To make a donation, visit drsearswellnessresearchfoundation.org, kimbrafoundation.org or call 561.784.7852.

A portion of the proceeds of the sale of Healing Herbs of Paradise go to the Kimbra Foundation through the Wellness Research Foundation.

DR. SEARS' ORDER FORM

Uniquely Qualified To Keep You Healthier For Life.
Start Your Journey and Take Back Control of Your Health — Starting Today!

Name: _____   Address: _____

City: _____   State: _____   Zip: _____

Phone: _____ (In case we have a question about your order.)

Important: please print your email address so we can email you your order and shipping
confirmation and information._____

ITEM #	PRODUCT NAME	QTY.	PRICE EACH	TOTAL PRICE

We Stand Behind Our Products With Our Money-Back Guarantee.

Subtotal	$_____
Shipping & Handling	$ 8.95
International Shipping Notice	$ 25.95
Grand Total	$_____

PAYMENT METHOD

☐ Enclosed is my check or money order payable to Wellness Research and Consulting, Inc.

☐ Charge my   VISA _____   Mastercard _____

                    American Express _____   Discover _____

NAME AS IT APPEARS ON THE CARD
CREDIT CARD #
CREDIT CARD BILLING ADDRESS
SIGNATURE

For faster service, call 866.895.8555 — Monday through Friday; 9 a.m. to 5 p.m. EST.

Mail in your order to: Wellness Research and Consulting, Inc.
Attn: Customer Support, 11905 Southern Blvd., Royal Palm Beach, FL 33411

Money-Back Guarantee
Order now and do it risk free. As always, you'll get Dr. Sears' NO-HASSLE, FULL PROTECTION Guarantee.
If you are not satisfied with your purchase for any reason, simply return your purchase within 90 days and I will
send you an immediate, complete, and total refund with no questions asked — including shipping and handling.

NOTES

NOTES

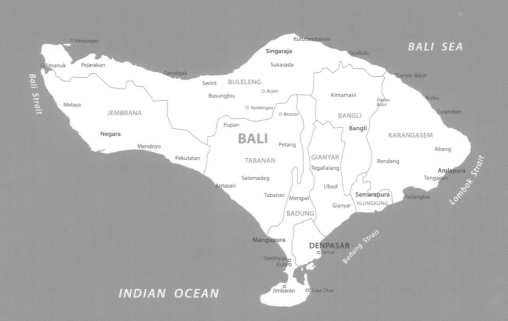

BALI SEA

P. Menjangan   Kututambahan

                                    Singaraja   Tejakula
Gilimanuk   Pejarakan   Sukasada

Bali Strait   Gerokgak

                              Seririt   BULELENG   Gianyar Barat

                              Busungbiu   *D. Buyan*   Kintamani   Kubu

                                              D. Tamblingan   *Danau*
                  JEMBRANA   *Batur*
      Melaya   *D. Beratan*   BANGLI   Tulamben

                                  Pupan   KARANGASEM
      Negara   **Bangli**

            Mendoyo   **BALI**   Petang   Abang

                  Pekutatan   Rendang
                              TABANAN   GIANYAR   **Amlapura**
                                              Tegallalang   Tengapan

            Antasari   Padangbai
                  Selemadeg   Ubud
                                                          Semarapura

                      Tabanan   Mengwi   Gianyar   KLUNGKUNG
                                                                              Lombok Strait

                                  BADUNG

                  Mangupura   **DENPASAR**
                                          Sanur
                        Seminyak
                          Kuta   Badung Strait

INDIAN OCEAN
                              Jimbaran   Nusa Dua